Grand Bargains

Fixing Health Care
and the Economy

By

David K. Cundiff, MD

Cover art provided by Eddie Young

Library of Congress Cataloging in Publication Data
Cundiff, David K.
Grand Bargains—Fixing Health Care and the Economy
by David K. Cundiff

ISBN 9780-9761571-2-8
    1. Medical care—United States.
    2. Health care reform—United States.
    3. Economics
    4. Health care economics—United States.

Dewey Decimal # pending 2015

Also by David K. Cundiff, MD

Euthanasia is Not the Answer:
A Hospice Physician's View

The Right Medicine:
How Make Health Care Reform Work Today

Money Driven Medicine:
Tests and Treatments That Don't Work

Whistleblower Doctor:
The Politics and Economics of Pain and Dying

Dedication

To my granddaughters Ruby Drew Thompson and Olivia Freemon. They are two good reasons for humanity to evolve along a healthful, peaceful, tolerant, and environmentally sustainable path.

Contents

INTRODUCTION IX

CHAPTER 1 GRAND BARGAINS OVERVIEW 1

CHAPTER 2 ACCOUNTABLE CARE COOPERATIVES 47

CHAPTER 3 DIRECT PRACTICE PCPs LEADING PATIENT-
CENTERED MEDICAL HOMES 62

CHAPTER 4 PREVENTIVE MEDICINE AND HEALTH PROMOTION ..78

CHAPTER 5 END-OF-LIFE CARE REFORM 85

CHAPTER 6 ADDITIONAL HEALTH AND SOCIAL SERVICES 109

CHAPTER 7 ACCs COMPETE TO PREVENT ABORTIONS 128

CHAPTER 8 EVIDENCE-BASED MEDICINE INFORMING
CLINICAL DECISIONS 133

CHAPTER 9 SELF-REGULATION FOR ACCs 151

CHAPTER 10 ACCs CAN BEST DELIVER SOCIAL SERVICES ... 163

CHAPTER 11 ENTERPRISE LIABILITY FOR MEDICAL
MALPRACTICE AND LEGAL SYSTEM REFORM ..179

CHAPTER 12 JOBS, JOBS, JOBS 201

CHAPTER 13 FOOD AND AGRICULTURE POLICY REFORM 220

CHAPTER 14 IMMIGRATION REFORM: A FOUNDATION FOR
ZERO POPULATION GROWTH 248

CHAPTER 15 PUBLIC INFRASTRUCTURE INVESTMENTS 270

CHAPTER 16 EDUCATION: ACCs TO FOSTER
EXPERIMENTATION 277

CHAPTER 17 ACC ENHANCED NATIONAL SECURITY:
INTERNATIONAL DEVELOPMENT AID 288

CHAPTER 18 ACC-BASED MEDICAL INSURANCE REFORM ...307

CHAPTER 19 PAYMENT REFORMS 324

CHAPTER 20 HEALTH CARE COST CONTROL 340

CHAPTER 21 TAX REFORM: FLAT INCOME TAX AND
CONSUMPTION TAXES 357

CHAPTER 22 ENERGY DIET FOR A SUSTAINABLE ECONOMY..387

CHAPTER 23 SOCIAL SECURITY AND OTHER
RETIREMENT PLANS..............................406

CHAPTER 24 PERSONAL AND NATIONAL FINANCIAL SECURITY..419

CHAPTER 25 BETTER CARE FOR SENIORS AND PEOPLE
WITH DISABILITIES..............................451

CHAPTER 26 GRAND BARGAINS: THE URGENCY OF NOW 458

REFERENCES 467

INDEX..............................537

ACKNOWLEDGMENTS 545

Introduction

"Lead and the leaders will follow." The *grand bargains* proposed in this book should be worthy of immediate widespread discussion. They embrace the spectrum of public policy concerns generated by the failures of well-meaning leaders from big government and the corporate world.

I define a grand bargain as a public policy approach capable of unifying diverse people with opposing legitimate interests in order to benefit people, the economy, and the environment.

Without a matrix of grand bargains to fix our dysfunctional health care system, we can't begin to fix our entire economy – and *vice versa*. Only in conjunction with comprehensive health system reform can we begin to address unemployment, the national debt, Social Security, increasing income inequality, undocumented immigrants, welfare, abortion, gun violence, tort reform, education, infrastructure, national defense, and the systemic risk in the financial system. These interrelated health and economic policy quandaries loom larger than ever and are the subjects of this book.

These issues are complex, and I don't claim to have all the answers. However, in this time of crisis with no consensus on a way forward for the nation, we need innovative game-changing ideas more than ever. Given the current intractable political stalemate, we shouldn't leave our fates to the politicians. With the leadership vacuum, we can and must now move public policy discussions forward as citizens. Please feel free to improve on the ideas in this book.

The effects of each of 29 grand bargains to be introduced will inject energy and sustenance for the affected groups of people, social institutions, and economic sectors. Consideration has been given to the likely consequences for all stakeholders—children, parents, students, workers, employers, taxpayers, patients, health care providers, the unemployed, residents of other countries, and the environment that allows the existence of all.

My proposals assume that, without a deep and broad restructuring and unifying of all interconnected aspects of our beleaguered but resourceful society, we cannot fix health care or any other major problem in the U.S. The multifaceted interrelationships between health care, welfare, and other dysfunctional sectors of the economy should lead us to a multi-dimensional solution—a network of grand bargains.

Strident voices say that economic system reform can only mean less government regulation and more free-market capitalism. Others point to widening wealth inequalities, and advocate moving toward socialistic approaches that give all people access to health care and redistribute the wealth. How about considering some of both?

To simultaneously deal with health, social, and economic outcomes, this book lays out a hybrid free-market/communitarian plan. Free-market capitalism will constitute roughly two-thirds of the projected $17.9 trillion gross domestic product (GDP) in 2016. This free-market capitalism will involve a downsized role of government and major benefits to both employees and employers.

Communitarianism is defined as a social and political philosophy that emphasizes the importance of community in the functioning of political life. This encompasses institutions as well as understanding human identity and well-being. A new society-wide institution, to be described shortly, will embody communitarianism in the plan. It is designed to complement free-market capitalism, improve wealth distribution, and social justice.

This hybrid free-market / communitarian proposal to improve health care and to reform the unsustainable overall economic system takes shape by utilizing 29 grand bargains. The bargaining will involve the interests of everyone: patients, health care providers, other workers, taxpayers, and other stakeholders. The overarching grand bargain consists of a woven tapestry of all the grand bargains. Once established, it will be an ongoing process of refinement and improvement for people on the local community level.

Few citizens may agree on every grand bargain on the list. However, the overarching grand bargain, with its many tradeoffs and compromises, is designed to have great appeal for stakeholders from all economic sectors (e.g., health care, finance, agriculture, manufacturing, government, etc.), areas of employment (e.g., laborers, managers, investors, entrepreneurs, etc.) and social institutions (e.g., families, universities, businesses, religions, etc.). These proposed public policy bargains will forever be a work in progress. My goal in producing this plan was to find politically and economically workable health care and economic policy prescriptions. They need to appeal, at least in part, to a broad spectrum of people. If conservatives think that they are too liberal and liberals think that they are too conservative, I have probably achieved a major part of my purpose.

Who is David Cundiff to Offer Fixes for Health Care and the Economy?

As a physician practicing internal medicine and palliative care/hospice medicine at the LA County + USC Medical Center, my interest in health policy arose in the early 1990s. Installments of the intense and partisan debate over President Bill Clinton's health care reform plan, lead by his wife Hillary, appeared daily in the newspapers, radio, and television.

Buoyed by the modest success of my book on the physician assisted suicide/euthanasia debate titled, *Euthanasia Is Not the Answer—A Hospice Physician's View*,[1] I jumped with my publisher's support for me to write a book on health care reform. With co-author Mary Ellen McCarthy, PhD, a Wall Street financial analyst, I published *The Right*

Medicine—How to Make Health Care Reform Work Today.[2] The book advocated universal health care funded entirely with "sin taxes" on the goods and services that contribute to diseases and injuries (i.e., tobacco, alcohol, fossil fuels, violent media, junk food, etc.). Unfortunately, the August 1994 date of publication was just before the midterm election landslide victory for the Republicans. This took health care reform off the radar for the next 10+ years.

While I enjoyed practicing medicine in a safety-net teaching hospital, I saw firsthand the dysfunction of money-driven medicine funded primarily by diverse public insurers. Although most of my patients had no insurance, I tried to give them the best possible care. The biggest challenges I encountered were not with the patients but with the medical bureaucracy.

For instance, a hospice nurse and I instituted the "Pain and Palliative Care Service" for terminally ill cancer and AIDS patients in 1987. It was very popular with patients, their families, nurses, and residents. However, the unhealthy financial bottom line doomed the Service. The Medicaid insurance that funded the LA County + USC Medical Center paid primarily for acute care days in hospital ($3800 per day in the late 1990s). The better my team's palliative care controlled pain and symptoms of advanced illness, the fewer patients needed to be in the hospital, and the more potential Medicaid funding the hospital lost. After my service cost the hospital an estimated $9 million in Medicaid revenue in 1994, the administration closed my service in 1995.

I then became a whistleblower concerning the poor state of pain management and palliative care for terminally ill patients and the dysfunctional and wasteful system of government funding for indigent patient care. The hospital administration retaliated by firing me and taking my medical license. My book, *Whistleblower Doctor—The Politics and Economics of Pain and Dying,*[3, 4] tells the story.

Being out of clinical medicine gave me the luxury of time to research and write about the pervasive dysfunction caused by financial special interests dominating medical orthodoxy. I documented over 70 medical tests and treatments funded by public and private insurance for which scientific evidence does not support efficacy or safety. Each year, these medical interventions kill at least 75,000 Americans and cost over $1 trillion. My next book, *Money Driven Medicine—Tests and Treatments that Don't Work,*[5] appeared in 2006.

Medical interventions that I challenged included medications for mild hypertension,[6] cholesterol lowering pills, tight control of type 2 diabetes, bypass surgery for coronary artery disease, screening mammograms, screening prostate specific antigen (PSA) tests, and anticoagulants for atrial fibrillation[7] and venous thromboembolism.[8]

This book, *Grand Bargains,* draws from my eye-opening experiences with patients in my medical practice. This book also derives from my firsthand knowledge of the dysfunction in health care system financing, and draws upon my interest in integrating health care reform with an institutional restructuring of the U.S. economy.

Obamacare, Political Polarization, and Changing the Public Policy Conversation

Implementing any change in health care, welfare, or the other sectors of the economy has been difficult because of conservative *versus* liberal polarization. For example, the Patient Protection and Affordable Care Act (i.e., Obamacare or the ACA) continues to be hotly debated among Democrats and Republicans. Policies on guns, abortions, welfare, entitlements (i.e., Social Security, Medicare, Medicaid, etc.), protecting nature, and national security are among many other divisive issues.

Concerning Obamacare and other polarizing political and economic issues, this book does not favor the positions of either major political party. Republicans can consider that my policy prescriptions amount to repealing and replacing Obamacare. Democrats can rightly believe that without their having passed the ACA the necessary fixes to and overhauling of Obamacare detailed in this book would have never been considered.

I hope this book changes the conversation from simply arguing whether Obamacare is good or bad. Starting from the reality that Obamacare is the law at least until 2017, this book is about imagining what public-policy grand bargains will help us to attain the best health care and healthy living on earth.

Many analysts have written excellent articles as well as books and delivered eloquent speeches detailing the dysfunctions of the health care and economic strategies in the U.S. I will recount only as little as necessary about what is wrong with the status quo medical and economic policies, in order to provide context for positive Grand-Bargains' prescriptions for fundamental reform.

By design, the policy solutions proposed here address talking-points from the right and the left. Both sides have valid insights to offer. Concerning the way forward for health care and the economy, we need innovative, outside-the-box, new approaches to the issues that conservatives, liberals, and others care about.

Few if any of the grand bargains proposed, taken as isolated policy suggestions, would stand much of a chance with a polarized, hyper-partisan Congress and electorate. However, consider these 29 grand bargains as a package or platform, containing ideas from the right, left, and center. Imagine how these ideas might lead people of good will to see solutions that will unite the long-divided and increasingly discouraged public.

For instance, few politicians favor raising the federal minimum wage to $15 per hour—a projected cost of $660 billion in 2016 or nearly 4% of the projected GDP. Fewer still would vote for eliminating the state and federal corporate income taxes ($557 billion in 2016) and freeing businesses from providing most employee benefits (saving businesses $1.6 trillion in 2016). Hardly anyone would vote for imposing almost $1.9 trillion in new taxes on goods and services that harm health, the economy, or the environment (e.g., tobacco, alcohol, fossil fuel, plastic products, guns, too big to fail banks, etc.). Only politicians on the far right would advocate for completely eliminating federal deficit spending ($530 billion projected for 2016) and beginning to pay down the

$18 trillion federal debt. Only left-leaning politicians would support finding over $3 trillion additional funds over the next decade for infrastructure expansion, repair, and rebuilding.

But consider enacting all of the above proposals *at the same time.* Businesses could afford the higher worker wages with money left over to hire millions more workers. Additional workers resulting from business-friendly policies and infrastructure-building will grow the GDP or, better yet, grow the economy *qualitatively.*

Consumption taxes on unhealthful products and services will reduce the damaging effects of those products and services. These targeted consumption taxes will reduce the need for income taxes and job-killing business taxes. This will allow us to add tens of millions of jobs and do away with deficit spending while heavily investing in our infrastructure.

And this is just the beginning: the end result can be a superior standard of living characterized by much wider accountability and stronger community for all to enjoy in health, safety and shared prosperity. In the book chapters that follow, I will briefly summarize the well-known problems that we face and then describe proposed grand bargains to optimize health, welfare, education, freedom, prosperity, security, and opportunity.

Don't expect a panacea with minimal societal disruption. Disruptions may be monumental and highly challenging, but less difficult to deal with than financial collapse and civil unrest.

As with any major change in society, individuals and groups may vie for self-interested policies. My suggested fixes are designed to be fair and flexible—not one-size-fits-all. They call for comprehensive policy changes in conjunction with hard work, sacrifice by all, and unity of purpose.

People who financially benefit from waste and dysfunction in various institutions of society will be challenged with undergoing changes in their careers and in their lives. Millions of displaced workers will be called to undergo life-affirming transformations to new occupations. This process will be facilitated by the resources, power, and flexibility of communities to bring about major institutional and societal changes. As this book will show, many more good jobs will be created than lost.

The first chapter of this book provides an overview of my initial 22 of the 29 grand bargains for health care and the economy. The subsequent chapters describe in more detail the background and rationale for the initial grand bargains and seven additional grand bargains. These chapters will also delineate the mutually supporting interaction of all 29 grand bargains into an overarching grand bargain for fixing health care and the economy.

In the larger sense, a culture change will result for lasting benefit to the individual, the community, the nation, and the planet.

We are *all* in this together, so let us use our collective power to create what we want for a better tomorrow, starting now.

Chapter 1
Grand Bargains Overview

O ur diverse society has found itself at the historic point of urgently needing to forthrightly address widely diverse health and economic crises. We are a nation of reasonable and aspiring people willing to share the burden to improve our collective lot in a changing world. Strategies, solutions, and fair compromises for intractable issues need to be allowed public hearing and debate. When ways forward are determined by consensus (or near consensus), they must be implemented immediately.

It is not hyperbole to say that success in comprehensive changes in our health care and economic systems is required for human survival as we know it on the planet.

Health policy experts and ordinary citizens almost uniformly agree that reforming our health care system means (1) improving health outcomes, (2) enhancing quality of care, (3) providing access to care for all, and (4) reducing the cost. Targeting those four goals simultaneously will be priority one of this book.

But health care reform in isolation is an impossibility. The connections between excellent health outcomes and economic well-being are too strong. Consequently, health care reform must go hand in hand with overhauling the entire economic system.

I define a well functioning, sustainable economic system as one that

1. supports full employment in jobs paying a living wage,
2. distributes resources equitably,

3. fosters environmental sustainability,
4. taxes fairly in support of good outcomes for health, the environment, and the economy,
5. requires no debt to be passed to future generations,
6. advances liberal democracy,
7. allocates sufficient resources to affordable education,
8. promotes entrepreneurial innovation, and
9. promotes sustainable development worldwide in our interdependent global community.

Studies show that low-income urban populations generally suffer poor health, especially if not sufficiently benefiting from a social safety net. Accordingly, some grand bargains proposed in this book seek to improve the various, root-causes of poverty and excessive wealth differences. Other grand bargains address the unmet needs of exceptionally capable, innovative, entrepreneurial people who are overregulated, overtaxed, overworked, and stressed.

Culture Change Necessary to Accompany Health System and Economic Changes

"Culture" has several definitions. I use the word to mean "the set of shared attitudes, values, goals, and practices that characterize an institution, organization, or group."[1] Our economic system, rooted in our culture and cultural practices, affects health and the attempt to prevent and treat diseases. The proposed grand bargains in this book will facilitate positive changes in cultural dynamics regarding health and the economy. And *vice versa*, beneficial cultural changes will enhance the positive effects on health and economic outcomes related to the 29 grand bargains proposed.

Most people would like to change our culture's acceptance of high-stress sedentary lifestyles, junk food diets, tobacco addiction, binge drinking, prescription drug abuse, materialism, high levels of debt, excessive low-quality electronic media, ever looming violence, and lax controls on environmental pollution. These destructive aspects of our society cause some acute medical problems and promote many preventable chronic diseases that account for about *75% of our chronic disease health care costs.*[2, 3]

The adverse health and economic consequences of aspects of our way of life call for culture change. These aspects and their root causes are determined by culture, in turn controlled by a society adhering to sometimes unacknowledged cultural forces. To enable the needed changes to come about, a deep shift in values is required, and has even been underway. We live in the advanced form of Western Civilization that has produced unprecedented material production and consumption. As the influence of materialism and focus on money grew, people's connections to nature and their forebears' traditions and skills have been all but severed. As the dominant culture has a hold on its members' minds, society and its problems and crises are an outgrowth of the culture.

To deal with our social, economic and environmental crises the people will be emphasizing culture-changing methods and experimentation such as strengthening cooperative and communitarian models. Deeper shifts should follow. This is not necessarily incompatible with free-market capitalism as will be shown.

Transformation and upheaval in society are challenging and not entirely predictable, but when rational and in the interests of the many, transformation and reforms should assist people in adopting healthful lifestyles and economic advantages that reduce chronic disease. Obesity, cardiovascular diseases, over-consumption, unsustainable personal debt, fossil fuel overreliance, failing schools, and welfare dependence confront us all in one way or another. There is no top-down, one-size-fits-all solution—no number of federal or state government programs to fix our problems. All these issues can be better addressed by local participatory institutions that reinvigorate community and earn citizen support.

Harnessing "soft power" is a Grand Bargains' approach for all of the above problems. Joseph Nye, PhD, Professor of International Relations of Harvard University defined "soft power" as "the ability to attract and co-opt rather than coerce, use force, or give money as a means of persuasion."[4] We need to combine financial and human resources together with soft power from diverse stakeholders to help drive beneficial cultural transformations.

Together with soft power, the grand bargains herein are designed to help us transition to a health-promoting, life-affirming, prosperous, sustainable culture.

Strategy for Health and Economic Policy Analysis

Americans are known for innovation, adaptability, and team work. We may have an historic political window of opportunity to use those attributes to discover the way forward to fix our health care and economic systems. Twenty-nine grand bargains will serve as a compass or blueprint. With this guidance on ways to better our lives and the lives of our children, Americans can strive together for common goals and succeed.

The grand bargains articulated here need vetting and refinements. Some of them may require significant changes. Our tools of democracy (free speech, debate, polls, compromise, legislation, etc.) can improve on what is here proposed.

Given the complexities of people, society, politics, markets, religion, and technology, many tradeoffs will be presented in this book. Compromises will involve all classes of society, regions of the country, and ideologies of the citizenry. Most of us might need to give up some of perceived advantages we may have in the status quo in order to achieve a better future for ourselves, our children, our communities, and society as a whole.

While our institutions of health care, welfare, finance, law, education, business, and national security require urgent overhauls, the workers in these professions are more heroes than villains. In truth, we are all villains and all heroes. Though we suffer greatly individually and as a country from the dysfunctions of our economic and political systems, there remains much good in our democratic form of government and capitalist economic system.

As Thomas Jefferson predicted over two centuries ago, periodic revolution, "at least once every 20 years," is "a medicine necessary for the sound health of government."[5] Our vibrant democracy needs peaceful revolutions in times of crisis so that it can evolve in ways that best serve the people and the country. One miracle of this democratic country is that educated, informed people can engage in open discussion of complex, seemingly intractable issues and find creative and effective solutions for individual and societal problems. As each new generation must learn, our precious democracy is a "use it or lose it" proposition. Using the tools and institutions of democracy to work together on our problems counteracts cynicism, malaise, and alienation.

Conservatives as well as liberals will see their hot button issues addressed within each grand bargain to be described. Each grand bargain relates to longstanding, unresolved, and interrelated problems. And they are all related to our health.

This first chapter will be divided into grand bargains that are related to health care and grand bargains throughout the rest of the economy.

Health Care Grand Bargains

The first 11 grand bargains are health care related. Eleven more grand bargains in this chapter will address economic issues in other economic sectors. Finally, seven additional grand bargains will be more thoroughly detailed in the chapters that follow.

Grand Bargain #1: Accountable Care Cooperatives (ACCs): Centerpiece of the Grand Bargains

Obamacare calls for health care grand bargains "accountable care organizations" (ACOs), owned by physicians, investors, and/or hospitals, to provide coordinated, cost effective, quality care for patients, emphasizing "patient-centered medical homes" (physician-led primary care teams, Chapter 3). Enhanced reimbursement rates for ACOs that follow the Obamacare prescriptions for saving money while providing quality care are the basic idea. However, studies of ACO performances have shown little or no improvement in quality of care or cost control compared with the status quo.[6] Americans need a new model for health care.

The *first grand bargain is to replace Obamacare's ACOs with "account-able care cooperatives" (ACCs)*. ACCs will be constituted as nonprofit cooperatives as defined by the International Co-operative Alliance's Statement on the Co-operative Identity: "autonomous associations of persons united voluntarily to meet their common economic, social, and cultural needs and aspirations through jointly owned and democratically controlled enterprises."[7] Most of the other 28 grand bargains require that ACCs replace ACOs in order to work.

Like Obamacare ACOs, ACCs will provide comprehensive health care and preventive medicine services within patient-centered medical homes (Chapter 2). Whereas Obamacare ACOs must all provide their members *identical* health care and preventive medical services, *diversity between ACCs* in medical practice guidelines and human services benefit packages is expected and encouraged (Chapter 9).

ACCs will have "global budgets" to fund all health and human services. A global budget is a fixed amount of money to provide all services (medical, social-safety-net, and other). ACCs will be self-regulating as far as what health care and other human services will be offered with the available financial and human resources.

Cooperatively owned ACCs will offer much more than health care and preventive medicine. In a fully integrated manner, ACCs will also provide social services (Chapter 10), job placement (Chapter 12), legal consultations and representation (Chapter 11), enhanced educational opportunities (Chapter 16), financial counseling and guidance (Chapter 24), and much more. They will promote innovation, flexibility, and solidarity within diverse communities. Successful ACCs will encourage cooperation, volunteerism, and mutual self-help in local neighborhoods, schools, social services agencies, and places of worship.

ACCs will be communitarian in that members of each ACC will likely, but not necessarily, share similar philosophies regarding health care, human services, religion, personal finances, and even politics. Members of an ACC will have access to similar services as other members of that ACC but not necessarily access to all services provided by other ACCs. Each ACC member will benefit to the degree that all other members receive high-quality health care, have good health outcomes, pay affordable health care premiums, avoid civil or criminal litigation, maintain meaningful employment, receive adequate wages, and give back to the other members of the ACC.

Members of ACCs will be encouraged and expected to provide input to ACC managers and each other about the policies and services of their cooperatives. Clinical practice guidelines and benefits packages of ACCs will be in a constant state of flux based on member input, new medical research findings, and health, social, and financial outcomes of ACC members and those reported by competing ACCs.

The creation and operation of ACCs are key to slashing government waste. Shifting various federal government programs to local ACC control results in less bureaucratic control over our lives by Washington, D.C.

The role of a much downsized government will be to move out of directly providing and dictating health and human services from Washington, and working to accommodate competing private ACCs to operate in a transparent free-market setting. This will provide the political, economic, and cultural environment for diverse groups of people to come up with their own unique health and human services solutions. Comparisons of health and social outcomes of different ACCs as related to clinical practice guidelines and benefit packages they offer will drive ACCs to copy successful models and lead to steady public health and economic progress.

Healthy Competition Between ACCs

ACCs will compete in devising strategies to help enrollees accomplish what most people want to do—improve their diets, avoid lifestyle-related chronic diseases, attain maximal wellness, conserve energy, steer clear of or handle litigation, find good jobs, obtain quality education, manage money, retire comfortably on Social Security and/or their pensions, support their communities, and assist in providing for the security and liberty of the country.

Funding for ACC services (about $4.26 trillion in 2016, about $13,000 allocated on average per member[a]) will come from government health and human services budgets and from member premiums. We start by shifting retirement savings (i.e., Social Security and pensions)

---

a $4.26 trillion (total revenue of ACCs) / 328 million (projected U.S. population in 2016[8]) ≈ $13,000

away from entrenched, inefficient and at times corrupt government and corporate bureaucracies. These funds will transfer over to ACC managers that are accountable to members (Chapters 19, 23, and 24). ACC-affiliated credit unions and Savings and Loan Banks will then manage about $1.72 trillion in 2016—about one-third of the gross domestic product (GDP).[b]

Given that ACCs will provide comprehensive services and receive a defined amount of funding, competition between ACCs will lead to reductions of institutionalized waste and inefficiency throughout health care and human services. Communitarian ACCs that compete in a free market will also greatly facilitate the restructuring of the other dysfunctional economic sectors.

Since ACCs will offer diverse health care and human services, they will charge different health care premiums accordingly. People who are dissatisfied with their ACCs will be able to change to other ACCs.

Expanding ACC Services

After I conceived of combining health care with social services within ACCs, a major impediment to the design of my health care reform plan arose—the world financial system meltdown. Beginning with the U.S. subprime home mortgage crisis in 2007, the still unresolved financial system crisis demonstrated that U.S. society faces multi-dimensional economic challenges. However, entrenched bureaucracies and corrupted special interests throughout the economy, enforced by our increasingly polarized and plutocratic government, make piecemeal reforms virtually impossible or ineffective.

Interrelated crises—wealth inequality, environmental degradation, unsustainable energy consumption, water shortages, lack of immigration reform, education quality problems, terrorism, wars of choice,

---

b $6 trillion (total revenue of ACCs: $4.26 trillion health and human services + $1.72 trillion retirement savings investments) / $17.9 trillion (estimated GDP in 2016[9]) = 33.5%

domestic gun violence, etc.—now threaten not only our economy but also our freedom and security. Consequently, optimal personal and population health outcomes require other sectors of the economy (i.e., education, finance, agriculture, food services, transportation, immigration, criminal justice, governance etc.) to function well. Thus, personal wellbeing and economic security require that fundamental restructurings extend throughout other institutions of society.

The new ACC key participants may well come from government or corporate managerial positions. However, in the less bureaucratic and more transparent ACCs, managers will be empowered to use flexibility, innovation, and experimentation. They will find it easier to help the people they serve than in entrenched government and corporate bureaucracies.

After the introduction of ACCs, medical insurance companies will become ACC-affiliated financial services companies. The change of terms is significant. The financial services company administrators will not make any decisions about allocation of medical and other services for enrollees (Chapter 18). ACCs will insure all the 300+ million U.S. residents that *voluntarily* choose to join them. As will be detailed in subsequent chapters, ACCs will provide affordable and universal access to health care and other human services. Consequently, an individual mandate to enroll in an ACC will not be needed or recommended.

Some ACCs will fail and their members will need to join better-run ACCs. Each ACC will keep funds in reserve to protect members against ACC bankruptcy.

To control health care and welfare entitlement spending over the long term, the government's contribution to ACCs will be frozen at the 2016 level.

Grand Bargain #2: "Direct Practice" Primary Care Providers for All

Rushed clinic visits to overly burdened primary care providers (PCPs: physicians, nurse practitioners, and physician assistants) do not serve patients or PCPs well. Unfortunately, Obamacare does not adequately address the crisis in primary care medicine. Many PCPs care for more than 2000 people—too many patients, too much bureaucracy: a prescription for burnout and substandard care.

Frustration of PCPs and patients with these conditions led to "direct practice" PCPs or direct primary care providers (previously called concierge or boutique physicians) emerging in the 1990s. Direct practice PCPs do not bill public or private insurance for services to patients. Instead, they charge the patients cash for more personal attention and additional services. They limit their practices to about 750 patients on average. Patients of direct practice PCPs receive added services such as 24-hour PCP access, PCP-accompanied specialist visits, longer clinic visits, house calls, and same day visits.

The second health care grand bargain proposed is for every U.S. resident to have a direct practice PCP.

The Grand Bargain #2 involves the government's commitment to fund the training of additional primary care physicians, nurse practitioners, and physician's assistants to provide for a ratio of patients to PCPs on average of 750/1 (i.e., ranging from 500 – 1000). Then everyone can have access to a direct practice PCP.

Coordination of care of individual patients will be facilitated by "patient-centered medical homes" (Grand Bargain #3) within ACCs. Direct practice PCPs, as leaders of patient-centered medical homes for patients will be primarily responsible for health services provided and cost control in each ACC (Chapter 20).

The relatively low cost of training the additional PCPs required to transition to direct-practice primary care will be recouped by the efficiencies of transitioning to a well coordinated health care system.

Grand Bargain #3: Direct Practice PCPs to Provide Primary Care in "Patient-Centered Medical Homes"

According to the National Center for Quality Assurance, the seven key facets of patient-centered medical homes include (1) enhanced access to clinicians after hours and on-line, (2) long-term patient and provider relationships, (3) shared decision making, (4) patient engagement on health and health care, (5) team-based care, (6) better quality and experience of care, (7) lower cost from reduced emergency department and hospital use.[10]

These seven key features are goals that have not necessarily been achieved by health care providers just because of the designation "patient-centered medical home." For instance, patient engagement in health and health care depends largely on the resources of the health care providers and the incentives for the patients to participate. Health industry bureaucrats writing guidelines and lists of requirements for patient-centered medical homes do not necessarily foster patient engagement or fewer emergency room visits.

As will be more fully detailed in later chapters, federal bureaucratic metrics for measuring quality of health care are not yet ready for prime time. Documentation of improved medical outcomes with current versions of patient-centered medical homes has not been consistently demonstrated. Reviews are mixed. Neither have overall cost savings or reduced emergency room visits been the typical experience of patients enrolled in National Center for Quality Assurance-designated patient-centered medical homes.[11, 12]

Fortunately, with ACC-based health care reform, the care provided by direct practice PCPs (Chapter 3) and allied health workers will be greatly enhanced with the shift to the model of care called "patient-centered medical homes."

The third grand bargain is that direct practice PCPs will lead teams of health care professionals, providing coordinated care for patients in patient-centered medical homes.

As will be detailed in subsequent grand bargains, a component of ACC-based reform is for PCPs to have major new responsibilities. Direct practice PCPs will lead patient-centered medical homes in which patients receive comprehensive medical treatment integrated with medical specialists' services and social services (Chapter 10). Preventive medicine services (Chapter 4), alternative treatments (Chapter 6), long-term care (Chapter 6), and end-of-life palliative care (Chapter 5) will also be major components of the patient-centered medical homes.

Cost control will be largely a PCP responsibility (Grand Bargain #4 and Chapter 20). Since the total funding of ACCs must include all enrollee services, PCPs and the rest of the patient-centered medical home teams will be responsible to their patients for eliminating unnecessary tests and treatments and specialist referrals. Money saved by cost-conscious medical practices will go to premium reductions and additional high-value services provided to enrollees by the ACCs. Health care professionals will not receive bonuses for denying care to patients, as is the common practice among medical insurance corporations.

Competition between ACCs will ensure cost-conscious efficiency and continuous innovations, to improve services of the PCP led patient-centered medical homes, specialists, and health care support-workers. As a result, ACCs will enhance the health outcomes of patients and the overall public health.

Grand Bargain #4: Direct Practice PCPs will Assume Responsibility for ACC Cost Control

Cost control initiatives in all sectors of medical care have all been failures for over half a century. We currently have neither a functioning medical market nor government price control. Nationally, health care costs have skyrocketed 479% since 1980 after adjusting for inflation.[13, 14] If we are to stop the unsustainable inflation in health care spending, an effective mechanism for cost control must be implemented.

People with private insurance cannot cost-consciously shop for value in purchasing health care services. There is a lack of transparency in the charges for health services. For instance, people with back aches or chest pain can greatly overpay for consultants if they have no guidance from a health care professional that understands orthopedics and cardiology and knows what local specialists are most skilled and what they charge for services.

To control costs, ACCs will need to provide all services with a set amount of money per member (or per capita)—i.e., under a capitated budget. "Capitated funding" means a designated amount of money to cover an entire population of patients (e.g., an ACC with more than 20 patient-centered medical home teams and more than 100,000 patients). Someone or some group inside of each ACC must be designated with the responsibility of controlling costs (Chapter 20).

The fourth grand bargain is to have direct practice PCPs become accountable to their patients and colleagues for overall ACC cost control.

Like Obamacare's ACOs, the proposed ACCs will have health care funded by member insurance premiums and by public insurance (i.e., transfers of funds from the government equal to 2016 budgets for Medicare, Medicaid, Veterans' Health Care, etc.). However, ACCs will be self-regulating and will not need to adhere to government guidelines about the allocation of medical services (Grand Bargain #5 and Chapter 9). Before making important financial or other policy decisions, PCPs and ACC managers will seek inputs from all stakeholders (patients, health care workers, medical researchers, taxpayers, and policy experts). With ACCs having capitated funding, all stakeholders will benefit by eliminating worthless or harmful tests and treatments as well as unnecessary bureaucracy in the delivery of excellent care.

Members' premium-charges will be set by ACC managers after input from all stakeholders. The amount of funding per person or per capita (capitation level) will vary according to the member premiums charged by ACCs. This kind of flexibility in payment system reform will be needed to help fix the financial aspects of our broken health care system (Chapters 18-20).

Grand Bargain #5: Replace Government Health Care Guidelines and Regulations with ACC Self-Regulation

Doctors increasingly make decisions about medical tests and treatments for their patients according to clinical practice guidelines. Highly influential academic physicians write clinical practice guidelines according to principles of "evidence-based medicine"—findings from randomized controlled trials and other scientific substantiation. However, drug and medical device producers generally fund the randomized controlled trials and employ the physicians that eventually end up conducting the trials and writing the clinical practice guidelines. Safeguards to eliminate biases only prevent the most blatant and obvious instances of the widespread inherent, related corruption.

Agencies of the U.S. Department of Health and Human Services have issued many of the guidelines. For example, the Food and Drug Administration (FDA) regulates drugs. The FDA determines what drugs to approve and which to keep off the market. The Center for Medicare and Medicaid Services decides which tests and treatments will be covered and what fees the government will pay Medicare and Medicaid providers for their services.

In reality, the identification of what works and what doesn't work in medicine is very frequently *controversial*. Examples abound of guideline-driven clinical practices followed for years by physicians that subsequent studies showed did harm to patients. Clinical guidelines change at a rapid pace, indicating that many guidelines were erroneous in the first place.

There has been widespread corruption in the development of many guidelines. Extensive harm to patients from following faulty guidelines has occurred, such as giving 100% oxygen to premature babies, which has lead to many instances of blindness.[15] Seeking rigid conformity in health care practices costs taxpayers and health insurance payers dearly.

What should we do?

We must abandon requiring universal compliance with health care guidelines and mandates coming from federal or state governments, insurance companies, or medical special interests.

Consequently, the fifth grand bargain is to replace universal health care guidelines by the government or expert authorities with ACC self-regulation.

Questions arise.

How should we monitor health care quality and safety without federal and/or state government experts telling physicians how to practice medicine? If the federal government isn't the entity that sanctions the metrics used to measure the performances of physicians and health care institutions (e.g., quality of care indicators), then who should do it?

We can incorporate the answers to these questions with an explanation of deregulation of health care.

Medical practice guidelines and benefit packages should still exist. However, they should be *decentralized*. They should be determined by physicians and other stakeholders of each ACC for that ACC.

Adhering to the status quo should be the default course of action regarding each clinical practice guideline. However, ACC managers, informed by collaborative input from all ACC stakeholders, should be able to make changes. They should be able to institute what they believe are interventions that will improve patient care and to eliminate coverage of what they deem to be unnecessary tests and treatments.

With decentralized clinical practice guidelines and different ACCs offering alternative benefit packages, research into the relationships of medical interventions and patient outcomes will be greatly enabled. Consequently, progress in finding more effective treatments can advance much faster than now. In this manner, a functioning health care marketplace will evolve. The marketplace will be characterized by intense competition, increasing efficiencies, and ongoing quality improvement. This free market in health care among private competing ACCs will spawn a race to the top in quality and a race to the bottom in cost.

Grand Bargain #6: ACCs to Provide Long-Term Care

Of about 16 million disabled Americans requiring long-term care, only approximately 1.6 million live in institutions. The rest remain at home receiving varying amounts of personal care (e.g., bathing, dressing, and preparing meals) delivered by about 46 million unpaid family members and friends, and about 1 million professional home health aides. The home health aides, primarily low-income women, are themselves unprotected by basic labor standards despite efforts in Congress to institute appropriate regulations. Consequently, low pay (averaging $9.62 per hour in 2007), long hours, provider burnout, and high turnover undermine the quality of long-term care.[16]

Grand Bargain #6 is for ACCs to provide comprehensive long-term care for frail elderly and disabled people (Chapter 6), and to provide for the caregivers' just compensation.

Grand Bargain #7: ACCs to Provide Oral Health Care

Dentistry is in crisis. More U.S. dental schools have closed than have opened in the past 25 years. The number of dentists who retire each year exceeds the number of dental school graduates by at least two thousand. Access to oral health care, particularly among the poor, is a major problem. Since the mid 1990s, oral health outcomes in the U.S. have not improved overall.[17, 18]

Grand Bargain #7 is for oral health care to be included in health services covered and delivered by ACCs (Chapter 6). This is no mere policy option, but something concrete that millions of us can sink our teeth into.

Grand Bargain #8: Merge ACC Health Care with Social Services

The availability of quality medical care explains only 10%–15% of the variation in the major health indices (i.e., preventable early deaths, infant mortality, longevity, quality of life, etc.). The "social indicators of health" (income, education, nutrition, social relationships, race, where someone lives, etc.) account for nearly 80% of health outcomes.[19] Genes account for less than 5% and the rest is attributable to the accessibility and quality of health care. Consequently, social services should be better integrated with health care.

Grand Bargain #8 is to combine our health care and social-safety-net (welfare) systems and allocate social services through ACCs.

I propose that federal, state, and local welfare-program administration and delivery be shifted to the ACCs. Within an ACC, there will be perhaps 20-5000 patient-centered medical homes (i.e., serving 100,000 – 25 million members). Each patient-centered medical home will serve its patients by coordinating diverse social service professionals (e.g., social workers, psychotherapists, child protective services providers, etc.) and volunteers (church groups, mutual support organizations, etc.) in delivering social services. Patient-centered medical homes within ACCs will deliver health care and social services in a free market, according to their own guidelines and benefit packages. Some social services professionals will be based in the offices of the patient-centered medical homes and others will be available for contracting as needed.

Funding for social-safety-net services will come primarily from block grants from the federal government. Due to controversies about block grants for social services from the federal government to states, block grants have been rarely utilized. The proposed greatly expanded block grants that will be detailed will equate to the "risk-adjusted" allocations of welfare funds determined according to socioeconomic statuses of ACC members (Chapter 10). "Risk-adjusted" means that more funds go for older, sicker, and more socio-economically disadvantaged people than those who are younger, healthier, and more affluent.

To control welfare spending over the long term, the government's social-safety-net budget will be frozen at the 2016 level. When people choose ACCs offering more or fewer services, this will be reflected in higher or lower monthly premiums. In this way, people in the medical marketplace will control their own costs by their choices of ACCs.

Grand Bargain #9: Comprehensive Payment System Reform with ACC Providers Deciding Medical Coverage

With medical benefit packages decentralized and clinical practice guidelines decided by each ACC, our medical insurance system will have to change.

The requirement for employers to be responsible for the health care insurance for their employees and their families is unraveling. The "employer mandate" for employee health insurance has been an uneven, unworkable policy and should end. The first change is for patients to choose their providers and pay their own premiums to an entity that will take responsibility for their employment opportunities (i.e., ACCs).

Secondly, the current system of private and public insurance companies deciding what medical tests and treatments to cover, and what not to cover, has well recognized problems. Grand Bargains' reform will end medical insurance companies as we know them. Yet, we still need someone to collect the premiums from ACC members and from government programs (i.e., Medicaid, Medicare, Children's Health Insurance Program, Veterans Administration Health Care, etc). Someone will also be needed to pay health-care and other providers for their services and to keep track of money received and spent.

Based on bad experiences of many people with insurance companies (public and private) that determine medical benefits for people, we need to have some entity other than the money collector & dispenser decide what medical interventions to fund and how much to pay for covered services. The PCPs of the ACCs, in collaboration with other patient-centered medical home members, with input from other stakeholders, are best positioned for that role.

Consequently, *Grand Bargain #9 is to have comprehensive payment system reform with ACCs—not insurance company administrators or government bureaucrats—making all decisions about funding for medical and other services for enrollees.*

As part of this grand bargain on medical payment reform, medical insurance companies will change to "financial services providers" and remain in business since they will be vitally needed for ACCs' functioning. Beginning in 2016, ACCs or their affiliated financial services providers will increase their number of enrollees to the entire population and expand their financial administration services to include social services, other human services, and entitlements (Grand Bargains #8, #12, #17, and #18).

Underwriting will not be needed to buy medical insurance. The amount of one's premium will depend only on his/her age. No matter what the health risks, the premium will not change. The ACCs rather than the insurance companies will deal with complaints about coverage of medical services. So ACC-affiliated financial services companies will be able to cover all U.S. residents with greatly expanded services for about the overhead costs medical insurance companies now incur providing a mind-numbing array of health insurance products for a little more than half of the people in the country.[c] The competition between ACCs will keep financial services executives from being excessively compensated.

To earn the privilege of working with ACCs, financial services companies will compete based on promptness, accuracy of service, and cost per enrollee for revenue management. Each ACC will contract with a financial services company to receive age-adjusted health care premiums from members (Chapter 18). The same financial services companies will also receive the government risk-adjusted health care funds totaling the personal health care costs that are projected for each year (about $3.3 trillion in 2016[20]-2025, i.e., frozen at the 2016 level). The ACCs' financial services companies will also receive government social services funds (about $500 billion in 2016[21]-2025). Government welfare programs (Medicaid, Obamacare, Children's Health Insurance Program, Head Start, Public Assistance, Government Subsidized Housing, Food Stamps, etc.) will then become administered in an integrated, efficient manner by specialists in health care and social services from ACCs. In this way, the federal, state, and local government services to the public are much decentralized and more locally accountable.

---

c   About 180 million U.S. residents covered by private medical insurance out of about 325 million residents.

Out of funds for health care and other human services received, the financial services companies will pay for products (e.g., medical devices) and services as directed by the ACC management. Decision-makers in each ACC will determine the amounts to pay providers of patient care and social services (e.g., salaries, consulting contracts, fee-for-service, etc.). Who in each ACC become decision-makers will be up to each ACC. However, ACC physicians and staff will not receive bonuses for limiting medical interventions as Obamacare proposes for ACOs.

Incentivized by medical marketplace discipline, comprehensive health care and other services delivered by ACCs will align the interests of patients, health care providers, and taxpayers. ACCs will seek the most efficient and least wasteful allocation of resources for medical care, preventive medicine, health promotion, alternative treatments, and social services to optimize health and social outcomes. This approach will incentivize health care and other services to be coordinated, innovative, and flexible.

ACCs will be able to adapt to local needs using local human and material resources. Savings from ACC efficiencies in administering health and social services funds will go to additional patient services and/or to reducing medical premiums for patients. Competition between all ACCs, as they are self-regulated, will attract patients and will be a major strategy for controlling the cost of enrollee premiums and health care overall.

Grand Bargain #10: Reduce Administrative Complexity in Health Care and Retrain Redundant Workers

According to the National Academy of Sciences, the health care industry employs 810 medical administrators per $1 billion in products and services versus 50 administrators per $1 billion for the average business.[22] For patients, providers, and taxpayers, decentralizing health care regulation and of reforming the health care payment systems as described in Grand Bargain #9 could save over $1 trillion per year without reducing valuable services.

Since health services will be provided by private competing ACCs with decentralized clinical practice guidelines, PCPs and specialists will no longer need to deal with excessive medical bureaucracy. The administrative integration of social services (Grand Bargain #8) and of disability benefits (Grand Bargain #12) into competing ACCs will further reduce paperwork and increase benefits to members.

Reducing all this administrative complexity will save lots of money to benefit all ACC stakeholders. However, out of about 21 million jobs in health care and social assistance today,[23] it will also make redundant up to a quarter of these workers. Consequently, the grand bargain to reduce administrative complexity calls for millions of medical administrators to be retrained in order to move to other careers. The ACCs of these displaced workers will be responsible for finding them other job opportunities.

With Grand Bargains-based reform, the businesses of health care and social services will be more about health care and social services and less about paperwork and money. This necessary downsizing of medical and social services bureaucracies will enable funding to train and employ millions more medical and social services professionals. These will include PCPs, other health care workers and human services providers including social workers, financial counselors, educators, legal advisors, employment counselors, community gardeners, environmental restoration teams, etc. ACCs will employ many of these workers within the ACCs or place them elsewhere in their communities.

Grand Bargain #11: ACCs to Adopt an "Enterprise Liability" Medical Malpractice System

Tragically, the career consequences of a medical malpractice case often lead practitioners not to admit errors. As a result, care providing teams of clinicians miss opportunities to learn from mistakes and improve system performance.

Medical errors causing harms to patients arise most commonly as medical system problems rather than solely as mistakes of individual practitioners. In a fair and just system, individual providers should not be assuming all responsibility for adverse patient outcomes.

Grand Bargain #11 is for comprehensive malpractice system reform to include ACCs' assuming responsibility for all medical errors causing patient harms. This type of medical malpractice system is called "enterprise liability."[24]

The responsibility for patient safety will lie with the ACC (the enterprise), so all physicians and allied health care workers will have joint responsibility. Exceptions will be with intentional harm inflicted by providers on patients, sexual misconduct, and adverse patient outcomes related to provider substance abuse. In those cases, providers could be sued in criminal or civil courts. For physicians and other health care workers that willfully harm patients or are deemed hopelessly incompetent or negligent by coworkers, ACC staff will have every reason to fire them and report them to legal authorities.

In most cases, ACCs will consider medical errors "system problems" rather than mistakes caused solely by individual practitioners. For instance, a physician writing the wrong dose for a medication should be noted and the physician alerted by a nurse or pharmacist reading the order. Each error causing an unfortunate patient outcome will become an opportunity to help spur the needed corrections in the system of health care delivery.

Enterprise liability will give each staff member of each ACC a stake in ensuring that all its PCPs, specialist consultants, and other ACC care providers are competent and diligent. It will provide a safeguard that the entire organization works collaboratively to reduce risks of harm to patients. Medical errors will be deterred because all ACC health care providers and other employees will be rewarded by good reputations for reducing the risk of errors.

For services authorized by ACCs, physicians and other health care providers will not need malpractice insurance. Safe medical practice and error avoidance will be the mutual responsibility of all ACC care providers. ACCs with providers that commit excessive errors that harm patients will have a hard time competing in the competitive market-place of ACCs. This kind of self-regulation of quality control will work much better than the often capricious and error-prone involvement of the medical malpractice system.

Grand Bargains in Non-Health Care Sectors

Health, health care, and outcomes of health care interventions are strongly influenced by what people eat, where they live, what work they do, whether they have legal troubles, if they have financial security, their educational opportunities, how they travel from place to place, and the stability and security of the community and the country. These next grand bargains will address all these issues that indirectly but hugely affect health care, health, and wellbeing.

Grand Bargain #12: ACCs to Provide Disability, Unemployment, and Workers' Compensation Benefits

Most of the disability claims projected to be paid in 2016 will be through government programs—Social Security Disability,[17] and Veterans Administration disability benefits.[19] Workers Compensation[18] and unemployment insurance benefits also help people in need of financial assistance due to employment issues. Complex medical problems, including malpractice allegations, may be involved in many cases. The bureaucratic processes in these overlapping disability and employment programs leads to a range of frustrating delays and unwarranted denials on the one hand, to unjustified wasteful payment allocations on the other.

To take enterprise liability a step further, Grand Bargain #12 *is to integrate disability, unemployment, and workers' compensation benefits into social-safety-net services provided by ACCs.*

As administrators of all public disability and unemployment insurance (Social Security Disability, Social Security Supplemental Insurance, Veterans Administration benefits, unemployment benefits, workers' compensation, etc.), ACCs will determine fair compensation for people who are disabled or otherwise not working for money. This will greatly simplify disability issues and the often related problem of unemployment. It won't matter what is the cause of the disability (e.g., medical malpractice or unfortunate accident). ACCs will have the resources and the flexibility to provide fair compensation and opportunities to offer rehabilitation and appropriate employment. This will not require adjudicating whether the problem was due to medical malpractice, to bad luck involving a medical intervention, or not caused by a medical system encounter. Ascertaining blame takes a lengthy, expensive, and error-prone litigation process that we have with the current broken system.

Instead, all payments for medical malpractice occurrences *and* any other disabilities will be the responsibility of the ACCs. ACC legal and social services teams will mediate prompt and fair compensation to patients for severe harm or disability by any cause.

ACCs will combine these overlapping disability benefits programs, and assign "human services" providers to manage them. PCPs will determine which enrollees are disabled and what disabled members can still do. As will be detailed in Grand Bargain #14, ACCs will assist all work-ready members to find jobs. For the most part, this will take the place of unemployment dole payments. Our unemployment system is broken, bureaucratic and inefficient. The ACCs will receive the unemployment revenue from the U.S. Treasury as part of welfare block grants. ACCs will provide the assistance to unemployed people in a manner that ACC stakeholders feel is most effective. For most people, finding a job or entering a job training program will be most desired.

Competition between ACCs will be, in part, around the fairness, equity, and flexibility in which they work with disabled and unemployed members, and with members hurt on the job or through their medical misfortune.

Grand Bargain #13: ACCs to Foster Legal System Reform

Torts and litigation in the U.S. consume about 2% of the GDP compared with about 1% of GDP in other developed countries.[21, 22] Our excessive litigation fees and unnecessarily high incarceration rates themselves constitute injustice. Many feel unprotected by our legal system and also feel that money unduly affects outcomes in legal proceedings. While providing public defenders for indigent people charged with crimes somewhat offsets corruption, discrimination, or incompetence in law enforcement, poor people are still often treated unfairly in the criminal justice system.

Grand Bargain #13 is for each ACC to provide prepaid basic legal services for its enrollees, including those involved in the criminal justice system.

Providing ACC members, especially youth, with educational, recreational, and employment opportunities will be among the methods used by legal services departments in partnering with other ACC departments to prevent criminal behavior. Successful legal services teams will substantially reduce the number of ACC enrollees sent to jail and the recidivism rates of those released from jail.

Out of money saved from efficiencies and innovations in health and social services, ACC managers will hire lawyers and paralegals charged with advising clients about legal matters. Whenever possible, disputes will be kept out of the courts. ACC legal teams will strive towards fairness, justice, mediation, rehabilitation, and minimizing legal costs. ACCs will not provide legal services for businesses of enrollees.

ACCs will compete with each other, in part, on the performances of their legal services departments in minimizing the legal liabilities, civil and criminal, of enrollees. With these ACC legal services in place, overall litigation costs in the U.S. will drop as will costs for law enforcement, prisons, and courts.

For legal system workers made redundant by legal system reform, it will be the responsibility of the ACCs to help them find other job opportunities.

Grand Bargain #14: ACCs to Provide Jobs for Members

Franklin Delanor Roosevelt's inaugural address was famous for the phrase: "The only thing we have to fear is fear itself." But, in that speech, he also said: "Our greatest primary task is to put people to work." And he said the country should treat that task "as we would treat the emergency of a war."[23] So it is in the U.S. today. Improving health care and health outcomes must involve dramatically increasing employment. The usual theories and remedies for doing this, such as "trickle down" economics and boosting monetary supply by the Federal Reserve, have not countered the ravages of recession or the sending of millions of U.S. jobs to other countries.

According to the "Employment Situation Summary" by the Bureau of Labor Statistics for October 2014, about 20 million U.S. residents were unemployed, working part-time for economic reasons, or wanting to work but too discouraged to actively seek a job.[24] Another 60+ million or more people work in very challenging non-paying jobs: parenting young children and/or caring for disabled friends or family members.

The Department of Labor projects that this miserable employment situation will be pretty much the same until 2022.[19] This is not good enough. We cannot let this become the new normal.

The way the U.S. economy is structured, businesses *do not* create jobs. Demand is what creates jobs.[22] Businesses have every reason to dispose of workers. The marketplace incentives to reduce jobs include high corporate income taxes, crushing medical insurance premiums, payroll taxes, workers' compensation, unemployment insurance, foreign competition with cheap labor, government regulation, and domestic competitors that overwork and underpay their workers.

We need multiple, complementary, game-changing grand bargains that address economic needs of the workers and the employers.

Consider workers first (later grand bargains in this book address employers' needs): *Grand Bargain #14 is for ACCs to provide jobs for unemployed members so as to achieve at least 98% employment.*

Each ACC will have a "jobs department." Staff members of ACC departments of employment will have the task of assisting every work-ready ACC member to find a job. Financial resources that will be available to ACC jobs departments to keep members employed will include the $500 billion federal and state welfare budgets (Grand Bargain #8) and roughly $64 billion that the U.S. Department of Labor's Employment and Training Administration spends trying to create jobs.[25] ACCs will also tap savings from reducing waste, inefficiency, and bureaucracy in health care, to create tens of millions of jobs which will stoke the economy.

ACCs will have the resources to pay up to 10 million (full-time equivalent) stay-at-home parents for their child care. Another 10 million (full-time equivalent) or more ACCs members will be employed to care for elderly or disabled relatives or friends.

As an incentive, ACCs keeping employment rates above 98% of the work force will receive additional federal welfare funds. With Grand Bargains' reform, welfare from government agencies—which often fosters dependency—will be replaced by assistance from ACCs that will be more flexible, accountable, innovative, and results-oriented.

Grand Bargain #15: Raise Minimum Wage to $15/Hour

Low-wage workers are increasingly resorting to public social services such as food stamps and Medicaid to make ends meet. Widespread public protests have advocated for a living minimum wage of $15 per hour.[26] Some cities are enacting this new standard. The protesters and local legislators make a valid point. Few can live on the current $7.25 per hour minimum wage and pay for essentials, let alone have any kind of quality of life.

Overall, 25% of workers supplement their incomes with public assistance. Over 50% of fast food workers rely, in part, on public social services.[27] This amounts to a subsidy from the taxpayers to low-wage businesses. While large corporations have more wealth than at any time in history, U.S. taxpayers—present and future—are bearing much of the hidden costs of Wall Street's boom. The solution is for employers to pay living wages.

Grand Bargain #15 will be for the federal minimum wage to be increased to $15 per hour.

For roughly 75 million workers that currently earn less than $15 per hour, the cost of raising the minimum wage to $15 per hour will be about $660 billion (Chapter 12). The minimum wage will be adjusted upward or downward depending on the cost of living in different areas of the country, using the MIT living wage calculator.[28] Businesses will have lots of help affording the higher minimum wage, according to several business-friendly grand bargains. Businesses will save a projected $557 billion by the elimination of corporate income taxes (Grand Bargain #19). Additionally, the responsibility for most employees' benefits will be shifted from employers to the ACCs (Grand Bargains #9 and #12), amounting to an additional over $900 billion saved by businesses (Chapter 21).

Grand Bargain #16: ACCs to Provide Members Financial Education and Counseling

Our culture is infected with "affluenza"—defined as "a painful, contagious, socially transmitted condition of overload, debt, anxiety, and waste resulting from the dogged pursuit of more."[29] Affluenza affects personal lives as well as our "consumer" economy. Trying to assign blame for our dysfunctional economic system tends to divide rather than unify people. At least to some extent, we are all villains and we are all victims. *Grand Bargains' reforms* focus more on answers than on identifying the villains responsible for our wasteful consumption, unsustainable debt, and economic mess.

The federal government Consumer Protection Agency is well intentioned, and employs very smart people. However, it has failed at teaching ordinary people to become financially literate. All the financial industry regulations enacted by Congress will not be enough to keep many financially illiterate people from excessive indebtedness, bankruptcy, and destitution.

A new public policy approach to foster widespread sound financial management, regular saving, frugal spending, and eventual financial security is what we need.

Grand Bargain #16 is to have financial education and counseling provided by ACCs to members.

The grand bargain of adding financial education services to the responsibilities of ACCs will be one of the game-changers to lead us out of wasteful ways. Using federal block-grant funds, ACCs will promote financial literacy and economic security for their members. While the top 1% in wealth may not need help, ACCs will be well positioned to aid the "99%" of middle and lower income people to become financially more secure. In the long run, this promotes stability and healing of society, thus benefiting even the 1% as well.

ACC financial experts will also provide individual counseling. These financial services specialists will aid members in shopping for value and affordability in food, transportation, housing, education, financial services, telecommunications services, energy, retirement plans, and investments. This will drive down prices, as overpaying becomes more rare. ACC financial counselors will help enrollees reign in debt, understand mortgages and other loans, avoid being victimized by fraud, manage their money, and save for a rainy day.

ACC will provide members with financial professionals charged with increasing the efficiency of and reducing the cost of member financial services. Consequently, the exorbitant aggregate cost of financial services will be reduced. The savings can go to high value economic activities that create jobs, strengthen communities, and help the environment.

Since major health and social problems arise more often in association with poverty and financial mismanagement, educating people on financial matters by ACC counselors will promote good member health and socioeconomic outcomes.

In an environment of ACCs competing in part on financial successes of enrollees, ACC financial services professionals will be incentivized to help enrollees utilize their financial services to full advantage. Experimentation in approaches to offering financial services will lead to steady improvements in financial security of ACC members.

Financial services workers that become redundant because of ACC related efficiencies in the reformed financial system will have ACC assistance in finding new jobs.

Grand Bargain #17: ACCs to Administer Social Security for Members

Nobel Prize winning economist Milton Friedman has called Social Security a "Ponzi scheme." Current entitlement spending, including Social Security, robs future generations while potentially leading the country towards insolvency. Economic reform to balance the federal budget without entitlement reorganization is an oxymoron. Simply cutting benefits without dealing with fraud, waste, and inefficiency in the government's administration of entitlements will increase wealth inequality and lead to social unrest. We need fair and equitable entitlement reform.

Grand Bargain #17 will transfer the management of Social Security to the ACCs.

The federal government will continue to collect Social Security payroll taxes. However, the Social Security Administration will transfer the money to ACC-affiliated credit unions/savings & loan banks (S&Ls). The credit unions/S&Ls will distribute Social Security benefits to members. Social Security will no longer be a responsibility of the federal government except to collect the payroll taxes and transfer the payroll tax revenue and the Social Security Trust Funds now in the U.S. Treasury to the ACCs (Chapter 23). ACC-affiliated credit unions/S&Ls will invest the Social Security in-reserve funds into home mortgages for members, foreclosed homes, other properties, job-creating social benefit businesses, and other investments.

Social Security benefits being administered by ACC-affiliated credit unions/S&Ls will accompany coordination of comprehensive financial and social services (Grand Bargains #6-#8, #12-#18, and #20-#22) for those currently receiving Social Security. Those who are now paying into Social Security will appreciate the ACCs' providing long-term stability and security that the funds will not run out or be diminished (Chapter 23). This entitlement reform will also bolster the solvency of the federal government. By distributing the Social Security Trust Funds to ACC-affiliated credit unions/S&Ls, ACC management of Social Security will enhance the health and sustainability of local economies throughout the country (Chapter 24).

Grand Bargain #18: ACCs to Administer Pension Plans for Members

The Pew Center for the States estimated that states' public pension plans across the U.S. were underfunded by $1.4 trillion in 2010.[30] Employee contributions into public pension funds dropped due to the difficult economic times of the Great Recession. State and local governments also decreased pension contributions as they struggled to maintain vital services with declining revenues. In an effort to make up for the huge pension fund deficits, public pension funds have been going into risky investments. Public pensions are doing somewhat better now, in part because of the five year bull market on Wall Street. However, another downturn in the economy could create another pension fund solvency crisis.

Assigning blame for unsustainable pension obligations for public sector employees does not help. Perhaps the system can be fixed with a plan acceptable to both liberals and conservatives. Shifting public servant pension obligations from government agencies to ACCs is the perfect fix.

Grand Bargain #18 is for ACCs to administer public and private sector pension plans.

Given the unsustainability of worker pension costs for many federal, state, and local government agencies,[31] ACC-affiliated financial services companies will take over management of new pension saving accounts of government workers and receive subsequent contributions. Existing pension accounts with investment funds will remain in place under the current management and closed to new contributions. As new ACC pension accounts are created, ACCs will negotiate with government employees or their unions about the terms and conditions of the eventual distributions of their ACC-managed pensions.

Agencies of the government will fund each employee pension by sending the monthly contribution of funds to the employee's account in the ACC-affiliated credit union/S&L. The ACCs will integrate pension disbursements into the social and financial services that members receive.

Since state and local governments will shift the responsibilities for funding health and human services to ACCs, the fiscal conditions of these governments will improve, allowing them to fully fund their pension programs for past and current employees. This will allow state and local governments to get back to solvency, to provide needed services, and to again take on important new projects for the public good.

Private sector pension plan defaults nearly made the Pensions Benefits Guarantee Corporation[a] become insolvent during the Great Recession.[32] Millions of workers took big cuts in their expected savings for retirement. Taxpayers will be at risk if another wave of private pension plan defaults occurs. For the security of private sector workers and taxpayers, Grand Bargains reform calls for private pensions to also be managed by ACC-affiliated credit union/S&Ls on a voluntary basis. Since this will be safer and easier for employers and employees, most workers and employers will choose ACC-managed pensions.

---

a   Pensions Benefits Guarantee Corporation is a federal government agency that serves as an insurance company for private corporate pension plans (Chapter 24).

Grand Bargain #19: Taxing Consumption More Than Income

Direct practice primary care providers, clinical practice guideline deregulation, and ACCs integrating health care with social, financial, legal, and employment services will have plenty of resources to improve public health. ACC-directed and -coordinated services will also begin to lower costs of health care, welfare, financial services, entitlements, and the government itself. However, tax reform will be needed to simultaneously further improve health outcomes, reduce income inequality, facilitate environmental sustainability, balance the federal government budget, incentivize job creation, and spur economic growth in terms of quality of products and services, not just quantity (as in the GDP).

Grand Bargain #19 is to restructure the federal and state tax systems to tax consumption more than income.

I propose almost $1.9 trillion per year of federal consumption taxes on the following commodities and services:

1. tobacco
2. alcohol
3. freshwater
4. plastics
5. trades of equities on the stock market
6. guns (Grand Bargain #29)
7. holdings of too big to fail banks
8. internet connection services
9. health and environmental imprint of imports
10. fossil fuels and nuclear energy

These new taxes will be offset by completely eliminating the federal and state corporate income taxes and the federal and state personal income taxes on individuals earning less than $60,000 per year or couples earning less than $120,000 per year. For the high earners (roughly 10% of current income tax filers), our current system with graduated tax rates and myriads of complicated deductions will be replaced with a revenue neutral flat tax of 25% of taxable income. Deductions will be eliminated. Filing tax returns will be easy.

Drastically reducing the number of income tax filers and the complexity of filing will reduce the cost of compliance with the Internal Revenue Service code by an estimated 90% (i.e., instead of $200 billion per year currently, it will cost no more than $20 billion). Administration of consumption taxes will be relatively simple, costing at most half of the current costs of income tax compliance (i.e., consumption tax compliance will cost no more than $100 billion in 2016). This will mean the loss of jobs involved with compliance with the IRS code. ACCs will retrain these people in other occupations and assist them in finding new jobs.

The Grand Bargains' consumption taxes will be levied on the above commodities and services that have negative health, economic, or environmental consequences (Table 1, Chapter 21). A tax on the labor of undocumented immigrants will also be levied (Grand Bargain #20 and Chapter 14), although they will be paid the new minimum wage of $15 per hour.

Eliminating the corporate income tax will have a major immediate benefit on jobs and the economy. Over a trillion dollars in tax sheltered overseas corporate income will be repatriated to create jobs and boost U.S. economic growth. Companies will save tax money by bringing their earning back to the U.S.

The new taxes will reduce federal deficit spending to zero. As a bonus, about $1 trillion per year will be saved by consumers by (1) decreasing the consumption of the highly taxed commodities and services, (2) by reducing health care costs associated with the taxed commodities, and (3) by reducing the cost of compliance with the tax code. Health care premiums will go down over time because reduced utilization of the items taxed will mean fewer diseases and injuries.

Table 1. Consumption and Undocumented Immigrant
Labor Taxes to be Levied and Money to be Saved

Item for the tax	Tax revenue generated ($billions)	Money saved by less consumption ($billions)	Other money saved ($billions)
Tobacco	$27	$14	$40
Alcohol	$75	$50	$60
Nonrenewable energy	$700	$343	$40
Water	$300	$130	-
Plastics	$150	$100	-
Equity trades	$150	$10	-
Guns	$50	-	$30
Systemic risk banks	$50	-	-
Electronic media	$120	-	-
Imported goods	$240	$120	-
Undocumented labor tax ($3/hr)	$60		
Income tax system compliance cost savings			$80
Total	$1922	$767	$250

Grand Bargain #20: Comprehensive Immigration Reform

If we could somehow suddenly deport all 11 million undocumented immigrants that are peaceably living and working among us,

the economy, particularly agriculture, would suffer greatly. Ongoing prosperity in the U.S. depends on attracting hard-working immigrants with skills and talents that we have in short supply. Both highly educated professionals and less educated agricultural, food service, and domestic workers can help our country prosper.

Grand Bargain #20 is to allow undocumented immigrants to remain in the U.S. with a path to citizenship. Employers of illegal immigrants will pay a tax of $3 per hour on their labor.

With this proposed grand bargain on immigration reform, immigrants (undocumented as well as legal) will be eligible to enroll in ACCs. However, they will need to pay the full costs of their insurance premiums and will not be eligible for social-safety-net funding until they become citizens. Only by paying taxes and ACC insurance premiums for all previous time spent in the U.S. will immigrants be eligible for eventual citizenship.

Retaining innovative, hard-working, highly-motivated immigrants will enhance our economy, our diversity, and our quality of life. Additionally, billions of dollars per year will be saved by less bureaucracy and policing/militarization of immigration, legal and illegal.

Grand Bargain #21: ACCs to Lead Experimentation with the Education System

People with more education live longer, earn more money, contribute more to their communities, and have a better quality of life. Educational achievement is a major social indicator of health. Highly educated people are less likely to receive welfare and will usually have smaller families. Prosperity—not necessarily defined entirely by money—depends on excellence in education.

Deficiencies in some aspects of our educational system threaten our competitiveness in the global economy. Politicians debate about whether more charter schools, more testing, higher pay for teachers, more of any of the current policy prescriptions of the Department of Education will fix our schools. Liberals complain that teachers are underpaid and undervalued. Conservatives gripe that teachers' unions and school system bureaucracies are out of control. Without taking sides on these polarized arguments, it's fair to say that here is no "one-size-fits-all" solution.

Grand Bargain #21 is to give ACCs an education mandate. U.S. Department of Education funds will be channeled through ACCs to communities, supplementing for society the financial and human resources of public and private schools. Along with the education funds comes the authorization for ACCs to find their own supplemental approaches to attaining educational excellence.

We need to experiment to achieve educational excellence. Different ACCs will try different approaches to enhance the education of students. This will require that ACCs employ educators to listen to and work with teachers, parents, students and school district administrators. The strategies that work will be replicated widely.

Since people will choose their ACCs, educational excellence and positive impacts of the use of ACC education funds will be part of the competition for members between ACCs.

As with other grand bargains, some people will be displaced from jobs. Public education system administrators made redundant by the shift of education funds to ACCs will be assisted in finding other jobs by their ACCs. Net employment in education and funding to education will be expected to increase substantially.

Grand Bargain #22: ACC Members to Enhance National Security as Development Workers

The mission of the Department of Defense has always been "to provide the military forces needed to deter war and to protect the security of our country."[31] However, the characterizations of threats to the security of the U.S. and the nature of military combat have both changed dramatically in the past 100 years. For instance, the threat due to terrorism has become transnational as well as domestic in the last decade. Consequently, we need to fundamentally reassess how best to protect ourselves from danger coming from outside and inside the U.S. borders.

To deter war and terrorism, we need to understand the causes of major conflicts at a deep level. Then we must proactively work to prevent social injustice, religious intolerance, prejudice, and inequity in economic opportunity. By addressing the breeding grounds for extremist ideologies, we can prevent incidents escalating into wars or acts of terrorism.

Deterring war and terrorism should be mainly about partnering with people around the world to help them develop. We can teach them strategies to combat poverty, facilitate education, institute sustainable farming methods, build clean drinking water systems, and promote public health. This will not only help stabilize and enrich their lives, but it will build good will towards us.

Grand Bargain #22 is to generously fund Third World development programs run by nonprofit organizations staffed, funded, and monitored through the ACCs.

An example of a suitable nonprofit to partner with ACCs in humanitarian aid work would be the United Nations Peacebuilding Commission that supports multidimensional peace efforts in countries emerging from conflict.[32] Their mission is to help prevent relapses into fighting. Success in this crucial field is underappreciated and rarely noticed. Development work is greatly underfunded.

The Congressional Budget Office projects a major decrease in national defense spending over the next decade as a proportion of the GDP. This national security grand bargain will more than offset the decline in spending and jobs in national defense. At a time that the military Joint Chiefs of Staff are planning to cut tens of thousands of men and women from the military service, this will be a huge job creator. The increases in spending will be exclusively for development in Third World countries.

ACC members' bolstering national security in foreign country development jobs completes the spectrum of services to be provided by the various departments of the ACCs.

The Big Picture of ACC-Based Health Care and Economic Reform

Figure 1 illustrates the relationship of ACC enrollees with professionals in the various ACC departments. Each ACC will provide comprehensive services to members. Flexibility and innovation will be incentivized. Staffing for the ACCs will come from current government workers from agencies that become downsized or eliminated and from providers of health and human services in the private sector. Since ACCs will manage about $6 trillion in 2016 (one-third of the economy), employees will have to number > 60 million (one-third of the workforce).

Table 2 shows the status quo sources of U.S. government revenue for 2016. Note that over half a trillion dollars will be borrowed. This high national debt (over $19 trillion in 2016) jeopardizes our national security and economic sustainability.

Table 3 details projected government revenue after a shift from a largely income-tax based system to less income tax and a predominantly consumption tax system. Federal government borrowing will be eliminated and over $400 billion of additional revenue will be raised to invest in long deferred infrastructure projects, pay some of the national debt, strengthen national defense, shift social taxes to federal block grants, and apply to other priorities.

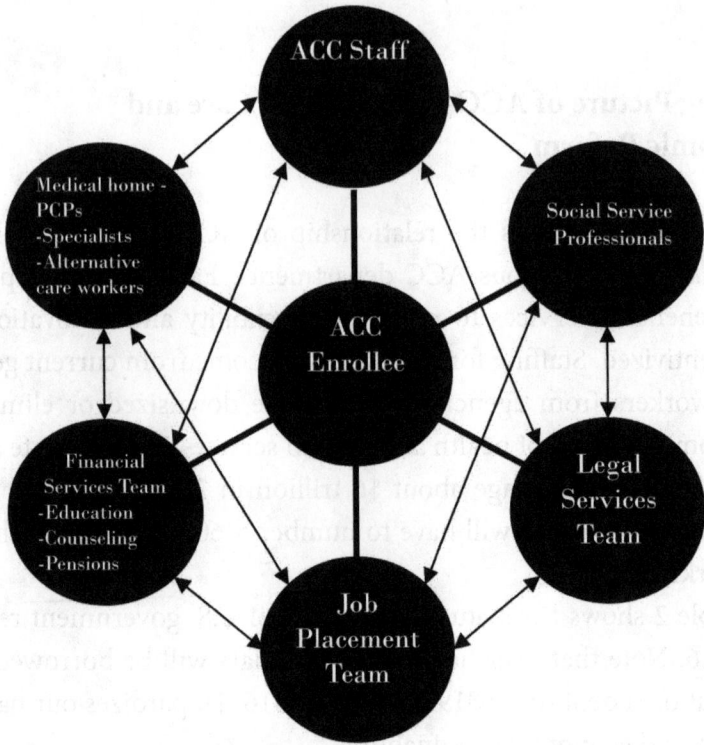

Figure 1. Relationships of ACC Enrollee to ACC Components

Table 2. U.S. Federal, State, and Local Government Status
Quo Revenues Projected for 2016 ($billions)[33]

Sources of U.S. government revenue	2016 projected revenue
Federal	4100
Taxes, fees, insurance	3570
Individual income	1648
Corporate income	502
Social insurance	1130
Old age and survivors	690
Disability (SSI)	120
Unemployment	60
Hospital insurance	250
Business and other	60
Ad valorem taxes	220
Excise	60
Transportation	50
Other	110
Borrowing	530
State and local revenue	2711
Individual income	336
Corporate income	55
Social insurance	380
Unemployment	80
Retirement	300
Business and other	370
Utility/liquor	150
Fees and charges	460
Health	150
Ad valorem taxes	1110
Excise	60
Sales	490
Property	420
Transportation	80
Licenses	50
U.S. government taxes + borrowing	6810

Table 3. U.S. Federal, State, and Local Government Revenues Projected
for 2016 ($billions) with ACCs and the Grand Bargains

Sources of U.S. government revenue	2016 revenue
Federal	4676
Taxes, fees, insurance	4676
Individual income	1400
Corporate income	0
Consumption taxes	1862
Trading equities	150
Nonrenewable energy	700
Plastics	150
Tobacco	27
Alcohol	75
Guns	50
Water	300
Systemic risk banks	50
Electronic media	120
Imported goods	240
Immigrant employment	60
Social insurance	1074
Old age	901
Disability (SSI)	173
Unemployment	0
Business & other	60
Ad valorem taxes	220
Excise	60
Transportation	50
Other	110
Borrowing	0
State and local revenue	2566
Individual income	326
Corporate income	0
Social insurance	300
Unemployment	0
Retirement	300
Business and other	370
Fees and charges	460
Health	0
Ad valorem taxes	1110
Excise	60
Sales	490
Property	420
Transportation	80
Licenses	50
Total U.S. Government revenue	7242

Competition between ACCs will reduce waste and inefficiency allowing for ever improving services.

Summary and Conclusion

Our democracy, with economic and political power concentrated in the federal and state governments, has served us well in many ways since the founding of the U.S. However, our systems of health care, welfare, and entitlements being provided by government bureaucracies have become dysfunctional and the increase in wasted resources is unsustainable. Political polarization, economic stagnation, increasing inequality, and unsustainable consumption of limited and pollution-generating resources now threaten our security and way of life. These intractable and increasingly urgent issues should lead us to consider fundamental system changes.

Partially decentralizing economic and political power into private, competing Accountable Care Cooperatives, comprising about one-third of the economy, will be a game-changer. ACCs, as communitarian organizations accountable to all members, will harness market forces to provide high quality health care that is universally accessible and affordable. Full integration of health and social services with self-regulated ACCs, a free-market health care environment will drive innovation and efficiencies. ACCs can reinvigorate our systems of health care, welfare, education, finance, law, government, and other sectors. They can bolster our economic and cultural strengths.

The grand bargains so far previewed will decentralize decision making and accountability in health and human services. They will empower individuals while strengthening democracy. Thousands of democratically run ACCs will provide an end run around the crippling polarization in our plutocratic, corporate-controlled, waste-ridden country. ACCs will unify the nation toward overcoming our formidable health-care, economic, and cultural challenges. They will also enable us to reform pockets of corruption, inefficiency, overconsumption, and waste interspersed throughout each of our economic sectors.

During the period of transition to ACCs, GDP may go up or down. However, long-term GDP growth will be driven by increasing employment by at least 40 million workers and fostering a business friendly environment. Millions of infrastructure project and national defense/ foreign development jobs will supercharge the productive economy. Since the corporate income tax will be gone and employee benefit costs drastically reduced, big corporations and small businesses will be able to afford higher employee pay.

Simplifying the tax system and shifting it more towards consumption taxes will create jobs and enhance entrepreneurism and innovation in business. As a result, over a trillion dollars in tax sheltered overseas corporate income will be repatriated to create jobs and boost U.S. economic growth.

Introducing communitarian ACCs to administer one-third of the economy will reduce wealth inequality while it spurs competition and entrepreneurial innovation. These culture-shifting moves will synergistically curb overconsumption and foster environmental and economic sustainability. The marked improvements in employment opportunities, the economy, and culture will also enable more time for family, community, and individual health promotion.

The best days will be ahead for people in the U.S.

Chapter 2
Accountable Care Cooperatives

I hailed the passage of the Patient Protection and Affordable Care Act (ACA or Obamacare) as a significant step toward improving our broken health care system. Without this law, we would remain stuck with the dysfunctional status quo in health care. However, I think most of the Republican criticisms of the ACA are well taken. Thankfully, the ACA probably will not be repealed over President Obama's veto until Democrats and Republicans collaborate to create something better to modify or replace it.

Unfortunately, the patient-centered medical home prescribed by Obamacare does nothing meaningful about controlling costs and too little to improve access to care and quality of health care services.[1] While Obamacare incentivizes adding social workers to patient-centered medical homes, it does too little to fully integrate social services with health care. Solutions to local clinical problem just don't magically appear due to top-down government mandates.

As mentioned in the Chapter 1, the central concept in this book is to replace the Obamacare "accountable care organizations" with "accountable care cooperatives" (ACCs). This chapter will explain in more detail how I envision ACCs, why we need them, and how they will facilitate reforms in health care as well as other sectors of the economy.

In 2016, thousands of private, competing ACCs will begin providing comprehensive health services. Just as ACCs turn out to be just the right institutions to reform health care, ACCs will provide social-safety-net services (welfare) and other human services. Given that

ACCs will be working with global budgets,[a] they will be mandated to control spending. Staff and members of ACCs will collaboratively determine their own priorities and methods to achieve fiscal discipline (Chapter 9). However, as the first priority, they will compete to achieve good patient outcomes in health, welfare, education, financial security, employment and in other spheres. Without good health and other outcomes for members, an ACC will risk losing members and going out of business.

ACCs will be disruptive to individuals, the society, and economy— but in a good way. At least 60 million people will need to start working on a new job or change jobs. An estimated 40 million more jobs will be created than will be lost.

Historically, disruptive influences on societies have caused job losses leading to crises in the lives of many people. However, many economic disruptions in the past have led to increased employment in more productive and fulfilling occupations, improvements in quality of life, and accelerated economic growth.

In the U.S. one hundred years ago, about 80% of people lived and worked on farms. Industrialization and technological innovations led to a mass exodus from the farms to factories and to blue collar and white collar service jobs in the cities. These radical changes disrupted the lives of many people. For example, my grandparents were the last of many generations to live on a farm in a small western Virginia village. However, the quality of life and the standards of living widely have vastly improved because of the disruption of industrialization. Many new jobs were created and productivity soared.

At the local community level, ACC staff and members will have both the resources and the mandates to work together in overcoming diverse and seemingly intractable challenges—diet related epidemics (e.g., obesity, cardiovascular disease, and cancer), poverty, food insecurity, wealth inequality, homelessness, excessive incarceration, barriers to educational opportunity, environmental *degradation*, etc.

---

a   Global budget: a defined amount of money from member premiums and government funding to provide all health and human services for all members

Given the roles of churches, temples, and mosques in helping those in need and in fostering ethical conduct, the religious community will likely take leading roles in ACCs. Integrated health care services providers that are currently operating (e.g., Kaiser Permanente, Mayo Clinic, etc.) will likely become ACCs and continue serving their members. However, they will offer greatly expanded programs and benefits.

Advantages of ACCs over Obamacare ACOs

Currently, most privately insured people have insurance through their employer, so the employer, not the employee, makes the choices of health care coverage and providers. Typically, employees may have one, two, or three choices of insurance companies. Those companies decide, often arbitrarily, what to cover and how much to pay. Even people who have a wide choice of insurers still have little choice in what health services their money is buying. However, many have no options but to remain with their employer-selected company or go without health care insurance.

Obamacare's ACOs offer choices between "Platinum, Gold, Silver, or Bronze" insurance, representing a confusing mixture of deductibles, co-payments, and other charges. Premiums will be highest with platinum level insurance and deductibles and co-payments lower. Bronze insurance with the lowest premiums will stick you with 40% copayments for expensive procedures (e.g., for a $20,000 hospitalization, an $8000 copayment). This hardly protects low income people from catastrophic bills. Obamacare is not designed to reduce out-of-pocket expenses of medically insured people.

With ACC-based reform, health care will be separated from employment—no more employer mandate to provide health care for employees. Patients will be able to choose between competing ACCs that offer care with significant differences in clinical practice guidelines and patient benefit packages. That is to say that ACCs will be self-regulating (Chapter 9). ACCs will provide comprehensive health coverage to all enrollees with much greater simplicity and transparency concerning premiums and co-payments.

Both ACCs and ACOs can consist of local networks of physicians, hospitals and their affiliated physicians, or fully integrated health systems like the Mayo Clinic or Kaiser Permanente (i.e., health maintenance organizations or HMOs). However, unlike ACOs, ACCs will be owned by members rather than by hospitals, doctors, and investors. For rare medical conditions with limited numbers of excellent care providers, ACCs will find it much easier to contract with subspecialists outside of their local networks. Indeed, subspecialists will endeavor to forge relationships and contracts with as many ACCs as possible.

Alternative therapies appeal to a large percentage of the population. ACOs typically do not cover alternative therapies (e.g., midwife assisted home births, platelet rich plasma injections for musculoskeletal pain, massage, acupuncture, etc). With the choice of competing ACCs, people can shop for the ACC that covers their alternative therapies of choice (Chapter 6).

Compared with ACOs, ACCs will have more financial and human resources to fully integrate social services with health care (Chapter 10). ACCs will be one-stop shopping for health care, alternative therapies, social services, and many other human services. People will be able to choose the ACC that gives them the most of what they want. In 2016, about one-third of the U.S. GDP (about $6 trillion) will be administered by ACCs that are responsible to their members. For instance, ACCs will have more flexibility and resources to provide poor people healthful food, affordable shelter, jobs, financial services, etc.

Reducing Administrative Waste with ACCs

The U.S. Department of Labor projects that jobs in health care supportive services will increase by 28% over the next decade, the greatest increase of any occupation.[2] However, we already have way too much paperwork in health care. We don't need more.

One example of excessive federal government regulation that un-necessarily increases administrative complexity is the "International Classification of Diseases, Ninth Revision, Clinical Modification (ICD-9-CM)." In order for physicians to bill Medicare for a service to a pa-tient, they must include the "clinical modification ICD-9 codes" for the diseases, signs and symptoms, abnormal findings, complaints, social circumstances, and external causes of injury or diseases. Additionally, there are ICD-9 *procedure codes* for doctors to utilize.

In October 2015, the Center for Medicare and Medicaid Services will require physicians to switch to the new ICD-10 codes. Whereas the ICD-9 codebook includes over 14,000 different coded items, ICD-10 will have over 68,000 codes. For instance, there will be two different codes for getting struck or bitten by a turkey (ICD-10 codes: W61.42 or W61.43).[3] There will be nearly as many chart coders as primary care physicians in the U.S.

As mentioned in Chapter 1, reducing the administrative complex-ity of health care and social services to that of the average business would save hundreds of billions of dollars a year. However, ACOs are not designed to reduce administrative waste. On the other hand, with ACC-based reform, competition between ACCs together with the elimination of government regulations will cause health care and social services paperwork to dramatically decrease.

With ACC-based reform, savings from reducing administrative complexity will go directly into reducing medical insurance premiums and providing more services that members want. Redundant medical administrators will be retrained for other jobs, including providing other services through the ACCs.

More Advantages of ACCs

As mentioned in the book overview (Chapter 1), ACCs will be owned cooperatively by the enrollees. Joint ownership of the ACCs by the members will increase trust in these cooperatives. Joint ownership will also foster a willingness to volunteer to help others for the sake of the common good.

According to the definition of "nonprofit cooperative," each ACC's enrollees will share "common economic, social, and cultural needs and aspirations."[4] ACC enrollees, staff, health care professionals, and other employees will all have a stake in aligning the interests of patients, health care providers, and taxpayers in reducing waste and maximizing valuable services. Patients, service providers, and administrators will all benefit from patient choice, transparency, efficiency, and accountability. Competition between ACCs will drive continuous quality improvement.

Constituting health care delivery organizations as self-regulating cooperatives will serve to counter the increasing cynicism about the corruption by special interests in medicine. If an ACC's health care costs become unaffordably high, ACC enrollees will not be able to blame their insurance company, the FDA, or health care special interest lobbyists in Washington, D.C. Instead, members will be able to work with ACC staff and service providers to obtain the spectrum of ACC health care and other services that best meets their needs at the prices they are willing to pay.

Cooperation, trust, evidence-based medical care, and altruism will be needed to address the tradeoffs that will continually arise. Disagreements and conflicts concerning covered health care interventions and other services will occur. These issues will not be settled by Congress or distant insurance company bureaucrats. Disagreements will be resolved according to the unique priorities of the members and staff of each cooperative.

Currently, FDA-approved drugs must be covered by Medicare. After extensive lobbying by drug companies, Congress forbade the Center for Medicare and Medicaid Services from negotiating prices with drug companies as is done in other countries. Drug companies may take advantage of guaranteed Medicare coverage with outrageous pricing. For instance, Gilead Sciences, of Foster City, Calif., charges $1000 a tablet for its new hepatitis C drug, sofosbuvir (Sovaldi).[5] Private insurance companies generally follow Medicare's lead with drug coverage, even with drugs of marginal benefit or medications in which controversy exists about whether the benefits justify the risks and costs.

With Grand Bargains-based reform, ACCs will negotiate drug prices with pharmaceutical companies. They will be able to barter for good prices either individually or as coalitions of ACCs. For sure, some ACCs will not agree to cover a $1000 per pill hepatitis C medication. Less expensive hepatitis C medications are available.

Free market competition between ACCs and between health services providers will spawn innovation and efficiency. Savings from ACC efficiencies will go to additional patient services and to reduce patients' premiums.

Doctors and Managers to Determine ACC Clinical Practice Guidelines and Benefit Packages

Reforming health care requires decreasing funding for worthless or marginally beneficial interventions and increasing funding for valuable tests and therapies. Our current top-down, one-size-fits-all public and private insurance coverage systems attempt to do that. However, any system with top-down decision making just does not fairly or efficiently utilize our precious health care dollars, for several reasons:

1. Official treatment guidelines are often fallible.
2. Powerful special interests (drug companies, etc.) may influence coverage decisions by public and private insurance companies.
3. Money may corrupt decision makers at the top who have no contact with patients.

Primary care providers (PCPs: physicians, nurse practitioners, and physicians' assistants) and other patient care providers (Chapter 3) are less likely to be corrupted by medical special interests that top-level bureaucrats. Consequently, reforming the health care system requires fundamentally changing the method of determining the scope of insurance coverage, putting PCPs and other health care workers in charge. Obamacare, with its ACOs, does not do this.

With the concept of ACOs as defined in Obamacare, providers should work together to provide high-quality, low-cost care that is in full compliance with government guidelines. The government's intent is for this to give health care providers a financial incentive to cooperate with each other in order to provide coordinated, cost-effective care. Medicare rewards ACOs that avoid "unnecessary" tests and treatments and comply with all government-endorsed clinical practice guidelines. With the money saved for avoiding unnecessary care, the ACO providers receive bonuses from Medicare. However, as payers and health services providers profit from limiting care, the ACO model will become unpopular with patients as happened with HMOs in the 1990s.

In contrast with ACOs, ACCs will leave the clinical practice guidelines and benefit packages up to the doctors and ACC staff serving the patients. ACC representatives will solicit input from patients and specialist health care providers. They will also study the scientific basis for the current standard guidelines before keeping or revising benefits and guidelines (Chapters 8 and 9).

Since medical research and new discoveries will be ongoing, ACC benefit packages and guidelines will be reviewed and changed periodically. ACCs will be held accountable by their members for health outcomes and for optimizing the use of financial and human resources. ACC physicians and staff will not receive bonuses for limiting or denying coverage of medical interventions. However, they will need to adopt practice patterns in accordance with what the members can afford to keep members happy.

As an important check on the processes of ACC guideline development and determination of benefit packages, patients will be empowered to choose ACCs that are in alignment with their values and priorities. Patients will also provide ongoing feedback to ACC managers about their preferences regarding covered and non-covered services.

ACC Practice Models

Currently, most physicians receive payments as fee-for-service, based on the volume of treatments and procedures they provide. Public and private medical insurers pay health care providers by tallying the volume of services, sometimes giving bonuses based on degree of compliance with orthodox treatment guidelines. However, neither more health care services provided nor a higher degree of compliance with orthodox guidelines necessarily translates to better health outcomes.

In the past, as Congress cut Medicare and Medicaid funding for physician services, physicians subsequently increased the volume of services making up for the loss of income. Health outcomes were not improved by the increased volume of services. Data show that quality of care is not improved by increasing the volume of professional services rendered.[6] Consequently, an emerging consensus of health policy experts supports a shift from paying for quantity of services to paying providers according to health outcomes, quality of care, and patient satisfaction.

ACCs will consist of local networks of physicians (PCPs and specialists), ancillary health care professionals and affiliated hospitals, or fully integrated health systems like Kaiser Permanente and the Mayo Clinic. Hospitals and their affiliated physicians will compete with each other to provide their services to ACCs. Direct practice PCPs (Chapter 3) will become leaders of ACCs, because they treat the whole person. In a well functioning health care system, PCPs typically get to know their patients better than specialists who focus on one particular organ or disease category.

Data on health interventions, costs, and health outcomes will be widely available to patients, care providers, and researchers under the ACC model. These data will constantly drive efficiencies and better quality of care. Within ACCs, the members will reap the benefits of the savings from not funding unnecessary tests and treatments. Patients will also receive the health- and safety-net-services that they want and less out-of-pocket costs. Where expensive and risky medical interventions are not included in benefit packages of ACCs, more conservative tests or treatments or lifestyle programs might be offered as alternatives.

ACCs could pay providers on a fee-for-service system, a salary model, or a mixed-payment scheme. Kaiser Permanente and other successful salary model health maintenance organizations (HMOs) could remain intact and adapt to creating their own treatment guidelines and benefit packages. Networks of physicians (PCPs and specialists) affiliated with a single ACC or physicians affiliated with a single community hospital that serves several ACCs could each determine whether fee-for-service or salary worked best for them. Contracting hospitals, specialists, and safety-net-services providers could compete for referrals from PCPs based on quality of care and cost.

Experiences of different ACCs using different models of health care worker-compensation will lead to innovations that will further improve health outcomes and patient satisfaction. The optimal payment system will incentivize PCPs and other providers to consider patient care and patient outcomes foremost. Financial considerations will be secondary in relationship to overall benefit to patients. Efficient and effective providers will benefit indirectly by attracting more patients. In the long run, the Grand Bargains' goal and result will be many fewer people needing medical interventions because of good preventive medicine.

ACCs Accommodating Religious and Cultural Diversity

Replacing government imposed standard guidelines and benefit packages with individual ACC guidelines and benefit packages will allow ACCs to serve sub-segments of the population by accommodating their unique preferences. In particular, religious groups could play big roles in influencing the services provided by ACCs that their members choose. Since religions generally promote altruism and service to humanity, they could join forces with local ACCs to provide social-safety-net services. Nothing will prohibit religious denominations from partnering with ACCs that enroll their members. Churches, temples, or mosques could negotiate with local ACCs and support those that are most in alignment with their philosophies.

For example, Seventh Day Adventists because of their religious and cultural practices (e.g., vegetarian diets) may not select ACCs that cover cholesterol lowering pills, angioplasty, or coronary artery bypass surgery. Instead, they may elect ACCs that cover lifestyle change programs for cardiac risk factor reduction (e.g., diet, exercise, and stress management). Christian Scientists could choose ACCs that covered prayer healing sessions on the same footing as medical interventions. Reimbursement for prayer healing sessions was included in some versions of Congressional health care reform legislation.[7] While imposing this provision on all taxpayers is open to constitutional challenge, there should be no reason that individual ACCs could not offer this benefit to attract Christian Scientists and other believers in the power of prayer.

Abortion opponents will be able to choose ACCs that do not fund abortions while pro-choice advocates select ACCs in alignment with their preferences (Chapter 7).

Options for Patients Denied Services by ACCs

If ACCs do not fund certain types of medical treatments, patients will be free to receive those services by paying out-of-pocket. Patients could also appeal the denial of their ACC's authorization for payment for health care services in two ways. For each ACC, a committee composed of ACC staff and patients will serve as an appeal board to review denials of payments for services. A majority or supermajority of appeal committee members would need to vote to overrule the ACC's denial of coverage for a disputed medical service. Alternately, a patient that was denied financial coverage for a medical service could appeal the ACC's decision by changing to an ACC that would approve payment. However, a patient would likely only switch ACCs only when he or she found a new ACC willing to assume their care and the expense of the disputed medical service. This will create a balance to make it possible but not easy to change ACCs over controversial issues.

ACC Transparency

ACCs will be required to post on the Internet and on their public premises their yearly allocations of health services, social services, other services, expenditures, and health outcomes by patient care category. Patients could provide feedback and could shop for ACCs according to, among other things, how well individual ACCs manage the resources for sickness care, health promotion, long-term care, and the social determinants of health (Chapter 10).

ACCs will operate on a prepaid basis within the budget from enrollee premiums and federal government risk-adjusted allocation for the enrollee population (Chapter 18). Paying the premiums will entitle members to all services provided by the ACCs. ACCs will compete, in part, by providing evidence-based services (Chapter 8) and avoiding payments for ineffective medical interventions. A high degree of transparency will be needed for patients, practitioners, and others to evaluate exactly what tests, treatments, and other services are provided by ACCs and what patient outcomes relate to those services.

ACCs as Administrators of Safety-Net Services

Allowing homelessness, malnutrition, and other poverty-related problems to cause preventable acute and chronic medical illnesses will be philosophically and financially unacceptable to ACCs. For the good of all patients in an ACC's practice, the PCPs and affiliated health care professionals will enlist interested enrolled members, on a paid or volunteer basis, to help provide safety-net services. To effectively compete, ACCs will strengthen the safety net by coordinating social services and giving members powerful incentives to help each other.

Each ACC will administer the risk-adjusted welfare funds from federal government agencies (Chapter 19) for members. ACCs will need to employ or contract with social workers, counselors, psychiatrists, vocational rehabilitation specialists, drug/alcohol rehabilitation workers, and others to provide the specific services needed for their patients (Chapter 10). Given these resources to help impoverished or disadvantaged patients, each ACC will be responsible for assuring that each of its patients has shelter, healthful food, job training, employment opportunities, and other appropriate social services.

All immigrants will be eligible to enroll in ACCs (Chapter 13). However, undocumented immigrants will not receive subsidies in paying their ACC insurance premiums. Given high employment in living wage jobs (Chapter 12), few citizens will require subsidies to pay premiums.

Continuous Quality Improvement

With this patient-centered, self-regulated system of determining practice guidelines and health benefits for ACCs, controversial medical interventions will be offered by some ACCs and not by others. With large populations of patients having differing health and social interventions, researchers will be able to study the risks and benefits of controversial medical tests and treatments. Researchers will also compare the overall health outcomes of patients in competing ACCs. ACCs with the best health outcomes will be emulated and those with poor outcomes will need to reconsider their guidelines and benefit packages.

Transparent data on health interventions and patient outcomes will be presented widely by expert health researchers, and this will drive continual improvements in all aspects of care.

Summary and Conclusion

Americans are increasingly prey to inefficient and corrupt government and corporate bureaucracies. In increasingly insidious ways, government agencies, affected by stalemates and gridlock, exert tremendous power over ordinary people. ACC-based reform will shift about one-third of the GDP away from these entrenched government and corporate bureaucracies, over to the ACC managers chosen by members. Americans will learn to depend on their local ACCs and on each other more than government administered services, entitlements, and subsidies. Shifting much of that power to communitarian, competing ACCs will be a game-changer.

Our health care system needs competing, innovative ACCs rather than government-guideline driven, bureaucratic ACOs. ACCs will be mandated to control spending but will have no agenda other than good patient outcomes. Just as ACCs turn out to be just the right institutions to reform health care and welfare, they can also be part of Grand Bargains reform of other economic sectors, including financial services, education, law, national defense, etc. ACC services in these areas will be detailed in subsequent chapters.

ACCs will have the authority to authorize insurance payment, with or without co-payments from patients, for any and all health care and social services (diagnostic tests, treatments, hospitalizations, medications, specialist consultations and services, preventive medicine strategies, drug/alcohol abuse rehabilitation programs, long-term care, food, disability payments, subsidized housing, etc.). ACCs providing health care and expanded safety-net services led by direct practice PCPs will:

- provide care in patient-centered medical homes (fully described in Chapter 3),
- integrate safety-net services with health care,
- reduce funding for non-beneficial services,
- cut administration costs,
- increase funding for underfunded health care and safety-net priorities, and
- promote patient choice, provider autonomy, and healthy competition among providers.

As you will find in subsequent chapters, ACCs will also compete on their success in strategies to help enrollees avoid or cope with litigation (Chapter 11), conserve energy (Chapter 22), find good jobs (Chapter 12), improve their diets (Chapter 13), integrate immigrants into society (Chapter 14), obtain quality educations (Chapter 16), live affordably on Social Security and/or their pensions (Chapter 23), manage money (Chapter 24), and assist in providing for the security of the country (Chapter 17).

Chapter 3
Direct Practice PCPs Leading Patient-Centered Medical Homes

As a member of the General Internal Medicine Service at Los Angeles County + University of Southern California Medical Center (LAC + USC Medical Center), I supervised and taught many internal medicine residents in the clinics and hospital wards of the Center. Almost all of the faculty and staff members teaching the residents, myself included, had medical subspecialty board certification and practiced subspecialties of internal medicine. The residents had few role models of real primary care physicians.

Residents attended one half-day general internal medicine clinic per week except when they were rotating in the intensive care unit and thus were excused. If the resident had been up all night admitting patients to the wards, he or she still had to attend the morning or afternoon clinic. I practiced before 2002 when the Accreditation Council for Graduate Medical Education limited work hours for residents to 80 hours per week (averaged over a four week period). I question whether residents have it any easier now.

In the clinics, patients typically waited several hours to see their resident doctor or medical student. Between clinic visits, patients had no mechanism to contact residents about medical problems. In the general internal medicine clinics that I attended, about one-third of patients missed their appointments. Clerks made no phone calls to patients reminding them of clinic appointments. If patients missed appointments, no one contacted them to find out why and to reschedule.

For a patient, phoning a clinic to schedule an appointment could take hours. The average wait for a new patient to get an appointment to see an internal medicine resident doctor was four months. Physician time with patients, most of whom had complicated medical histories, was limited.

In an outpatient clinic, I supervised up to 12 internal medicine residents and medical students. Between them, they saw up to 50 patients in a typical half-day general internal medicine clinic. Consequently, I had little time with each resident to go over a patient's history, physical findings, and lab results. Nor was there much time to draw on my experience to teach the residents and students some important medical lessons related to their cases. I rarely had time to see the patients myself, so I usually had to depend on the patient presentations given by residents or students.

Due to the time pressures, the residents and medical students focused mainly on checking laboratory test results, monitoring medications for chronic illnesses (i.e., adding or stopping drugs, adjusting doses and checking for side effects), and referring patients to subspecialty clinics. Although most patients had lifestyle related diseases (obesity, diabetes, hypertension, coronary disease, etc.), the residents had little time to counsel patients about lifestyle change approaches to benefit their medical problems. We had too few dietitians to routinely refer clinic patients for nutrition counseling.

With each new crop of smart, hard-working physicians in training, I would survey the interns for their knowledge of nutrition and their favored dietary recommendations for patients. Less than 25% of the medical interns in my clinics had ever taken a clinical nutrition course in medical school. Less than 50% knew how many calories were in a gram of fat, protein, or carbohydrate. Few could figure out the percentage of fat calories in whole milk. Fewer still knew what was in the recommended diets of the American Diabetes Association, the American Heart Association, or the American Cancer Society. Not one had an opinion about whether they agreed or disagreed with the dietary recommendations of those organizations.

After discussing a patient with a resident or medical student, I generally asked what diet he or she was recommending and why. Usually, they admitted that they gave no dietary recommendation. I always suggested that they order a plant-based high fiber diet (Chapters 4 and 13). Sometimes they complied and other times they ignored my suggestion. Once, a patient that had adopted a plant-based diet on my recommendation sought me out in clinic to thank me. She was amazed by how much it helped with her bowel symptoms.

For the patients, continuity of care with the same resident was unusual. When residents missed their medical clinics due to vacations, intensive care unit rotations, or illness, their patients would see other residents or medical students.

Many, if not most, of the practicing physicians in the U.S. have been trained in settings similar to the LAC + USC Medical Center. The setting was unpleasant and unnecessarily stressful for both patients and physicians in training. This is the norm in U.S. hospitals and clinics. It will need to change for us to address the crisis in primary care medicine in the U.S. Unfortunately, Obamacare does not offer much hope in its present form.

Few Medical Students Seek Primary Care Careers

Among U.S. medical students and physicians in training I taught and supervised in the 1980s and 1990s, primary care as a career was not very popular. Most of them aspired to fellowships in medical subspecialties that would pay more money and be less demanding of time than being a general internist. The situation for general internists is even bleaker now due to more government and insurance company bureaucratic hassles and less time to see patients. Since 1997, increased administrative burdens on PCPs and skewed financial incentives favoring specialists have led to a greater than 50% drop in U.S. medical school graduates planning careers in primary care.[1]

An often quoted poll of medical student career preferences published in *JAMA* (formerly *Journal of the American Medical Association*) found that only 2% of students planned careers in primary care internal medicine (PCPs for adults). In this poll, 274 out of 1177 students (23.2%) planned careers in internal medicine but only 24 (2.0%) as primary care physicians. Most aspired to careers in subspecialties of internal medicine (e.g., cardiology, infectious disease, cancer, etc.).[2] I was the same way, specializing in medical oncology and hematology (i.e., cancer and blood disorders). Less than 1% of medical students preferred careers in general pediatrics.

The Current Status of Primary Care Medicine in the U.S.

Health care from "any willing practitioner" tends to become fragmented, inefficient, and overly expensive.[3] Almost all health policy analysts agree that health care reform requires strengthening primary care medicine.

Relative to medical specialists, PCPs have been chronically underpaid in the U.S. by public and private insurers. Even more than medical specialists, PCPs suffer with administrative hassles due to insurers' bureaucratically intense but largely ineffective attempts at cost control. The stresses of overwork and the administrative hassles have led many PCPs to burnout and take early retirements.

Compared with many other developed countries, our primary care system does not function very well. This accounts, in part, for our poor showing in international health outcome rankings. In the U.S., areas with strong primary care services (e.g., affluent suburbs) have better health outcomes (e.g., infant mortality and longevity) than places with fewer PCPs per capita (e.g., poor inner city and rural areas). These significant benefits associated with a strong primary care system remain after adjusting for the better health outcomes of affluent versus poor people due to factors other than availability of PCPs. Public health researchers see this pattern in countries around the world. On the other hand, increasing the number of specialists does not improve health outcomes in the U.S. or other developed countries.[4] The implications of this fact go beyond the need for more primary care physicians. American doctors and patients tend to give or seek referrals for expensive solutions for health problems rather than to first focus on common sense diet and lifestyle change strategies that PCPs can prescribe.

American primary care physicians work as hard as or harder than specialists, make less money, and have less prestige. Managed care organizations allow PCPs inadequate time for patient visits, and patient/PCP relationships are often transitory. Battles with insurance companies over treatment denials and pre-authorizations for procedures add to the frustration. The "hassle-factor" of dealing with bureaucrats from Medicare, Medicaid, health maintenance organizations (HMOs), preferred provider organizations (PPOs), and insurance companies wears down many PCPs. The administrative burdens of PCP practices grow every year while malpractice concerns are always looming.

Physician burnout tied to a spate of early retirements of primary care doctors threatens to make access to PCPs even less available in coming years. A survey conducted by the Physicians' Foundation found that almost half of primary care physicians (about 150,000) plan to quit or reduce their practice load in the next three years if they have the opportunity.[5] A large increase in PCPs, including family doctors, internists, pediatricians, physicians' assistants and primary care nurse practitioners, will be needed not only to keep pace with population growth and the retirement of practicing PCPs, but also to reduce the patient load of each PCP.

President Obama addressed the shortage of PCPs inadequately. He suggested increasing PCP reimbursement for preventive care and providing financial aid for medical students who choose primary care. An on-line poll found that only 16% of physicians, nurses, and pharmacists thought that those measures would be sufficient to attract more physicians to primary care.[6] Timid financial measures will do nothing. Working conditions, job satisfaction, and the status of careers in primary care must be improved.

Much of the dysfunction of our current health care system is due to the fragmentation of care. Because of fragmented care, quality of care is spotty, our health outcomes compare poorly with other developed countries, and costs are high. Without many more PCPs, we will continue to have fragmented care.

What do we want from our PCPs?

My friend Barbara Starfield, MD, MPH, now deceased, was a Professor at the Johns Hopkins School of Public Health and longtime advocate of strengthening our primary care system. She described what kind of physicians and allied providers our primary care training system should produce.

> "Primary care" doesn't only mean having a certain kind of physician as one's "regular source of care." It means having a doctor who functions in certain ways. This means providing access to services such that people seek care from that doctor whenever they have a new need for care or preventive services. It means having a strong relationship with that doctor, such that the doctor understands people's needs and people feel comfortable telling the doctor about those needs. It means providing care for ALL needs that are common in the population and referring to specialists when the problem is too unusual or uncommon for the primary care practitioner to manage. It also means coordinating care so that when people do have to be referred elsewhere, the advice received is integrated into total care so that

there are no conflicting recommendations that could cause harm. Many studies confirm the benefits of these four characteristics of primary care.

For successful and sustainable health care reform, we need to train the kind of doctors and other PCPs that Dr. Starfield described. To do this, the number of PCPs being trained must be increased, working conditions in primary care must be improved, and PCPs must be allowed to spend more time with patients.

"Direct Practice" PCPs

Because of dissatisfactions with primary care by PCPs and their patients, direct practice PCPs (formerly termed "concierge" or "boutique" PCPs) have emerged. As briefly described in Chapter 1, direct practice PCPs charge a yearly cash retainer in exchange for more personal attention and services. These PCPs provide unhurried yearly physical exams, 24-hour phone call access, email consultations, expedited scheduling of tests and consultations, little or no waiting for appointments, health reviews, nutritional counseling, and electronic medical records with up-to-date medical histories and test results for patients to carry with them.[7] These direct practice PCPs may have 500–1000 patients and charge each $1500–$10,000 per year for services not covered by Medicare or private insurers. Since both patients and PCPs are generally happy with the arrangement, this practice is rapidly growing more popular.[8]

Among other things, direct practice means much less administrative paperwork is required because payment is by cash. With direct practice PCPs in ACCs, time will be available for clinical teams to focus on preventive medicine, health promotion, chronic disease management, and palliative care (e.g., hospice for terminally ill patients).

Critics of direct practice care state that it creates a two-class system of medicine. This is true. The optimal solution to this valid criticism is for health care reform to extend this superior form of primary care to everyone. Only with first-rate primary care medicine will it be possible to coordinate care of patients, reduce waste on unnecessary tests and treatments, and increase funding for currently under-funded health services. Only with a strong primary care system can quality of care and patient satisfaction go up while costs come down.

Also in the reformed health care system, medical insurance, rather than out-of-pocket payments of patients, should pay for direct practice PCPs.

Give Everyone a "Patient-Centered Medical Home"

The "patient-centered medical home" has been suggested as a means of better coordinating care. Four organizations representing primary care providers collaborated to issue "Joint Principles of the Patient-Centered Medical Home." The first four principles of this document give the essence of the definition of medical home.[9]

1. Personal physician—each patient has an ongoing relationship with a personal physician trained to provide first contact and continuous and comprehensive care.
2. Physician directed medical practice—the personal physician leads a team of individuals at the practice level that collectively take responsibility for the ongoing care of patients.
3. Whole person orientation—the personal physician is responsible for providing for all the patient's health care needs or taking responsibility for appropriately arranging care with other qualified professionals. This includes care for all stages of life—acute care, chronic care, preventive services, and end-of-life care.
4. Care is coordinated and/or integrated across all elements of the complex health care system (e.g., subspecialty care, hospitals, home health agencies, nursing homes) and the patient's community (e.g., family, public and private community-based services).

Other important aspects of a patient-centered medical home are that evidence-based medicine principles guide decisions (Chapter 8), physicians in the practice accept accountability for continuous quality improvement, and patients actively participate in decision-making and feedback.

The creation of a true patient-centered medical home network depends on improving the working conditions for primary providers. Instead of 2000–3000 patients per "gatekeeper" PCP, a true patient-centered medical home requires direct practice PCPs that each care for between 500 and 1500 patients (average ≈ 750). This will allow PCPs to really know their patients and handle many medical problems that they now refer to specialists.

Patient-Centered Medical Homes to Coordinate Health Care Services

While there are several practice models possible that provide co-ordinated care, they all must have certain ingredients. There must be a commitment to continuity of care in a patient-centered medical home. The health care delivery system must standardize office processes to facilitate care coordination. The payment system must support care coordination, continuity of care, and appropriate information technologies for patient care.[5]

Nationwide, only about 15% of health services are provided in a coordinated fashion by integrated health services organizations like the Mayo Clinic or Kaiser Permanente Health System. The other 85% of health services are delivered in a fragmented manner by solo practitioners and small group practices will little or no coordination of care between PCPs, hospitals, and specialists.

Medical care is rapidly changing from delivery by physician-owned practices to delivery by bigger health care organizations. While larger organizations can perhaps provide more coordinated care, the value of longstanding doctor/patient relationships may be sacrificed. The push toward electronic medical records is partly responsible for the trend toward care by larger health care organizations. While these computerized systems improve patient safety and the efficiency and quality of care, large organizations rather than small medical practices benefit financially by installing these expensive and cumbersome systems.[6]

We need both the intimacy of long-standing doctor/patient relationships and the efficiency of large organizations in coordinating care delivery. The need for the large medical organization is as important as the patient-centered medical homes and direct practice PCPs. Optimally, we need a health care delivery system led by direct practice PCPs practicing in patient-centered medical homes within private, competing ACCs, as described in Chapters 1 and 2.

Patient-Centered Medical Home Certification is Premature

The visions that health policy wonks from the National Committee for Quality Assurance (NCQA) have about optimizing primary care make sense:[10]

- Creating new ways to improve access to care.
- Improving coordination of care between all the health care providers caring for patients.
- Giving providers more tools to improve quality.

The NCQA touts the benefits of patient-centered medical home certification:

1. improved patient experience,
2. reduced clinician burnout,
3. reduced hospitalization rates,
4. reduced ER visits,
5. increased savings per patient,
6. higher quality of care, and
7. reduced cost of care.[11]

It costs \$23,000 – \$90,000 per physician for this certification.[12] Yet, none of the claimed benefits of certification have been consistently demonstrated.

To efficiently provide superior care, a medical clinic must do more than go through a series of administrative hoops and pay a sizable fee to the NCQA to receive a patient-centered medical home designation. Becoming designated a patient-centered medical home does not insulate PCPs and other medical team members from the brutalizing administrative hassles of a profoundly dysfunctional health care system. This designation does nothing about the fee-for-service orientation of U.S. health care that rewards volume of tests, treatments, and patient encounters provided rather than patient outcomes. Indeed, a survey performed by the American Academy of Family Physicians of PCPs and other practitioners moving into certified patient-centered medical home environments showed increased workloads and higher rates of symptoms of burnout.[13]

Despite the lack of proof of efficacy, the NCQA commoditized this unproven formula into a certification process. This certification process creates huge bureaucratic hurdles for providers while generating a nice revenue stream for the NCQA. Concerning the patient-centered medical home certification initiative of the NCQA, Medicare Payment Advisory Commission Chairman Glenn Hackbarth, JD said, "In order to meet all the National Committee for Quality Assurance requirements, there are a lot of bells and whistles that have been added. My impression is that not all of them have really been validated as added value, but they add cost. I'm worried that maybe the medical home model has a real cost disadvantage."[14]

The term "patient-centered medical home" should not be allowed to be co-opted by the NCQA or any other health care special interest. The value of transitioning to patient-centered medical homes should be validated by the marketplace and not by regulators, whether they are self-appointed like those from the NCQA or bureaucrats from government agencies.

Most would agree that Kaiser Permanente Medical Care coordinates care as well or better than providers with the NCQA designation of patient-centered medical homes. Kaiser has long embraced the principles of patient-centered medical care. However, Kaiser does not pay the money or go through the bureaucratic hassles of becoming designated officially by the NCQA.

To summarize, NCQA patient-centered medical care certification is not a necessary ingredient of reforming health care. However, providing excellent care requires reforming the education of physicians and shifting to direct practice PCPs working in patient-centered medical homes.

Changing the Culture of Physician Training

The pressures on physicians in training lead to an increased risk of suicide. While medical students enter medical school with mental health profiles similar to those of other college graduates, they soon experience higher rates of depression, burnout, and other mental illnesses.[15] They are more likely to drink heavily, become addicted to drugs, and get divorced.

Dr. Liselotte N. Dyrbye, an associate professor of medicine at the Mayo Clinic in Rochester, MN and lead author of a study looking at the mental health of physicians in training, said, "There's no arguing anymore over whether there's a high prevalence of distress. What's important now is that we hold a mirror up to ourselves and ask why this is happening, because it is clearly not what we medical educators have intended."[16]

Due to constant pressure, medical students that are depressed often believe they are viewed as inadequate and incompetent by those around them. According to Dr. Thomas L. Schwenk, a professor of family medicine at the University of Michigan, "While depression can cause individuals to have negative and distorted views of their surroundings, the culture of medical school makes these students also feel like they can't be vulnerable or less than perfect."[17]

In my experience, the doctors with the most empathy are also the most vulnerable. Unfortunately, the "survival of the fittest" mentality can eat away at a young doctor's empathy. To produce less distressed and more empathic doctors, we need to change the training system.

Based on my nine years of training in medicine and 20+ years of supervising medical students and post graduate trainees, the changes I envision in medical education and post graduate training should make the art and science of medicine much better for doctors and their patients.

Proposed Changes in the Education of PCP Physicians

In 1971, the Hollywood movie, "Doctors' Wives," attempted to inject humor, drama, and satire into the problems with medical marriages. The tag line was, "Doctors' wives have everything ... except husbands."[18] Over my clinical career, I saw numerous colleagues with marital problems related to the demands of their careers. It is said that medicine is a jealous mistress. The unreasonable time demand of my career was one contributor to my divorce after 38 years of marriage.

Current postgraduate training programs for PCPs and other physicians are still brutally hard on doctors. Even with the work limit for a resident now reduced to 80 hours per week averaged over a four week period, medical practices and physicians personally pay a huge price because of the unreasonable training demands. Postgraduate physicians should average no more than 60 hours of clinical work per week.

To prepare PCPs for the expanded role of optimizing the utilization of health care resources, PCP training and primary care continuing education programs should focus more on what is most important. These programs should emphasize evidence-based medicine (Chapter 8), health promotion practices (Chapter 4), and alternative health modalities (Chapter 6).

Palliative care/hospice training of PCPs should facilitate improved quality of life of terminally ill people. PCPs and their palliative care specialist consultants should provide these people with better symptom management and compassionate care while decreasing high-tech procedures given to those with far advanced chronic diseases (Chapter 5).

Training should educate future direct practice PCPs about options for cardiovascular disease patients to participate in intensive diet, exercise, and stress management programs in lieu of expensive, risky, high-tech medical interventions. A person with chest pain (angina) who wants to reduce the chance of a heart attack should be able to access insurance funds for a plant-based diet, exercise, and lifestyle change program to reverse coronary artery disease such as the evidence-based program of Dr. Dean Ornish[19-21] (Chapter 4). PCPs in training don't usually learn about this.

Training for a career as a PCP should begin in the first year of medical school. After spending a month or so learning what questions to ask in a medical history and how to perform a physical examination, first year medical students should spend a half-day per week in the office of PCPs (usually medical school faculty member PCPs) seeing patients. Each week, freshman and sophomore medical students should do a thorough evaluation of one new patient to the practice—initially younger, low-risk patients with uncomplicated health histories. They should also see their previous patients for any follow-up visits.

In the third and fourth years of medical school, primary care oriented students should spend at least two half-days per week in clinic and evaluate two new patients per week. With the supervision of faculty PCPs, those patients should be the responsibility of the medical students for the duration of medical school. By graduation, medical students would be providing primary care under supervision for about 300 patients. Ideally, students should associate with groups of PCPs, so that they can learn from physicians with a variety of interests and practice styles.

It should be a priority for the student doctors to study the medical literature concerning all the medical problems of all their patients. They should learn the evidence supporting (or not supporting) any tests or treatments that they may order for their patients and find out what is the cost of the care that they provide. When a patient needs to see a specialist, the medical student should accompany his/her patient on the visit. With the help of the specialist, the student should research the evidence basis for any recommended tests and treatments, challenging medical orthodoxy when indicated. If a patient of a student needs to be admitted to a hospital, the student should see that patient in the hospital.

After medical school graduation, if the new doctor remains in the same city, he/she should continue to follow the same patients as during medical school. During internship and residency, primary-care-bound doctors in training (i.e., internal medicine, family practice, and pediatrics) should average at least four half-days per week in out-patient clinics seeing patients under the supervision of experienced PCPs— possibly some of the same ones they had as professors as in medical school. On average, they should be assigned four new patients per week while continuing to see their previous patients as needed.

During hospital clinical assignments or rotations (e.g., surgery, cardiology, medicine, etc.), when they encounter admitted patients without PCPs, they could become the PCP for those patients. If medical school and residency are in the same city, they may finish with 800 – 900 patients. Post graduate PCP residents that do not remain in the same city as medical school would follow about 600 patients by the end of a three year residency.

This approach should be mutually beneficial for patients and doctors in training. The patients will have the extra attention that trainees typically provide. The medical students/physicians in training will have continuous primary care responsibilities for their patients for years rather than the fragmented experiences with patients that are now the norm.

For nurse practitioners and physician assistants, a two year primary care residency should be required that is similar to the training experiences of primary care physicians.

Summary and Conclusion

Primary care in the U.S. is in crisis. Without a patient-centered medical home, no one is responsible for coordinating care, reducing unnecessary tests and treatments, and increasing access to valuable medical and social-safety-net services.

An expensive bureaucratic process of certifying patient-centered medical homes by the National Center for Quality Assurance or other self appointed nonprofit or for profit company or government agency is unnecessary. With ACC-based reform including direct practice PCPs, competition between ACCs and individual health care providers will lead to the patient care and health outcomes that NCQA certification cannot guarantee.

A "gatekeeper" PCP caring for 2000–3000 patients cannot give sufficient attention to each patient. Burnout and demoralization result and quality of care suffers. To avoid further fragmentation of medical care, the PCP training process, working conditions, relative pay, and prestige must improve. ACC-based health care reform will begin with improving the attractiveness of primary care careers. Only then can we train PCPs that love their jobs and have the time and resources to really care for their patients.

An important goal of health care reform should be a patient-centered medical home with a direct practice PCP for everyone. The process of accomplishing that goal can be healing and enjoyable for both physicians and patients.

Chapter 4
Preventive Medicine and Health Promotion

D r. Dean Ornish showed that a combination of a plant-based diet, daily aerobic exercise, hatha yoga, meditation, and a psychological support group reduced complications from coronary disease. In a medical breakthrough study; heart attacks, angina pain, bypass surgeries, and deaths decreased by about 50% over a five year period.[1] *The Dr. Dean Ornish's Program to Reverse Heart Disease*,[2] published in 1990, inspired many people to fundamentally change their lifestyles to prevent cardiovascular disease.

In 1991, I directed a small pilot project based on the Ornish program. Under the auspices of the LA County Department of Health Services, I did medical examinations and re-examinations with the help of my friend, Dr. George Haber. The former Buffum Downtown Long Beach YMCA provided the site for the classes. Faculty for the project included a registered dietitian, a hatha yoga instructor, a meditation instructor, a marriage and family therapist, an aerobic teacher, a YMCA administrator, Dr. Haber, and me. We volunteered our services in return for participation in the overall program.

We recruited participants with heart disease risk factors from the YMCA's membership and from the overall community. Of 16 initial participants, only two had already been diagnosed as having coronary artery disease, but most had one or more risk factors such as high blood pressure, high blood cholesterol, obesity, or diabetes. They paid for the use of the YMCA facility, plus nominal fees for lab tests, a health risk appraisal, and a physician office visit. We had no other funding of any kind, so we did not do coronary angiograms or other expensive tests.

This health promotion program was quite successful. After three months, re-evaluation showed that the average participant had lost over four pounds, had shown a drop in systolic blood pressure of seven points and diastolic blood pressure of five points, and experienced a reduction in low density cholesterol (the "bad" cholesterol) of 15 points. One highly motivated person reduced his cholesterol from 280 mg/dL to 220 mg/dL and his blood pressure from 160/100 to 120/70.

I greatly enjoyed helping these people improve their health. In all my years of medical practice, I have never taken pleasure in anything more than seeing my patients make positive lifestyle changes. The subjective benefits of this short program were just as impressive. People felt better overall and handled stress with more equanimity. Some greatly appreciated not having to take medication to control high blood pressure.

Dr. Dean Ornish Program in 2014

The Dr. Dean Ornish program with the plant-based diet continues to win adherents today. Dr. Kim A. Williams, a cardiologist at Rush University in Chicago and the president of the American College of Cardiology learned about the program from one of his patients. Since Dr. Williams' own LDL cholesterol was 170 mm Hg (moderately high), he adopted a plant-based diet and brought the LDL cholesterol down to 90 mm Hg in six weeks.[3] Dr. Ornish congratulated Dr. Williams for his courage and leadership.[4] MedPage Today, the publisher of these articles by Drs. Williams and Ornish, then conducted an online survey with the question: "Is there enough evidence to recommend that patients eat a vegan (plant-based) diet to prevent and reverse heart disease?" They found that 58% of physicians and others responded, "yes."[5]

Healthful School Lunches: A Political Football

First Lady Michelle Obama champions healthful school lunches for children as part of her push to combat childhood obesity. She advocates more fruits, vegetables, and whole grains. French fried potatoes and tomato paste are on her foods to be avoided list. She wants kids and adults eating foods with less salt, fat, and sugar.

Ms. Obama successfully lobbied her husband and Congress to allocate over $3 billion to make school lunches more nutritious. Many Republicans, especially from farm states, opposed her effort. After a "food fight" in Congress, conservatives succeeded in keeping French fries and pizza on the menu at the behest of food industry lobbyists.[6,7]

Four years after the rollout of the "Healthy, Hunger-Free Kids Act of 2010," critics and defenders of the program have again become very outspoken.[8] School districts receive about $0.06 per lunch extra to comply with the new U.S. Department of Agriculture (USDA) school nutrition guidelines, which they complain is not nearly enough to cover increased costs. Many in Congress are pushing to repeal the new standards to save money. The School Nutrition Association and the GOP want to see the legislation repealed. Both had supported the bill initially.

A *Los Angeles Times* investigation reported that Los Angeles Unified School District students waste an estimated $100,000 per day of their school lunches. Asked for a solution to the problem, David Binkle, the district's food services director, said, "We can stop forcing children to take food they don't like and throw in the garbage."[9]

Defenders of the Obama-USDA school lunch standards rallied 100 pediatricians to Capitol Hill to defend the program. Supporters of strict standards for school lunches cited a study that they claimed verified that more healthful food in the lunches contributes to reducing obesity in children.[10] The study was quite weak in my opinion.[a]

---

a   The study monitored the childhood obesity rates in states with "healthier" school lunch standards versus those with looser standards. The authors reported an association of healthier standards with a 12% drop in obesity. Many confounders

This exemplifies the top-down one-size-fits-all approach to health and public health. Many people just don't like folks in Washington, D.C. coercing them to change their lifestyles.

The promoters of the Healthy, Hunger-Free Kids Act of 2010 have the best of intentions. However, instead of dictating to public schools all over the county what kids should eat, maybe people might appreciate help in figuring out how to deal with preventing and treating obesity for themselves.

Consider giving school districts financial incentives to institute their own healthful school lunch programs and to monitor the results. Competition between school districts in keeping kids healthy will do more improve diets and health habits in kids than dictates from the White House and Congress.[11]

Health Promotion and Preventive Medicine Strategies

Increased funding for preventive medicine interventions polls well in surveys of Americans. Most people believe that eating a healthful diet will prevent a variety of expensive chronic diseases. However, based on 599 studies published between 2000 and 2005, spending money on prevention of disease *increased* overall medical spending over 80% of the time.[12] Other studies questioned whether preventive medicine interventions as reported in studies are cost effective.[13, 14] From a population health standpoint, previous public health approaches to prevent chronic diseases in general, and dietary change strategies in particular, have not improved health outcomes or lowered health care costs. Then again, none of these studies included diet and lifestyle changes as significant as the Ornish program.

Maybe our preventive medicine strategies have been faulty. For example, rigorous research shows that the Ornish program and similar multifaceted health promotion interventions do clearly reduce adverse

could have skewed these results. For instance, obesity in parents strongly correlates with obesity in children. The study authors failed to consider this obvious confounder.

health events and save money. Only after 20 years of Dr. Ornish's presenting data to the Center for Medicare and Medicaid Services did Medicare approve funding for the Ornish program in 2010.[15]

Just like diagnostic and treatment interventions for diseases, preventive medicine interventions–such as the Ornish program and Ms. Obama's healthy school lunches–should be rigorously researched and tested for efficacy in improving health outcomes. Some preventive medicine approaches work and others do no good, and may even do harm. Wasting money on ineffective preventive medicine programs takes away from funding strategies that will optimize health and wellness.

With ACC-based health care reform, ACC leaders will have the responsibility of determining which prevention approaches to offer to enrollees. Undoubtedly, the coverage of preventive medicine interventions will differ between ACCs. Consequently, with computerized medical record data from most of the population, research on prevention strategies and health outcomes of the population will be able to guide ACC staff members and their enrollees to determine which types of prevention approaches to fund in the future. The interventions that greatly reduce heart disease, cancer, type 2 diabetes, and obesity will be copied. The ineffective programs will be discarded.

Comparisons of Government-Determined versus ACC-Directed Health Promotion

Obamacare allows companies to discount insurance premiums by as much as 30% if employees meet certain health benchmarks (i.e., weight, blood pressure, cholesterol, etc.).[16] However, instead of promoting health for high-risk people, this is likely to price them out of health care insurance.[17]

With ACC-based health and social services on the other hand, ACCs will receive risk-adjusted money from the government (Chapter 18). Consequently, they will have no incentive to avoid sick people. Indeed, ACCs will be quite successful if they enroll poor people with government health insurance who are at high risk for bad health outcomes. They will have a chance to help those people change their lifestyles to reduce health risks. Patients, health care workers, and taxpayers will all benefit from innovations in lifestyle change programs fostered by competition between ACCs.

Obamacare mandates that medical insurance companies cover all screenings, preventive care, and vaccines recommended by the U.S. Preventive Services Task Force,[18] without charging co-payments or deductibles. Former Secretary of Health and Human Services Director Nancy Sebelius called on U.S. doctors to order the following government-endorsed but controversial preventive medicine measures on their patients:[12, 19]

1. colorectal cancer screening (e.g., colonoscopy),
2. mammography screening for breast cancer,
3. flu vaccines,
4. human papilloma virus vaccines for girls nine to 26 years old, and
5. aspirin therapy to prevent heart disease.

In contrast to the government's top-down approach, with ACC-based health care reform, preventive medicine interventions will be used only to the extent that they are deemed effective by ACC staff members and enrollees (Chapter 8). It will not matter if they are favored by politicians or government bureaucrats that were lobbied by special interests.

Summary and Conclusion

The determination of the optimal preventive medicine and health promotion strategies for Americans is way too important to leave to federal government bureaucrats and their expert advisors representing medical special interests. The U.S. Department of Health and Human Services Director, a political appointee, should not be in charge of what your doctor orders for you to prevent illnesses and promote wellness.

Financial incentives for ACCs to significantly increase funding and resources for preventive medicine and health promotion will evolve naturally as a consequence of instituting the financial components of ACC-based health care reform. For each ACC, the allocation of money and resources for disease prevention will be a decision of the doctors and managers with input from staff, patients, appropriate experts, and other stakeholders. ACCs will undoubtedly differ from one ACC to another in their determination of funding for preventive medicine interventions. Correspondingly, health outcomes of patients from different ACCs will vary as some enrollees will maintain healthy lifestyle habits better than others.

ACCs will revolutionize preventive medicine. They will feature the essential ingredient for success—experimentation. This will be in conjunction with careful monitoring of health interventions and health outcomes together with financial incentives for patients, providers, and payers. All stakeholders will be aligned toward the goal of promoting health.

Based on preventive medicine outcome studies and other factors, owners of each ACC (i.e., the enrollees) together with ACC health care workers and staff will continually revise their strategies to promote health and prevent diseases. Innovation in health promotion approaches will involve collaboration between ACC enrollees, doctors, and staff. It will also require competition between ACCs that leads to ever more effective health promotion programs and improved patient health outcomes.

Chapter 5
End-of-Life Care Reform

Mary, my only sibling, a younger sister, called me in the spring of 2010 with news that she had been ill with pneumonia that wasn't getting better. I arrived to visit her in an emergency room just as a radiologist was explaining to Mary and her husband about a procedure to diagnose cancer. A thoracentesis (removal of fluid from the pleural space in the chest) diagnosed her condition as lung cancer. A liver scan revealed liver metastases, meaning that the disease was advanced and incurable. I shared in the grief of the family.

After Mary's family practitioner consulted a medical oncologist, I called the cancer specialist to discuss my sister's case. I told the oncologist that I was a former oncologist, myself. He said that he planned chemotherapy, after ordering MRIs of the abdomen and pelvis.

Given Mary's diagnosis and prognosis, I asked him, "Why MRIs before the chemo?" He responded saying, "If you want to take her to Southern California and find another oncologist to treat her, Dr. Cundiff, you are welcome to do so." He went on to say that he was trained at the Memorial Sloan Kettering Cancer Center in New York and was taught to be thorough. He added that he wondered if she had a second cancer in addition to lung cancer—advanced, incurable lung cancer, I might add.

We didn't hit it off in our one and only conversation.

Chemotherapy stopped the accumulation of pleural fluid and reduced her shortness of breath. However, Mary still required oxygen for minimal exertion around the house. Moderate pain in her liver area went away after the first course of chemo, and she stopped taking hydrocodone pain pills.

I read about a randomized clinical trial from Harvard that compared palliative care initiated upon diagnosis of incurable lung cancer in conjunction with anti-tumor treatment (chemotherapy, radiation, etc.) versus waiting to transition the patient to palliative care/hospice after chemotherapy failed. Patients lived about two months longer on average when palliative care began right at the beginning.[1,2] I asked Mary to bring this study to the attention of her oncologist. She did and he either didn't know about it or disregarded it.

After about four months I called Mary on a Saturday and she told me about a new pain in her hip. She had restarted the hydrocodone, but it relieved pain only about two hours before it recurred. She said that she had told the oncologist about the pain on the previous Monday but did nothing. When Mary mentioned it to the visiting nurse, the nurse wrote it in her notes but nothing happened.

Through the hospital operator, I paged the on-call nurse practitioner covering for the oncologist that Saturday evening. No response. I paged again and still no answer. I then paged the visiting nurse. She called back and apologized that the doctor had not prescribed stronger pain medications. I asked her to page the nurse practitioner (a man) covering the service to get orders for additional pain medications. The visiting nurse said she would page the nurse practitioner, but if she did, he didn't answer her either. Mary received no new medications until her oncology clinic visit the following Monday. The oncologist offered no apology or explanation.

Unfortunately, the oncologist and his associates had inadequate expertise in using opioids in pain management. For long lasting pain control, he prescribed another opioid drug, fentanyl, by means of a patch on her skin. Unfortunately, the hydrocodone pill for breakthrough pain was dosed too low to be effective. No laxatives were initially prescribed, so constipation and the associated nausea and vomiting quickly stopped her ability to stomach any pain pills.

A computed tomography scan determined that the pain was caused by tumor obstructing one of Mary's kidneys. After she suffered a nightmarish week in hospital, the doctor diagnosed kidney failure. Without explaining the poor prognosis with tumor progression despite chemotherapy, or presenting hospice as an alternative course, the oncologist ordered Mary transferred for kidney dialysis to a better-equipped hospital 60 miles away.

At this point, I recommended hospice to Mary and her husband. They agreed. The kidney specialist consulted to perform dialysis was not disappointed. He told Mary that she had only a 10% chance of living significantly longer with the dialysis. Kidney dialysis certainly wouldn't have made the rotten management of her pain any better.

I arrived at Mary's bedside at the hospital shortly before an ambulance transferred her to a beautiful, state-of-the-art inpatient hospice nearby. Nurses quickly helped my sister settle into a bed in a hotel-like room, looking out on a lovely landscape.

The ward clerk told us that hospice volunteers and a singing chaplain regularly visited patients. Shortly thereafter, I spotted a black man carrying a guitar and asked if he was the chaplain. When he said, "yes," I asked if he would come to my sister's room and sing for her. When he came into the room, Mary was still anxious and upset about all the dramatic changes in her condition, fearing the implications of being a hospice patient.

As soon as the chaplain began to play and sing "Amazing Grace," she seemed to settle and become more comfortable. Soon, she was swaying to the music. Mary lifted one hand high, as was commonly done in her charismatic Christian church.

My sister surprised everyone and lived 17 days. Although she was comatose for the last eight days, the chaplain still came by each day and sang her spirituals and other songs.

At Mary's memorial service, my brother-in-law asked that any donations in his wife's memory go to the hospice facility. He told me that when he retires from his job, he will look into volunteering at the hospice. He also said that when his time comes, he would like to be in the same hospice.

Not all patients with terminal illnesses have the benefits of excellent hospice care. Another case that illustrates how far we have to go in improving palliative care involves a man that I saw at the LA County + USC Medical Center in 1991.

An Illegal Immigrant Requests Euthanasia

One busy day an intern called me saying that he had a cancer patient in the intensive care unit (ICU) screaming for euthanasia. By begging for death, the patient, a 52-year-old Korean man who I will call Mr. Kim (a pseudonym), made the young doctor and his colleagues very uncomfortable. As director of the Pain and Palliative Care Service, I listened to the intern's description of Mr. Kim's surgery in Seoul, Korea for stomach cancer 13 months earlier. I learned more of the patient's history from reviewing his three week ICU course in the very thick chart.

Since the cancer had already spread to the liver and elsewhere, his Korean surgeons infused chemotherapy into Mr. Kim's abdomen during the operation. Korean medical oncologists followed that by giving conventional outpatient chemotherapy.

Seeking a second opinion, Mr. Kim came to the United States and stayed with relatives. As an outpatient at the LA County + USC Medical Oncology Clinic, he received an experimental chemotherapy drug for six months. This failed to control his disease. The drug toxicity lowered his blood platelet count, which increased his chances of bleeding from the remaining abdominal tumors. He received multiple transfusions of blood because of constant hemorrhaging through his gastrointestinal tract.

One bleeding episode required hospitalization to achieve control. During that admission, after discussing it with his doctor, Mr. Kim agreed to a "do-not-resuscitate" order. Upon discharge from hospital, he was, unfortunately, not referred to a visiting nurse association hospice program or to my Pain and Palliative Care Service for comprehensive care in the terminal phase of his disease.

Three weeks later when Mr. Kim was again vomiting blood, his family rushed him to our emergency room. The emergency room doctors immediately transfused him with blood and moved him to what was then a new, ultramodern ICU. When bleeding persisted, he underwent angiography of his abdominal blood vessels (i.e., an X-ray study in which dye is introduced through a catheter threaded into an artery). An attempt to stop the bleeding by injecting plastic pellets into the stomach artery through the angiogram catheter failed. Undaunted, the specialists in interventional radiology later repeated this procedure because of persistent bleeding—again unsuccessful.

Because the cancer was so advanced and the patient was unable to take food while the bleeding persisted, the intensive care unit physicians ordered total parenteral nutrition (TPN) to prevent malnutrition. This consisted of over three liters of intravenous fluid per day containing about 3000 calories of nutrients delivered into a large vein near his heart.

Days later Mr. Kim developed a fever. His doctors promptly ordered antibiotics. When the fever persisted and blood cultures showed infection with resistant bacteria, they switched him to more powerful antibiotics.

On the 10th hospital day, a new intensive care unit doctor discussed with Mr. Kim and his family the seriousness of his condition. Mr. Kim again requested not to be resuscitated if his heart stopped beating. The doctor dutifully noted this in the chart.

Abdominal pain had been a big problem even before this hospitalization. Mr. Kim had taken prolonged-release morphine pills for pain for at least six months. While in intensive care, his pain had increased despite institution of an intravenous morphine infusion and raising the dose to 20 milligrams per hour (a high dose).

Mr. Kim's doctor asked the anesthesiology pain service to give a nerve block with a long needle into the nerves in the back of his abdomen in order to better control his severe pain. After deliberation for several days, the anesthesiologists declined to carry out the nerve block procedure for fear of causing internal bleeding and possibly shortening Mr. Kim's life.

On the 21st day in the ICU, with Mr. Kim now screaming for euthanasia, the intern called on me asking for new suggestions for the management of his pain. The young doctor had observed that a marked accumulation of fluid in Mr. Kim's abdomen appeared to contribute to the pain.

This case offered me an excellent opportunity to teach the intern and ICU team some of the basics of palliative care (pain and symptom management). I explained that, for a terminally ill patient in this situation, although we cannot honor a request for euthanasia, physicians are under no legal, moral, or other obligation to continue therapies designed to prolong life, such as blood transfusions, total parenteral nutrition, angiographies, and antibiotics. However, we are duty bound to control pain and other bothersome symptoms and to relieve suffering.

I suggested that they remove abdominal fluid (i.e., perform a "paracentesis") to decrease the pressure in Mr. Kim's abdomen. I also requested that the intravenous fluids, including the total parenteral nutrition, be stopped in order to prevent further misery from the accumulation of more fluid in his abdomen. Finally, I recommended an increase in the morphine infusion dose from 20 to 30 milligrams per hour, to better control his pain.

The next day when I saw Mr. Kim he was in coma and the morphine infusion had been stopped. Very distraught relatives filed in and out of his room for short visits, making their way between the hospital staff and the life-support technology.

Checking the chart, I noted that the paracentesis had not been done, again for fear of causing bleeding and shortening Mr. Kim's life. The doctors continued two intravenous antibiotics, total parenteral nutrition feedings, and frequent insulin injections. Cultures drawn two or three days earlier showed that two types of bacteria were growing in his blood despite the antibiotics. The doctors still ordered daily or more frequent laboratory blood tests.

I spoke at length with the intern and resident concerning palliative care in this type of situation and what to do if abdominal or other pain returned. During the following night, Mr. Kim woke up enough to express pain. A morphine injection was given intravenously, but initially did not work. Instead of giving Mr. Kim higher doses of morphine, the doctors injected Valium, a tranquillizer, which only quieted him down.

In the morning, the staff suddenly became concerned about the inappropriate utilization of the hospital's resources (the ICU bed) and ordered Mr. Kim's transfer to the regular ward. The total parenteral nutrition, antibiotics, and insulin could all be continued on the regular ward, but the morphine infusion pump could not because of hospital regulations.

The intern wrote an order for prolonged-release morphine sulfate tablets to be crushed and given through the stomach feeding tube. I pointed out to the staff that crushing prolonged-release morphine converts it into immediate-release morphine. In someone with tense fluid throughout the abdomen and acutely ill with sepsis (blood infection), as well as low blood pressure, oral medications would hardly be absorbed from the gastrointestinal tract. Plus, the dose of one 30 milligram prolonged-release morphine tablet every 12 hours was about 1/36th the equivalent of the 30 milligram per hour infusion he had previously received.

The nursing administration agreed to make an exception and allow the morphine pump for his final hours. However, the pump was not turned on, since Mr. Kim never came out of coma. The nurses and doctors were trained to wait for the patient to have pain before giving the pain medicine. This approach gives poor pain control to cancer patients with chronic pain particularly during the active dying process.

I wish there was a happy ending to this story, but there is not. When Mr. Kim died, the doctors told the family that they had done all they could medically to save him. No one could be charged with malpractice since this is not unusual treatment of the dying in the U.S.

Multiple obstacles in our medical care system and a lack of training in care of the dying had prevented even rudimentary pain and symptom control measures for Mr. Kim. The system provided virtually no help for him and his family with the psychological and emotional process of preparing for his death.

For Mr. Kim and many others who have received inappropriately aggressive high-tech interventions for advanced terminal diseases, the treatment was much worse than useless. It greatly increased the pain, suffering, and psychological distress during the dying process. This three-week stay in the ICU served only to magnify his pain and suffering enough for him to beg for euthanasia.

For Mr. Kim, euthanasia was not the answer. Physician training in palliative care and hospice medicine offered a far better solution. To date, post-graduate physicians and medical students at most teaching hospitals still do not receive adequate palliative care training.

In a time of dire shortages of health care funding for the poor, including illegal immigrants like Mr. Kim, we need health care reform to include reform of the care of the dying. Mr. Kim's futile treatment for three weeks in the ICU cost taxpayers over $50,000 in 1991. The cost would be over four times that in 2016.[3, 4]

My Proposal for a Hospice Ward at My Hospital

Weeks after Mr. Kim's death, I submitted a request to LA County administrators for an inpatient hospice ward at LA County + USC Medical Center. I brought Mr. Kim's case to the attention of Dr. Jonathan Weisbuch, medical director of the LA County–Department of Health Services. Dr. Weisbuch strongly supported my recommendation to start a hospice ward and arranged for me to present my proposal to the Chief of the Medicaid Policy Section of the California State Department of Health Services, T. George Wilson, MD, and his staff in Sacramento.

Dr. Wilson and his staff supported my proposed inpatient hospice to provide an alternative for patients like Mr. Kim. Dr. Wilson's boss,

Sally Lee, Chief of Medicaid Operations Division (Medi-Cal in California), wrote a letter of support to Dr. Weisbuch with copies to the director of the LA County Department of Health Services and other medical administrators.[5] Unfortunately, the proposed inpatient hospice ward would have reduced Medi-Cal funding for the LA County + USC Medical Center by decreasing the number of patient days in hospital. Consequently, no action was taken.

"Death Panels"

In the run up to the passage of the Affordable Care Act (ACA), detractors of Obamacare found a fear mongering talking point with the concept of "death panels." Rumors, spread by talk-show hosts like Rush Limbaugh and Glenn Beck, suggested that the bill empowered "death panels" to "euthanize" elderly Americans. Conservatives found a case to spotlight. ABC News reported on Ms. Barbara Wagner, a woman with recurrent lung cancer, who received a denial of a $4000 a month cancer drug from her insurer, the Oregon Health Plan. However, the Plan would pay for a $50 drug that could be used for assisted suicide.[6]

The Oregon Health Plan provided "basic" insurance to people on Medicaid, and to other poor people that earned too much money to qualify for Medicaid. The Oregon Legislature and Governor determined what the benefits included. Ms. Wagner's primary care physician had no say. This case illustrates why top-down insurance coverage decision-making by insurance company or government bureaucrats is unraveling.

Obamacare legislation included provisions for Medicare and private insurers to pay for optional consultations with doctors regarding hospice or palliative care benefits. Palliative care has come to mean pain and symptom management given concurrently while a patient still undergoes active life prolonging treatments (e.g., chemotherapy, radiation, etc.). Legislators eventually removed the provisions for paying doctors to do consultations about hospice and palliative care. However, the U.S. Department of Health and Human Services regulators snuck it back in as part of the ACA provision for Medicare to cover annual wellness visits to physicians.

The new rule allows doctors to discuss "voluntary advance care planning." The federal regulation provides a Medicare billing code for physicians to be paid to give information to patients on how to prepare an "advance directive," concerning the patient's wishes for or against heroic life support measures if they are terminally ill.[7]

I'm sorry, but the U.S. Congress, the Department of Health and Human Services, individual state legislatures, and insurance company administrators have no business practicing medicine. What outrages me is the implication that the practice of medicine consists of whatever Congress and medical insurance companies deem worthy of reimbursement. Increasingly, Congress and insurance companies are controlling the practices of physicians. Instead, physicians should have the autonomy to practice medicine while legislators govern and insurance companies just deal with paying the bills. Patients, then, could choose their physicians based on how different doctors practice medicine.

Underutilization of Hospice and Palliative Care Services

Ask yourself the question, "If I had a terminal illness, would I rather die at home or in the hospital?" In many lectures on pain and symptom management, I have polled audiences on this question. Almost everyone would prefer to die at home or in a supportive hospice environment. However, over half of terminally ill Americans die in hospitals, many in pain and with unnecessary suffering. The major reason for this paradox is the lack of training of physicians in counseling seriously ill patients and in treating the pain and other symptoms associated with advanced diseases. Few physicians-in-training do clinical rotations with hospice teams, which is the best place to learn to treat severe pain and distressing symptoms of people with terminal illness.

In three years of my hematology/oncology fellowship, I had no clinical rotation in hospice care and pain management. However, by spending the last clinical rotation of my fellowship in hematology/oncology working in hospices in England (Oxford, London, and Worthing), I made an unexpected discovery. I learned that I didn't know that I didn't know how to treat pain and other symptoms of terminally ill cancer patients. I resolved to spend my career trying to improve the situation.

The second major reason that so many terminally ill people die in hospital rather than at home is money. It costs much more to die in hospital. Not surprisingly to some, clinical practices follow financial incentives. While hospital doctors and staff may be very compassionate and want what is best for their patients, they work in a system driven by money. To be enabled to die at home instead takes a great deal of planning and preparation.

Helping people with the complex task of remaining at home in comfort for the duration of a terminal illness is not well reimbursed relative to having patients occupy hospital beds. And few doctors are well trained in undertaking the complexities of coordinating hospice-at-home care. The involvement of a hospice team is essential. As the system now works for terminally ill people, the default option is to die in hospital—where insurance companies will pay $5000 per day and up instead of maybe $200 per day for home hospice.

To have better end-of-life patient outcomes, physician training in palliative care/hospice and financial incentives of the health care system have to change.

The Pain and Palliative Care Service at the LA County + USC Medical Center

I served as Chief of the Pain and Palliative Care Service at the LA County + USC Medical Center from 1987–1995, caring for cancer and AIDS patients with severe pain. Over that period of time, a nurse, internal medicine residents, and I consulted on over 2000 patients. You could say that I acted as the "direct practice" physician (Chapter 3) for these people, usually following about 150 patients at any given time. I also worked as attending physician for teams of internal medicine residents and medical students that admitted patients to the hospital wards. About 20% of the general internal medicine patients my team admitted to my hospital ward service had pain and symptoms of advanced cancer or AIDS. One of those patients was Mrs. Brown (a pseudonym).

Mrs. Brown—a Woman with Far Advanced AIDS

While serving as attending physician for an admitting internal medicine team, Mrs. Brown, a black woman in her 60s, was admitted to my service. She was in coma from brain complications of AIDS. Mrs. Brown lived in the central California valley with a large supportive family. The local physicians had treated her over several years with the appropriate antiviral medications for AIDS, yet she had progressed to the end stage of the disease.

Once Mrs. Brown lapsed into coma in a hospital, the local physicians told the family that a transfer to an intensive care unit (ICU) would be futile and recommended no further anti-AIDS treatment. The family objected violently and asked for the ICU transfer and life support machines. Prolonged discussions between the outside hospital physicians and family members did not resolve the dispute.

Finally, the family paid $5000 to charter an airplane to Los Angeles where a waiting ambulance transported her to the LA County + USC Medical Center emergency room and from there to my admitting team. A brilliant and compassionate senior resident was in charge of the patient's care. He had been up all night with the usual 12–20 admissions but still called me at home to discuss Mrs. Brown. After he told me her story, I told him that I recommended palliative care on the AIDS ward rather than transfer to the ICU. He felt the same way. However, he wanted to clear it with me before meeting with Mrs. Brown's family about her condition.

After the meeting with her family, he called me at home again, saying he was unable to convince the family that it would be better for their mother to have comfort care on the AIDS ward than to be on a mechanical ventilator receiving aggressive life support measures in the ICU. He said that at least a half dozen family members were adamant about the ICU transfer. They hadn't flown her to LA to have symptomatic treatment alone.

I asked the resident to tell the spokesperson for the family—the patient's son—to call me at home. When the son, John (not his real name), called, he initially expressed a belligerent tone. John made it clear at the outset that he and the family were insisting on an ICU transfer so that everything possible could be done to save his mother.

Rather than argue with him, I asked him to tell me about his mother's illness. John said that his mother contracted HIV from a blood transfusion and not from sex or IV drug abuse. He and the family wanted everyone caring for her to know the origin of her infection. I commiserated with him about the tragedy of his mother becoming infected.

John told me that throughout the illness the family had supported his mother and that they all had a lot of love for her. He said that the demonstration of their love for her was chartering a plane to Los Angeles when the central valley doctors said they had no more treatments to give her. When John seemed to run out of things to say about his mother, I prompted him for further information until he fully expressed the family's sentiments.

During this 30-minute+ phone conversation, John's tone changed from hostile and belligerent to conciliatory. He seemed to be coming to an understanding that I cared about his mother and his family.

Before beginning my explanation of our treatment recommendations, I congratulated John and his family for all they had done out of love in her behalf. I told him that it was apparent to me that the family all wanted the best possible care to be given to his mother. He agreed.

I pointed out that she was on the AIDS ward, which had an excellent reputation for state-of-the-art treatment and for nursing care. I said that our doctors and nurses are some of the most experienced in the world in treating people with AIDS.

I asked him if he wanted to know what I thought was the best treatment for his mother. He said, "Yes."

I said that while we don't have a cure for her AIDS, we have good treatment for her. We could allay any discomfort or suffering that she may experience. I said that to hook her up to a breathing machine in an ICU would be needlessly increasing her suffering.

The belligerent tone returned somewhat, and John said that the whole family wanted her in the ICU. I said that, if she were my mother or someone I loved, I wouldn't want that for her. I repeated that she was very lucky to have such a loving family and that I was sure they all wanted what was best for her.

John finally agreed to having his mother remain in a regular ward bed rather than going to the ICU. I said that he and his family were welcome to be with her day and night as much as they liked. He thanked me. I called my resident to tell him about my conversation with the son. He thanked me effusively.

The patient died peacefully on the AIDS ward about three days later with her family in attendance.

Hope

Hope means different things to different people, and it changes as medical conditions change. A hope for a cure can morph into a hope for freedom from pain and suffering or that a relationship can be mended. For many people, hope and faith are inextricably linked. People may pray ceaselessly for a miracle for their terminally ill loved one, but then accept death when it comes as "God's will."

Physicians should tell the truth with kindness, but never try to take away the patient's hope. I never told any patient, "I have nothing more to offer you." Frequently, I told terminally ill patients something like, "While we don't have a cure for your condition, we have good treatment for the pain and symptoms. My staff and I will always be available to help you no matter what happens. No one knows how long you have to live. Whatever time you have, we can help you remain a comfortable as possible, whether at home or in the hospital."

Dr. Susan D. Block, a palliative care physician at Harvard Medical School, said it well, "Hope lives inside a patient and the physician's behavior can either bring it out or suppress it. When a patient has goals, it's impossible to be hopeless. And when a physician can help a patient define them, you feel like a healer, even when the patient is dying."[8]

Hospice Care for a Friend's Demented Mother

Thelma, the 85-year-old mother of Louise, a friend of mine, had advanced dementia. She lived in a home with other patients receiving around-the-clock nursing care. Thelma was incontinent, could speak only occasional random words, and required assistance with eating and other activities of daily living. After Thelma had a difficult hospitalization for a pelvic fracture, Louise enrolled Thelma with a provider of the Medicare hospice benefit at my suggestion. Both Thelma and Louise liked the care much better, and things stabilized for nearly a year. However, Thelma's condition was so stable that the hospice administrator notified Louise that Thelma would no longer be able to receive hospice care because of Medicare regulations. Congress designed the hospice benefit in 1981 to be available for terminally ill people with less than six months to live.

By not dying within six months of enrolling into the hospice benefit, Thelma was putting the hospice providers at some risk of being charged with fraud by Medicare. Indeed, in the 1990s, Center for Medicare and Medicaid Services administrators did analyze the lengths of stays of hospice patients around the county. Some hospice programs were cited because they had too many patients living longer than the Congressional regulation designated six months. Some of those hospices had to return some of the Medicare reimbursements and pay fines.[9]

Reluctantly, Thelma's hospice transferred her back to regular Medicare services and stopped visiting her. Since 24-hour emergency care was no longer available through the hospice, the care home felt that complying with federal regulations meant transporting Thelma to an emergency room for a sudden change in health status. I told Louise that Thelma was stuck with Congressionally-mandated, very dysfunctional regulations. I offered to help as much as possible.

A few hours before Louise was leaving on a trip to Eastern Europe, Thelma fell off of the commode and hurt her ankle at the care home. The attending nurse called an ambulance even before notifying Louise. Louise then informed me. I phoned the emergency room and asked for the physician assigned to Thelma. The ER doc had no chart and no one to give him his patient's history. He described an acutely agitated, completely incoherent, naked woman wildly moving all four extremities without apparent limitation.

I summarized Thelma's history for the grateful ER physician. He said that x-raying the ankle would require heavy sedation. He also wondered about the need to send her urine for bacterial culture to rule out a urinary tract infection causing the acute delirium. He asked me what to do.

I told the ER doctor not to order an ankle x-ray or a urine culture. I recommended that he immediately send Thelma back to the care home. Attempting some humor in this stressful situation, I asked him to order an emergency hospice consult. He didn't understand my joke and asked me to explain. I said that the poor woman should never have been forced by the federal government to leave her previous hospice care. He followed my recommendations.

As a slight consolation for Thelma, the Medicare hospice benefit law allows people like Thelma to re-qualify for hospice after an ER visit or hospitalization. Louise saw Thelma safely returned to the care home and hospice re-established. With her mother safe, Louise made her plane to Eastern Europe.

Thelma's ankle healed with time on its own, and she could walk with assistance after a couple of weeks. Over the next four to five months, she gradually deteriorated further. Her weight dropped from over 150 pounds when healthy to under 90 pounds. Louise took my advice and declined the insertion of a feeding tube. A few weeks before potentially timing out of the Medicare hospice benefit for a second time, Thelma died in the care home with Louise and her husband in attendance. Louise was very grateful for the hospice and for my assistance.

Palliative Care Appropriate for People with Dementia

Unfortunately, many people with dementia, like Thelma, have burdensome treatments during their final months on earth.

A study of 323 people with advanced dementia in nursing homes by Harvard researchers found that more than half of the patients died within 18-months. During the last three months of life, 132 patients received at least one inappropriate treatment, like transport to an emergency room, hospitalization, feeding tubes, or intravenous treatments.[9]

The investigators found marked differences in the inappropriate treatments based on what family members knew about dementia. When family members understood that dementia is progressive and terminal, few patients received aggressive care. Conversely, when family members did not understand the nature of the disease, most patients had unnecessarily burdensome treatments.

A report from the Alzheimer's Association showed that 71% of nursing home residents with advanced dementia died within six months of admission, yet only 11% were referred to hospice care.[10] This represents a failure of our health care system—particularly the primary care component—resulting in worse care and higher costs. Without proper counseling, grieving family members, who often struggle with guilt, do not stop aggressive treatment for fear of abandoning their loved one.

The answer is strengthening the primary care component of our health care system (Chapter 3) and better training of all physicians in palliative care and hospice.

Physician-Assisted Suicide California Campaign 1992

Following the lead of Oregon, advocates of physician-assisted suicide in California placed an initiative on the ballot in 1992 to legalize the practice. I joined the coalition of organizations formed to campaign *against* this ballot referendum. The opposing organizations included the Catholic Church, California Medical Association, California Nursing Association, and American Association of Retired People.

At the first meeting of the coalition to defeat the California physician-assisted-suicide initiative, I appealed for a campaign to educate physicians in pain control and palliative care for the terminally ill. The members all responded positively. The representatives from the Catholic Church and the California Medical Association promised to work on strategies to educate physicians in hospice medicine after defeating the assisted-suicide initiative.

When pollsters and politicians joined the coalition to defeat the assisted-suicide initiative, they advised the group to avoid mentioning that physicians are not trained to properly care for the dying. Without conducting focus groups on the issue, they probably rightly figured that the public would be confused on hearing that their doctors lacked training in proper pain and symptom management.

Instead, the campaign to defeat the assisted-suicide initiative focused on saturating the airwaves with 30-second sound bites designed to scare people about aspects of the initiative. The sound bites highlighted the lack of a required waiting period after a patient asked for assisted suicide. They mentioned that the family and friends need not be notified when someone is about to receive physician-assisted suicide. They also pointed out that non-clinician physicians, like pathologist and euthanasia crusader Dr. Jack Kevorkian, could assist suicide instead of treating doctors.

After voters defeated the initiative 54%–46%, none of the members of the coalition worked on improving physician education in pain and symptom management.

Book: Euthanasia is Not the Answer—
A Hospice Physician's View

In order to be more involved in the debate, I wrote my first book, *Euthanasia is Not the Answer—A Hospice Physician's View* (Humana Press, 1992).[11] The premise of the book was that terminally ill people receiving good hospice medical treatment with pain and symptom control do not want to be euthanized or to commit suicide. In order to eliminate the demand for euthanasia and physician-assisted suicide, physicians, especially those treating cancer and AIDS patients, should be trained in the principles and techniques of hospice medicine.

Much of the material for the book came from my experiences as chief of the LA County + USC Medical Center Pain and Palliative Care Service. By 1992, I had cared for over 1000 terminally ill patients. Only 12 of those patients had brought up the subject of assisted suicide or euthanasia. In all those cases, the patients mentioned to a nurse or other staff member rather than to me that they wanted help with dying. In 10 of the cases, the patients changed their minds after pain and disease-related distressing symptoms were relieved.

In one patient with lung cancer and pain in the neck from bony metastases, massive doses of morphine and other pain medicines did not bring the pain down to tolerable levels. I asked the anesthesia pain consultant to place a catheter next to the man's cervical spine so opioid drugs infused near the tumor could control the pain. At that time, the anesthesia pain consultant did not have the necessary high-tech equipment, so he did not do it. Unfortunately, the patient suffered and asked for euthanasia until he died from the tumor. I felt badly that the hospital could not muster the resources to help us control the pain. I saw the problem as a medical system failure rather than a reason to sanction euthanasia or assisted suicide.

One patient followed by our service with AIDS and depression, did commit suicide by overdosing on his prescribe medications. He lived in a downtown Los Angeles single-room occupancy apartment and had very little, if any, contact with family or friends. I felt that our palliative care services failed him because we did not have the resources to help him get sufficient social and psychological support.

Variations in Medicare Spending for End-of-Life Care

Cost-of-care for Medicare patients varies widely in different regions of the country. Quality-of-care is not better in high spending areas. Patients in regions with greater overall end-of-life spending do not live longer, have better quality of care, or patient satisfaction.[12] However, higher-spending regions do have a greater regional supply of specialists,[13] hospitals, ICU beds,[14-16] and sophisticated technologies.[17] When physicians are presented with terminally ill patients described in structured vignettes, those doctors that practice in high-intensity regions have a greater tendency to recommend tests, make referrals, and prescribe treatments, and are less likely to refer to hospice.[18, 19]

A nationwide study of care for Medicare recipients in the last six months of life compared the lowest spending quintile (one-fifth of patients) with the highest spending quintile. The authors found that patients in the highest spending areas underwent

- 1.8 times the number of days in hospital,
- 2.2 times the number of days in the ICU,
- 2.6 times the number of resuscitation attempts, and
- 2.9 times the number of feeding tubes inserted.

Patients in high-spending regions had many more expensive and uncomfortable procedures. However, their length of survival and most other outcomes did not differ significantly from those in low-spending areas. The satisfaction with care, however, was significantly lower in the highest-spending quintile compared with the lowest-spending quintile.[12]

The huge variations in spending—reflected by the above differences in days of aggressive treatment—for end-of-life care are not because patients in some geographical regions of the country demand more high-tech interventions than people in other areas. A published survey of 2515 Medicare beneficiaries all over the U.S. reported no significant differences in end-of-life care preferences between high and low spending regions:[20]

1. Patients concerned about getting too little end-of-life treatment—39.6% in the lowest spending quintile versus 41.2% in the highest

2. Patients concerned about getting too much end-of-life treatment—44.2% in lowest spending quintile versus 45.1% in the highest

3. At the end of life, patient preferences for spending their last days in a hospital—8.4% in the lowest spending quintile versus 8.5% in the highest

4. Patient preferences for potentially life-prolonging drugs that made them feel worse all the time—14.4% in lowest spending quintile versus 16.5% in the highest

5. Patient preferences for palliative drugs, even if they might be life-shortening—77.7% in lowest spending quintile versus 73.4% in the highest

6. Patient preference for mechanical ventilation if it would extend their life by one month—21% in lowest spending quintile versus 21.4% in the highest: or by one week—12.1% versus 11.7%

Most people want state-of-the-art palliative care at the end of life, but too few people receive it. The result is much unnecessary suffering and the waste of tens of billions of dollars.

Grand Junction, CO: Top Quality End-of-Life Care, Low Cost

The New Yorker magazine ran an article by Dr. Atul Gawande about health care costs in various cities.[21] This article caught the attention of White House and Congressional health policy experts, leading many to believe that $500 billion could be saved from Medicare over 10 years without reductions in necessary services. The article contrasted Medicare costs and quality of care in McAllen, Texas with those in Grand Junction, Colorado. The cost of the last six months of life for Medicare recipients in Grand Junction was $8366 and in McAllen was $21,123.[20] Dying Medicare patients in McAllen had over five times the IUC days as those in Grand Junction. Only 16.7% of Grand Junction patients died in an acute care hospital, compared with 45.1% in McAllen.[22]

In contrast with McAllen and other high medical spending areas of the U.S., the Grand Junction medical providers have fostered a culture of cooperation and innovation in the provision of excellent medical care at relatively low cost.[23] While Grand Junction medical providers are not administratively integrated into a single health maintenance organization, they have formed the equivalent of some components of an accountable care cooperative.

The Grand Junction community hospice provider, "Hospice and Palliative Care of Western Colorado," serves everyone regardless of insurance payer. It provides innovative end-of-life care and maintains a state-of-the-art inpatient facility for times when hospice patients cannot remain at home.

PCPs encourage advanced planning and communication. They assist specialists both in caring for the hospice patient and in talking to families at the appropriate time. Compared with hospices throughout the country, Grand Junction hospice patients spend significantly fewer days in the hospital, more days on the hospice benefit, and are more likely to die at home than in the hospital.[24]

Grand Bargain for Good Hospice/Palliative Care: ACCs

With Grand Bargains-based health care reform, the ACC of each person's choice will determine the medical benefits provided, including hospice and palliative care.

With ACC care, doctors of Ms. Wagner (the Oregon cancer patient on Medicaid insurance) would have decided the insurance coverage. Depending on the benefit package of the ACC, she might or might not have been offered chemotherapy. If not, reasons may include that the side effects caused by the drug, together with the highly questionable survival benefit claimed from drug-company funded trials, did not justify the treatment in the opinion of ACC physicians. Instead, she might have been offered nontoxic alternative anticancer therapies and palliative care. If she wanted to appeal the denial of the chemotherapy drug by ACC decision-makers, she could have taken the case to a committee of ACC staff and other members of the ACC.

The fear that bean-counting Washington, D.C. bureaucrats on "death panels" will decide what treatments you will or will not be offered in life or death situations will be resolved by **putting each person's chosen doctors and their ACC managers in charge of insurance funding decisions.**

Summary and Conclusion

A measure of the effectiveness of any health care reform proposal is whether it leads to better care of terminally ill people. A patient's PCP should stay actively involved in providing end-of-life care. The PCP is best suited to integrate active and palliative care as required throughout the course of a serious illness. For a person with an advanced terminal disease, appropriate and timely referral to a local hospice/palliative care organization by the PCP is the best way to improve quality of life.

With ACCs administering medical education funds for medical students and postgraduate physicians-in-training, the philosophy and techniques of hospice and palliative care medicine will be emphasized. Medical school educational curricula and postgraduate training programs will teach future PCPs and other physicians-in-training the art and science of end-of-life care (Chapter 19).

With proper training, PCPs will soon learn when patients with advanced incurable illnesses are best served by intensive supportive care—at home if possible—rather than futile hospitalizations and hugely expensive intensive care unit nightmares. Hospice programs with well-trained physicians and nurses should be available to people in need throughout the country.

Grand Bargains based payment reform will incentivize rather than discourage excellent end-of-life care. Early referral for terminally ill people to palliative care or hospice services will improve care, save money, and likely extend life modestly.

Excellent end-of-life care means better quality of life for patients while they are living, bereavement services for surviving family members and friends, and more affordable health services for all.

Chapter 6
Additional Health and Social Services

With ACC-based health care reform, ACCs will be in charge of allocating all health and social-safety-net funding (Chapter 2). ACC decision makers will have great flexibility in funding what they think are the most beneficial and innovative health and social-safety-net services for their enrolled patients. Alternative and/or additional services beyond what insurers now cover include (1) health promotion and preventive medicine (2) hospice and palliative care, and (3) child care, all of which are addressed in Chapters 4, 5, and 12, respectively. This chapter will address mental health care, experimental treatments, long-term care, oral health care, and what have come to be called alternative and complementary treatments.

Michael: My Mentally Ill, Substance-Abusing Friend

Over the last five years or so, I have gotten to know a 30 year old man, Michael (not his real name), diagnosed with mental illness, alcoholism, and drug abuse. A next door neighbor and friend introduced me to Michael when Michael showed up on his doorstep homeless and hungry. Michael is the nephew of a close friend of my neighbor.

Michael was allowed to sleep on my friend's living room floor for a few days while I tried to hook Michael into Alcoholics Anonymous and a local drug-alcohol rehabilitation program. I spent time with Michael getting to know him. I fed him, taught him a little about cooking and baking, and tried to use my skills of persuasion to convince him to become serious about getting sober.

Michael grew up in a dysfunctional family. His father and a brother had both been to prison. His parents divorced when Michael was young. At least two of his siblings also struggled with substance abuse. Michael dropped out of high school in the ninth grade to do construction work. He spent the money that he earned for drugs and alcohol. Despite great efforts by his mother and an uncle to help him get treatment for substance abuse and mental illness, Michael periodically found himself homeless and living on the street. He would enter drug and alcohol detoxification and rehabilitation programs only to quit within days or weeks.

Some friends of mine and I donated money to a local environmental cleanup nonprofit organization to employ Michael cleaning up local wetlands. He said that he would try it, but he never showed up for work. Owners of two sober living homes kicked Michael out while I was trying to help him.

One spring day, Michael showed up at the house, again without prior notification. This time Martha, a five-months-pregnant girlfriend, accompanied him. She admitted to being addicted to methamphetamine and lived on the streets like Michael. This was to be her second child. Her mother took care of a two year old toddler in a nearby city.

After they crashed on the floor in the garage for the night, I offered them breakfast and did my best to convince Martha to go into a shelter for homeless, pregnant women. I appealed to her for the sake of the baby. I referred her to the homeless crisis agency that I had found with an online search. Unfortunately, the pull of the drugs won. Michael and Martha departed for the streets shortly after breakfast.

A couple of weeks later, Michael appeared back at my front door, alone. He said that Martha had gone into a shelter for homeless women the day after our encounter. I was happy about that. He had told her good-bye and had no knowledge of whether she stayed in the shelter, stayed sober, or how she and the fetus were doing.

Michael said that he wanted to get into Alcoholics Anonymous meetings and asked me to find the local times and places for meetings. However, after I found him the local available alcohol rehabilitation programs, it was apparent that he had no real interest in attending.

I offered him a meal and listened to more of his story. He made it clear that his depression and chaotic family situation were his main problems. These led him to abuse drugs and alcohol as a teenager. Intermittently, he would have weeks or months of sobriety. Then he would get lonely and depressed. He would meet up with drug abusing friends and the cycle would repeat.

Michael's mother helped him access counselors and therapists beginning in high school. She worked the system and helped him get onto Social Security Disability. At first, she was his conservator and monitored his government checks. However, she tired of his constant nagging and finally withdrew from being the conservator. Inexplicably, the social services administrators allowed Michael to manage his own Social Security Disability payments.

Generally, he spent his government check on drugs and alcohol over a few days at the beginning of each month. No physician, medical social worker, or other health professional monitored his behavior. Michael said that more and more of his friends and acquaintances on the street were receiving government disability checks. It's frightening that Michael and presumably other addicts and alcoholics use disability checks for drugs and alcohol and have little or no professional monitoring.

He shared that he thought he would die young. He said before he died, he wanted to get back at the people that had done him wrong. Michael had some grudges against some family members and others.

He said he had read a lot about the so called the "night stalker," a serial killer and rapist named Richard Ramirez. Michael indicated that he identified with the loneliness that Ramirez felt that supposedly led him to his killing rampages. Michael read that Ramirez corresponded with and married a woman while in prison. Michael expressed some envy about that.

I had lots of concerns about Michael's troubled thoughts and feelings of anger and hatred. I wish to this day that there was a way to get him professional help with his mental illness and substance abuse. I worry that he might have a potential for violence.

Michael is big and strong. He had some training in martial arts while in his teens and during periods of sobriety. He told me that he has had to use his karate occasionally on the street when he got jumped. As far as I know from my neighbor and from Michael's uncle, Michael has never been arrested for a violent crime. Aside from 30 days in jail on a marijuana bust, he had never been in jail.

If I were to estimate Michael's risk of a major violent act of attacking someone or even a group of people he felt had done him wrong, I would guess it might be higher than the average person. I just hope that he never manages to obtain a gun.

How many Michaels are out there wandering the streets in your town? Don't you wish they were all in effective treatment programs?

In trying to help Michael, I decided to use a substance abuse counseling technique that I had read about called "motivational interviewing." According to Bill Miller, who introduced motivational interviewing to psychotherapists, "It's part of the therapist's job to help addicts find the motivation within themselves to change." Miller's most recent definition of motivational interviewing is ". . . a collaborative, person-centered form of guiding to elicit and strengthen motivation for change."[1]

Instead of dictating to the substance abuser what he should do, the professional is trying to help the patient find the motivation for change within. By using motivational interviewing, the therapist listens to the patient and asks questions. The therapist attempts to guide substance abusers to consider their options. This approach is meant to avoid the usual anger and defensiveness that addicts have when lectured about how bad their situation is and about what they need to do to become sober. The therapist endeavors to illicit in the patient a willingness to continue exploring the possibilities for change in a collaborative, hopeful, energizing manner.

I will continue to be there for Michael when he shows up for my support. I don't have money to give him, and I wouldn't give him money if I had it. However, I know that, if he is ever to get into recovery from his substance abuse, he will need people that care about him and wish for something meaningful for him to do with his life. I will do what I can in those regards. I wish it could be more.

The Broken U.S. Mental Health System

Michael's case may serve as a good point of departure for discussing gun violence. I hope he never owns a gun or uses one to hurt anyone. No one can say if he ever will. However, having thousands of Michaels on the streets with no mental health or substance abuse treatment is a recipe for violent crime.

Our epidemic of shooting rampages can't be stopped simply by more laws banning assault weapons or by requiring background checks before selling guns to people. Regulations restricting access to guns or more police with militarized weaponry will accomplish little or nothing. Reforming our mental health system needs to lead the way to preventing gun violence. Expanding insurance coverage to include mental illness treatment, as written into the ACA, is an important but small piece of the solution.

In the wake of the Newtown, Connecticut massacre at Sandy Hook Elementary School, Rep. Tim Murphy, PhD (R-Pa.), a clinical psychologist, introduced the "Helping Families in Mental Health Crisis Act." This was a step in the right direction for reducing mass shootings and other violence. Congressman Murphy pointed out that many of the 11 million Americans with schizophrenia, bipolar disorder, and major depression are going without treatment while their families struggle to find care for loved ones. For many of these most vulnerable people, the U.S. mental health system, consisting of a chaotic hodgepodge of inadequate and uncoordinated programs, spanning numerous agencies, is broken.[2, 3]

In his book *How Evil Works*, David Kupelian documented that most perpetrators of recent mass murders were either taking – or just recently stopped taking – psychiatric medications.[4] Regarding the Sandy Hook massacre, he noted that the media and public attention focused largely on the guns used by Adam Lanza, while the details of his psychiatric medication history have not been reported to this day.[5, 6] Regarding Lanza and others, it is important to understand that selective serotonin reuptake inhibitors (SSRIs: e.g., Prozac and Paxil) and other psychiatric medications under some circumstances may increase the chances of self-harm and violence towards others.

Our patchwork approach to mental illness, with an overemphasis on drugs, needs to be revamped. It does not optimize the therapeutic modalities available. We need more coordinated, holistic care. Additionally, better social welfare programs will keep people from descending into unhealthful living situations that only add to mental instability and depression.

The National Institute of Mental Health and other federal government health agencies have not had the resources to bring successful mental health treatment to vulnerable populations. Mentally ill people too often end up homeless or in the criminal justice system instead of getting effective treatment. A mentally ill person gunning down other people is one result of the failed mental health system.

With our very diverse country, I expect that the most effective answer to fixing our mental health system will probably vary in different communities and among different populations within those communities. Consequently, centralized mental health policies, procedures, and payment systems financially dependent on the U.S. Department of Health and Human Services and/or state and local government health agencies are not only wasteful but are impediments to reform.

We know the desired results of mental health system reform—good outcomes for mentally ill people receiving treatment, effective mental illness prevention strategies, and much lower rate of gun violence. However, we have no consensus about the method to achieve it. Consequently, we need to experiment.

Grand Bargain #29 Part 1: ACCs' Preventing Violence by Fixing Mental Health Care

For each and every U.S. resident, we need to have an ACC-affiliated team available comprised of mental health services professionals. This team will have full responsibility for prevention of mental illness and treatment of people with anxiety, depression, schizophrenia, and other psychological problems. These teams must have the human and financial resources necessary to find the people early who are at risk for violence and to establish mental wellness-promotion programs that work for the people at high risk. When psychological treatment is necessary, it needs to go well beyond pills, talk therapy, and psychiatric hospitalization. Experimenting with treatment approaches and documenting and publishing the outcomes will help us find better answers.

We may find that part of the solution to gun violence is to sharply curtail the use of psychiatric drugs and substitute cognitive behavioral therapy and/or other therapies. Physical exercise, meaningful work, volunteering opportunities, connections with peers, communing with nature, and spiritual practices—all of which are proven to give mental-health benefits—may play important roles.

The allocation of disability benefits to people with mental illnesses needs to be reformed in conjunction with psychological disease prevention and treatment reform. Disability benefits for the mentally ill should be delivered with great flexibility under the auspices of the same ACC-affiliated teams that provide mental-health prevention and treatment services. Obviously, no one should receive disability checks from Social Security for mental illness and substance abuse without being monitored—like Michael was.

Yet, unless family bonds are strengthened in the U.S.—some say the nation with the weakest family bonds and weakest sense of community—countless people will join the isolated, unsupported people struggling today in this country. This is why ACCs as cooperatives—offering more than just medical insurance—are vital for a society needing a stronger, healthier social fabric.

One major goal needs to be enhanced socialization of patients in society. Whenever possible, employment should also be a goal. For those who dropped out of high school, obtaining high school equivalency certification is almost always an important step toward rehabilitation.

The grand bargain for mental health reform and violence prevention will involve ACCs' providing the strategies to promote mental wellness, treat psychiatric illness, and prevent violence. Patient-centered medical homes within ACCs, with comprehensive health and human services, will ably serve people at risk for or who are already suffering with mental illness and/or substance abuse. For the wide spectrum of needs of these people, ACC medical home team members will call in psychologists, psychiatrists, substance abuse program experts, educators, financial counselors, job placement specialists, legal counselors, clergy, and any other needed consultants.

We also need to think outside the box. For some troubled citizens feeling cast aside or disenchanted with the "rat race," temporary respite and opportunities for growth may be found in the health promotion retreat centers recommended in Chapter 20. In such centers, especially ones in rural settings, mentally troubled people may well respond to opportunities for physical labor, recreation, communing with nature, social interactions, art, music, singing, healthful eating, and experiential learning all guided and monitored by mental health professionals.

ACCs will compete, in part, on how well they serve their members in fostering mental wellness, managing mental illness and encouraging healthier, happier lifestyles. Consequently, ACC's will need to employ innovative strategies to achieve optimal mental health outcomes:

- low incarceration rates
- no homelessness
- effective sobriety programs
- educational achievement
- full employment of all members able to work
- integration of parolees back into society and employment without recidivism

- the lowest possible level of violence
- options and opportunities for meaningful community volunteering and careers

ACCs will be adversely impacted financially and in their reputations if excessive numbers of members become homeless, incarcerated, unemployed, underemployed, or violent due to mental illness. Early interventions will improve outcomes and save money. Providing holistic mental health care (psychological, social, employment, exercise, nutritional, spiritual, environmental, psychiatric, etc.) within communities can help patients and the community, while reducing the costs of hospitalization and incarceration.

As Part 2 of this mental-health-system-reform grand bargain, I propose taxes on the purchase of any gun and a yearly licensing fee for ownership of each gun. These ideas will be detailed in Chapter 21 with the consumption taxes.

ACC-Based Mental Health Treatment Parity

Risk-adjustment formulas to allocate the federal government's health care funding to ACCs for their enrollees will consider diagnoses of mental illnesses on a par with physical diagnoses. Resources for mental health care will be allocated according to determinations of need by the ACCs. ACCs that provide resources for excellent treatment of mental illnesses will probably be preferred because poor treatment of mentally ill people will cost everyone.

Patients, PCPs, and their ACCs will all benefit from the emphasis on behavioral or lifestyle change approaches in addition to or in place of drug treatments for depression, anxiety, attention deficit disorder, and other psychological illnesses. Some ACCs might even try behavioral/lifestyle approaches to schizophrenia in some cases.[7] However, the PCPs will always be able to choose to fund the drugs that they and their psychiatrist colleagues think appropriate.

Jiddu Krishnamurti, a speaker and writer on philosophical and spiritual subjects, famously pointed out that adjusting to and fitting into society is not necessarily an indication of mental health: "It is no measure of health to be well adjusted to a profoundly sick society."[8] Some ACCs more than others would recognize that non-conformity and perceived eccentricity are not necessarily features of mental illness. Indeed, instead of drugs and talk therapies striving to bring about conformity to societal norms, originality and not fitting in to a sick society should be tolerated and, when appropriate, rewarded.

ACC-Based Addiction Treatment and Prevention

Alcohol and drug addiction need to be treated as medical conditions not as moral failings or law enforcement problems.

An effectively reorganized health care system must provide the estimated 10 million alcohol and drug addicts in the U.S. and our health care providers with financial incentives favoring rehabilitation over merely episodic acute care. Appropriate risk-adjusted allocations to ACCs for treatment of addicts and alcoholics by the federal government will assure that these patients are welcomed for intensive, holistic treatment by ACCs.

While our government spends relatively little on drug and alcohol abuse prevention and treatment,[a][9] the complications of substance abuse impact just about everyone. We must be creative in providing resources for rehabilitation of addicts. Younger addicts may need 6–12 months in residential rehabilitation centers rather than the current standard of 1–3 months.[10] State and federal bureaucrats will not be involved with administering the addiction prevention / treatment funds. ACCs will contract for prevention and rehabilitation services for their patients directly from local providers in their communities.

---

a   Addition rehabilitation funding is only $11 billion per year ($\approx$ 0.3% of government spending on personal health care)

In general, effective programs depend on helping addicts find employment and cultivating meaningful relationships with families, friends, and social services providers. Innovation in treatment programs will be tracked to learn the most effective approaches. The most effective programs will be widely copied.

Electronic Medical Records

With the current predominantly fee-for-service health care system that has poor patient care coordination, health care providers have major financial disincentives to investments in information technology. When new technologies reduce duplication of tests and unnecessary days in the hospital, the financial benefits go to insurers and patients and the costs go predominantly to providers. Creating a net savings from these technologies for providers will depend on a concurrent change from predominantly fee-for-service reimbursement to a payment system based on quality of care and health outcomes.

According to the Institute of Medicine, many preventable deaths in the U.S. stem from antiquated information systems in hospitals and doctors' offices.[11] If the electronic health records of all U.S. residents were available in secure computer networks that safeguarded patient privacy, health care providers would always have complete records for their patients. They could deal with emergencies faster and better. They would no longer have to re-order tests that have already been done.

Analysts predict that instituting electronic medical records throughout the country will be expensive.[b] It is far from clear that they will save money or save many lives. However, they do disrupt the doctor-patient relationship due to the time the doctor spends staring at the computer screen and entering data.[14] Many patients wonder if the doctor is listening to them. Doctors feel distracted and pressured by the requirement to constantly multitask.

---

b   A comprehensive electronic medical record system will cost over $200 billion (about $20 billion per year for a decade) to fully implement throughout the country.[12, 13]

Ironically, diet and exercise data is not being routinely collected about patients in the electronic medical records. While individual doctors may gather this data, Medicare keeps no national database of what patients eat and how much they exercise. They do nutrition and lifestyle surveys with limited potential to drive major health care policy changes. This makes no sense because 75% of deaths and disabilities of Americans relate to diet and exercise.

Perhaps we will need individual ACCs to innovatively experiment with electronic medical records to find what will work best to improve patient outcomes and lower costs.

Alternative and Complementary Services in ACCs

Given the rapid changes in medical science, the distinction between orthodox therapy and alternative treatment will remain fluid in all areas of medicine. Most alternative treatments are unproven because randomized controlled trials have not been done. In most cases, it is not because appropriate trials have demonstrated that these treatments are ineffective. For instance, how would you do a randomized controlled trial of fasting? How would you know if fasting might help a specific health condition if most people with that condition would not agree to be part of a randomized trial in order to test the efficacy of fasting? Not all beneficial health interventions are amenable to verification by randomized trials.

My book, *Money Driven Medicine—Tests and Treatments That Don't Work*,[15] discussed several therapies that are evidence-based to provide patient benefits that remain "alternative" because of medical politics. Some of these effective therapies that could be prescribed by physicians in some ACCs include:

- physician, nurse, or lay midwife-assisted home births,[16]
- prolotherapy for musculo-skeletal pain,[17, 18]
- lifestyle change programs like the "Dr. Dean Ornish Program

to Reverse Heart Disease," (covered by Medicare as of 2010 but not by many private insurers),[19] and

- autism spectrum disorder intensive treatments.[20, 21]

ACCs could also allocate funding for alternative approaches for which studies have not been done or have not shown benefit. Since alternative treatments are generally less expensive than medical establishment endorsed treatments, more funding than is the case now should arguably be allocated to alternative treatments. For many conditions, evidence-based treatment does not exist, so alternative treatments and experimental therapies are the only options.

Acupuncture is one of many examples of alternative and complementary treatments.

Acupuncture

The National Center for Complementary and Alternative Medicine, a unit of the National Institutes of Health, conducted a survey in 2007 showing that 3.1 million adults reported using acupuncture in the previous 12 months, up from 2.1 million in a 2002 survey. Indications for acupuncture include chronic headaches, osteoarthritis, depression in pregnancy, and low back pain. Insurers vary in their coverage of acupuncture and generally limit visits according to specific conditions.[22]

With ACC care, people could choose their ACCs, in part, by whether acupuncture or other alternative treatments were or were not included in the benefits package. People wanting acupuncture will be able to choose ACCs offering to cover the costs, and those not believing in acupuncture might select ACCs that do not cover this procedure, saving funds for other treatment modalities.

Comparison studies could assess whether people in ACCs covering acupuncture suffered less pain and other symptoms than those in ACCs not covering it.

Experimental Treatments

An outcry has arisen over the lack of experimental drug availability to patients for treatment of advanced cancer.[23] Dying patients and their supporters advocate for less rigid criteria for use of experimental drugs when there is no time to wait for the results of randomized controlled trials. Few cancer patients enter randomized trials anyway because of the possibility of receiving a placebo. Similar problems with access to experimental treatments occur in patients with fibromyalgia,[24] multiple sclerosis,[25] and other conditions.

As mentioned in Chapter 8, many more randomized trials involving drugs and other medical interventions will be available with ACC-based reform. ACCs, with their entire patient populations, rather than individual patients could be randomized to receive or not receive the experimental treatment. All experimental interventions used and the associated health outcomes will be tracked. Comparisons will be made of health outcomes in patients with and without access to each specific experimental intervention. With data continuously flowing in about patients receiving and not receiving experimental treatments for various conditions, efficacy of the experimental treatments will be ascertained much faster than by relying only on traditional randomized controlled clinical trials.

Companies with new drugs or medical devices will offer them free to ACCs conducting randomized trials of patients with various conditions. Once drugs or devices gain Food and Drug Administration approval because of data generated from early ACC studies, the companies can begin charging money for their products in the ACCs that decide to cover those products.

Grand Bargain #6: ACCs to Provide Long-Term Care

When my elderly and disabled father and stepmother required long-term care, I could utilize the equity in their house to hire compassionate and competent caregivers to keep them at home and out of an institution until they died. Considering the wonderful care the caregivers provided, their services didn't cost very much. Most Americans are not as fortunate as my parents and me in their options concerning long-term care.

According to survey data compiled by Strength for Caring, an organization that advocates for caregivers, approximately 46 million Americans are providing care to adult relatives or friends (over 30 million full-time equivalent jobs). More than 138 million Americans believe they will need to provide care to someone in the future. Caregivers suffer high stress, increased rates of anxiety and depression, and major financial and personal sacrifices. Based on this analysis and many other studies, advocates for long-term care have repeatedly called for the government to provide financial relief by tax credits or otherwise for caregivers of non-institutionalized disabled people. Despite pleas based on compassion and economic justice for caregivers, Congress has not responded.

Now that the economy is in seeming decline or characterized by growth benefiting only the very rich, consider the economic effect of providing caretakers money for caring for their frail elderly and/or disabled friends or family members. Up to 10 million full-time equivalent jobs budgeted through ACCs could be divided into many more half-time and quarter-time jobs. In 2016, caretaker jobs paying minimum wages ($15 per hour: Chapter 12) to family and friends of 10 million disabled people would cost about $330 billion.[c] In future years, this might be expanded to more caregivers.

These up to 10 million full-time equivalent paid jobs could be created immediately. This will be what the doctor ordered to provide long-term care while helping families, reduce income inequalities, and stimulate the economy. Much of the money will be immediately returned to taxpayers, because paying these health care workers will mean they will

---

c   10 million caring jobs x $15 per hour for wages x 1.062 (6.2% additional for Social Security payroll tax) x 2080 hours/year (including pay for vacations, sick leave, and holidays) = $331 billion.

not require public assistance. Much of the money will go back to ACCs as health care premiums (Chapter 18), retirement savings, and Social Security payments) and to consumption taxes (Chapters 21 and 22). The collateral economic benefit of the money these workers will spend for necessities will be multiplied, creating more jobs.

Paying home-care providers will also give financial incentives to move some of the 1.6 million Americans living in nursing homes or assisted living back home to their families and friends. For each nursing home resident moved back to home, about $50,000 per year will be saved.[d]

ACCs will administer this common-sense economical approach to long-term care without federal or state bureaucracies being involved. Disabled and elderly people will be the biggest winners, but formerly unpaid caregivers and the overall economy will also win.

My detailed suggestions about paying health-care aids to jump start the economy were published in the *Health Beat Blog*.[27]

Oral Health Care Faltering

The status of oral health has improved dramatically since the post World War II era. Fluoridation has been given much of the credit, but credit also goes to the dental profession and dental hygienists for treatment advances and educating individuals to take care of their teeth.

The obstacles to access dental care for over 100 million Americans that lack dental insurance relate primarily to money. Because of lack of access to dental care by the poor, progress in oral health outcomes (e.g., rates of lost teeth) has stagnated.

Since 1990, the number of dentists in the United States has remained at about 150,000 to 160,000, with more dentists working part time. For the next decade, the number of graduating dentists will likely be fewer

---

d $110,000 per year on average projected for nursing home care in 2016[26] – $60,000 for 69 hours per week of home care on average = $50,000.

than those retiring from dental practice.[28] The cost of going into dental practice is high.[e]

In more than 50 other countries, technicians called dental therapists are permitted to drill and fill cavities, usually in children. However, the American Dental Association and other dental organizations have successfully opposed the licensing of dental therapists in the U.S. Likewise, state boards of dentists and the American Dental Association, the main lobbying group for dentists, continue to fight the use dental hygienists and other non-dentists to provide basic care to people who do not have access to dentists.[28]

Many working poor families cannot afford to bring their children to dentists. While Medicaid and the Children's Health Care Program provide dental care to many children and adults, coverage varies among the states.[f] Many cash-strapped states are resisting further increases in Medicaid spending on dentistry.

The Affordable Care Act does not mandate dental care for adults as an essential health benefit. However, it does include oral health care as an essential health benefit for those under age 19. Obviously, this lack of essential dental care coverage is another reason for ACCs and the Grand Bargain approach.

Separation of Medicine and Dentistry

To the detriment of patients, dental providers, and the country, medicine and dentistry have been separated. This is unfortunate since research findings point to associations between chronic oral infections and diabetes, heart and lung diseases, stroke, and low-birth-weight, premature births. As emphasized in the Surgeon General's Report on Oral Health, *"oral health is integral to general health."*[30]

---

e The average loan payback for a dental school graduate is at least $200,000. The cost of setting up an office can run $150,000 to $200,000.[29]

f Medicaid spending on dental services grew at an annual rate of 11.2% between 1975 and 2002. Of that increase, 40% was due to an increase in recipients, primarily children. The rest was due to increases in costs of treatment and administration.

While most employers that provide health insurance also pay for dental coverage, workers that retire at age 65 with Medicare insurance do not automatically receive dental insurance. With the passage of Medicare in 1965, the dental profession chose not to participate. Dentists largely worked on a fee-for-service basis and did not want government interference in their profession. At that time, dental care was relatively inexpensive, so separating medical and dental insurance was not strongly resisted.

The cost of dental procedures has escalated at a much higher rate than overall inflation. Most dental plans have a maximum cap of yearly expenditures, usually set between $1500 and $2500. Major dental expenses, such as crowns and root canals, are just partially covered by insurance.

Grand Bargain #7: ACCs to Provide Oral Health Care

ACCs will guarantee access to affordable oral health care. ACCs will compete in part on how well they provide excellent oral health preventive and treatment services to members. The rate of caries in children and other dental outcomes will be reported online. For potential ACC members, the quality of the dental care may be a consideration in choosing an ACC. ACCs will have the prerogative to hire or contract with dental professionals as they wish. However, they will likely move to a capitated basis for reimbursement for dental services (set amount of money to provide all dental services for a population of patients). This will greatly increase the emphasis on preventive dentistry.

Summary and Conclusion

Under-funded components of the U.S. health care and social services systems include health promotion and preventive medicine (Chapter 4), hospice and palliative care (Chapter 5), mental health, substance abuse prevention and treatment, experimental treatments, alternative and complimentary treatments, child care (Chapter 12), dentistry, and long-term care (Chapter 25). None of these under-funded health and social services related issues can be successfully resolved in isolation. All of them require better integration of health and social services. All entail additional resources for services. However, health care already costs too much in the U.S.

Finding money for these important additional health care needs requires that we eliminate funding for tests and treatments that do not work (Chapter 8), reduce administrative costs (Chapters 18-20), and more efficiently use our limited welfare funds (Chapter 10). ACCs operating in a free market of health services will allow for us to provide appropriate resources to address all these issues while driving down the portion of the GDP going to health care and welfare.

Chapter 7
ACCs Compete to Prevent Abortions

Former President Jimmy Carter faced a great moral dilemma. He pledged to uphold the law of the land, including the *Roe versus Wade* Supreme Court ruling allowing abortion. However, he had to answer to his conscience, which opposed abortion. He noted that, in Scandinavian countries like Sweden, Norway, and Denmark, there were no restrictions on abortions, yet the rate of fetuses terminated was about one-third that in the U.S. On further study of opportunities for women in both countries, he concluded that a much more generous set of social services available to Scandinavian women with unplanned pregnancies encouraged more of them to keep their babies.[1]

As a consequence of his findings, President Carter championed greater funding for social services for single mothers, such as the Women, Infants, and Children (WIC) Nutrition Program. WIC provides food, nutrition education, breastfeeding support, and referral for health care and social services for low-income, nutritionally at risk, pregnant, and postpartum women, and for infants and children under the age of five.[2]

According to the Guttmacher Institute, a New York-based abortion research group, abortions in teens decreased from 33% to 17% from 1974 to 2004. However, abortions are still about three times as high in Latinas and black women as in whites. And Sweden, Denmark, and Norway continue to have about one-fourth the rate of teen pregnancies as U.S. women and girls.[3] This suggests that socio-economic disparities continue to be major factors in deciding whether to keep or abort a fetus.[4]

Obamacare's requirement for insurance coverage for birth control by employers has been challenged successfully in the Supreme Court in the Hobby Lobby case (Chapter 9).[5, 6] It is a particularly polarizing part of Obamacare.

An abortion-neutral component of health care reform should focus on prevention of unwanted pregnancies and should support ambivalent women that decide to keep their babies or put them up for adoption.

Frances Kissling, Former President of Catholics for Choice

"On Being," a radio show hosted by Krista Tibbett, featured a broadcast entitled, "Listening Beyond Life and Choice" about the abortion debate. Krista Tibbett interviewed Frances Kissling the former president of "Catholics for Choice."[7]

After a life dedicated to advocacy for access to abortion for mostly poor women, Ms. Kissling indicated that she didn't believe there was much promise of partisans concerning an issue finding common ground with people whose views and ideologies they fundamentally oppose. In her many polarized debates, she felt: "the pressure of coming to agreement works against really understanding each other." However, in recent years, Ms. Kissling has modified her relationships with those on the pro-life side of the abortion debate. She has sought to break down the gulf between partisans on the abortion issue with a willingness to be courageous and also to be vulnerable:[7]

> ...when people who disagree with each other come together with a goal of gaining a better understanding of why the other believes what they do, good things come of that. ... I have changed my views on some aspects of abortion over the last ten years based upon having a deeper understanding of the values and concerns of

people who disagree with me. And I have an interest in trying to find a way that I can honor some of their values without giving up mine.

At the center of the abortion debate, the freedoms of poor, disadvantaged women are colliding with the freedoms and the rights of fetuses. Both pro-choice advocates and pro-life proponents want women to have support, education, and resources that would prevent unwanted pregnancies. As she stated, Ms. Kissling now seeks to look for and acknowledge the validity of feelings on the pro-choice side of the debate.

David Gushee, PhD, Pro-Life Advocate and Christian Ethicist

As a Christian ethicist, moral teacher, and writer in a university, Dr. David Gushee frequently addresses hot-button issues like abortion, health care, war, torture, and gay rights. In discussions about abortion with Ms. Kissling and others, Dr. Gushee now seeks a more civil tone and a better understanding of the other side:[7]

> Over the years, I have tried to do something a little different when I engage difficult issues such as abortion. I try to play neither academic nor political games. I instead try to discern what it might mean to deal with the substance of the issue as if every person involved is sacred in God's sight, and I likewise try to deal with my dialogue partners as if the same were true.
>
> I do sense that decades of defending the rights and needs of the pregnant woman have trained many in the pro-choice side to avert their eyes from the child. But I also recognize on the part of many pro-lifers the parallel averting of gaze away from the woman and her situation as she experiences it. Decades of advocacy in a polarized

debate have caused both sides to miss the intertwined sacredness of woman and child. And it is certainly clear to me that the only way those whose gaze is fixed on the child will succeed in saving more of them is if they learn not only to look at the woman, but to love her.

Grand Bargain #27: Right to Life Proponents and Right to Choose Advocates May Choose ACCs in Accordance with Their Beliefs.

Acknowledging the feelings of everyone including the unborn, the ACC approach to the pro-life versus pro-choice issue will be for the ACC leaders to use all possible resources to make abortions as rare as possible.

ACCs could offer funding for abortions or not. If an ACC covers abortion, it would be fair that no taxpayers' funds would be used to pay for the procedure. Funding should come from the woman's payments of premiums toward her health care.

Pursuant to current law, if an ACC elects not to cover abortions, patients will be able to pay out-of-pocket for the service from specialists in the procedure.

ACCs affiliated with the Catholic Church or many other religions will undoubtedly decline to cover abortions. Secular ACCs will likely pay for it. This mirrors the divide in public opinion on the topic.

ACCs will compete, in part, on preventing unwanted pregnancies. As with other health interventions, the methods used (e.g., sex education programs, peer counseling, etc.) and costs will be documented along with the outcomes (rates of abortion and of healthy, wanted, cared-for children). The methods of those ACCs with the lowest unplanned pregnancy rates and abortion rates will likely be emulated by the others. People will choose ACCs in part to be in alignment with their preferences as pro-life or pro-choice.

In any case, the needs of single mothers and their young children will be met by all ACCs (e.g., nutrition, education, child care, housing, etc.). Where feasible, social support to help the father stay involved in raising the child will also be important.

Conclusion

People will choose ACCs, in part, based on the pro-life or pro-choice policies of competing ACCs. ACCs will compete to achieve low unwanted pregnancy and abortion rates.

Sex education methods will be determined by parents in conjunction with their caregivers from patient-centered medical homes as well as school educators (Chapter 16). Taxpayer funds will not be used to fund abortions.

For women in ACCs that do not fund abortions, any abortions will need to be funded out-of-pocket. ACCs will have resources and the mandate to support parents in caring for their children.

Chapter 8
Evidence-Based Medicine
Informing Clinical Decisions

Most of the time, people with illnesses recover without medical intervention. With illnesses destined to resolve on their own, if a doctor prescribes a drug or treatment and the patient gets better, the cure may wrongly be attributed to the medical intervention. If the ineffective drug or other treatment carries a risk of injury or death and is expensive, some patients may be harmed although most get better.

In determining whether a treatment works or not, one of the most important considerations is the patient's response to a placebo (inactive substance). The placebo response can be considered as the influence of the faith of the patient and/or caregivers or other factors to cause a favorable response to an inactive medication or treatment. An inert or ineffective medicine given to a patient who believes that it will work actually has a favorable response in many studies, averaging about 30% of the time.[1]

From ancient times, standard medical treatment in a community has been based on consensus. Consensus-based medicine means accepting the opinions of the majority of leading practitioners as valid concerning the value of medical tests and treatments. Given the power of the placebo response and how it may bias opinions of doctors about the efficacies of treatments, consensus-based medicine is often unscientific.

Doctors have been known to come to consensuses that were later found to be dead wrong. In colonial America doctors treated heart failure by bleeding the patient. The consensus of obstetricians in the 19th Century was that they didn't have to wash their hands before delivering a baby.

Regarding the value of many medical tests and treatments, thought leaders have disagreed. Consensus about a medical intervention in one country or state may radically differ from that in another. Consensuses change rapidly over time as treatments go in and out of fashion.

Remarkably, it is relatively recent in medical history that physicians appreciated that we need a better form of medical evidence to base clinical decisions than recalling outcomes from anecdotal cases from their past practices or the consensus of medical thought leaders.

Evidence-based Medicine versus Evidence-based Health Care

With the increasing realization of the shortcomings of consensus-based medicine, evidence-based medicine was introduced in the last half of the 20th century. It aims to apply the best available evidence gained from the scientific method to medical decision making.[2] One researcher said, "Evidence-based medicine challenges the medical profession by disputing what and how physicians know."[3]

The "gold standard" method used by evidence-based medicine researchers is the randomized controlled clinical trial. With this research design, patients with a medical ailment are randomly assigned to the experimental treatment versus standard treatment or a placebo. Statisticians determine if the experimental intervention has significantly better outcomes than a comparison treatment.

Evidence-based medicine has two distinct and somewhat conflicting meanings.[4]

1. Evidence-based individual decision making: evidence-based medicine as interpreted and practiced by the individual health care provider

2. Evidence-based guidelines: evidence-based medicine at the

organizational or institutional level as determined by a consensus of expert opinion leaders that all study the randomized trials and other clinical evidence. This includes the production of guidelines, policies, and regulations. This approach has also been called "evidence-based health care."[5]

Using evidence-based medicine methods of determining the efficacies of health care interventions is essential to improving health outcomes and for controlling costs. However, qualified experts often differ about the value of many medical tests and treatments, and the consensus among expert opinion leaders' changes over time. In reality, the foundation of evidence-based health care practice guidelines drafted by expert opinion leaders is consensus-based medicine of physician leaders.

Practicing doctors that do not conduct medical research trials or teach in medical schools rarely participate in drafting the guidelines sponsored by government agencies or special interest organizations. However, all practicing doctors are supposed to abide by these guidelines in their practices.

Doctors That Draft Evidence-Based Medicine Guidelines

How do physicians rise to the status of writing practice guidelines for all other physicians? Typically, they choose a career in a subspecialty of internal medicine, surgery, pediatrics, or other field. They then join a medical school faculty to teach, conduct research, and practice. They win contracts with drug companies, medical product manufacturers, or other health industry sponsors to conduct randomized trials with patients. These physicians compete with each other to publish their research in peer-reviewed medical journals. This competition has been dubbed, "publish or perish."

The proportion of medical research contracts funded by the government has fallen dramatically over the past 30 years. To succeed in academic medicine research, physicians usually need to conduct studies for drug companies, medical device manufacturers, or other commercial entities. If they don't win enough research grants and contracts, they don't make it in academic medicine and have to practice elsewhere.

The academic physician researchers who succeed with a steady flow of sponsored studies give lectures to medical students and other doctors about the results and implications of their research. If the results of the research are favorable to the interests of the financial sponsor of the research, that sponsor may pay the physician researcher to give lectures widely. This happened with my research on long-acting opioids for the treatment of pain in cancer and AIDS patients. Over about a 10-year period, I gave at least 100 drug-company-sponsored lectures to medical audiences about pain management for cancer and AIDS patients.

At some point, the physician researcher may be invited to be on a Food and Drug Administration (FDA) drug evaluation panel or a guidelines drafting committee in his/her specialty of medicine.

Given this typical background of an academic researcher entering the policy arena, one major problem with evidence-based health care drafted by a consensus of elite medical experts is that financial and other conflicts of interests may bias the treatment guidelines that are drafted. Worthless or harmful treatments may then become institutionalized as the standards of care. Due to corruption in research or in the interpretation of research results, some patients may be harmed and medical cost may go up for everyone.

The Power of Medical Industry Money

When pharmaceutical companies contract with researchers to submit articles to medical journals for publication, the articles go to peer reviewers that usually have also been hired by the pharmaceutical industry to conduct similar studies. Medical journals compete with each other to publish the important clinical efficacy trials. Reprint sales may be lucrative. Medical journal employees also depend on revenue from advertising drugs and medical services to stay in business.

Medical advocacy nonprofit organizations frequently rely heavily on drug company or other special interest funding. For example, Senator Charles Grassley of Iowa, Chair of the Senate Finance Committee, discovered that the National Alliance on Mental Illness (NAMI) receives about two-thirds of its money from drug companies. NAMI would risk losing much of its funding by warning patients against using certain psychiatric medications with life-threatening side effects.[6] Ethical conflicts like this are not uncommon.

In reporting on drug research, the medical media depends almost exclusively on sources with financial conflicts of interest. As an occasional exception, they may quote a drug company critic like Dr. Sidney Wolfe from the Public Citizen Health Research Group. He is lead author of the book *Worse Pills, Best Pills*.[7] However, in general, industry critics are marginalized, if not completely excluded, from public discussion.

Controversy about the Value of Many Medical Interventions

When giving a medical school commencement talk, Dr. C. Sidney Burwell, dean of Harvard Medical School from 1935 to 1949, said, "Half of what we have taught you is wrong. Unfortunately, we don't know which half."[8] The same is pretty much true today.

Intelligent well-meaning physicians may disagree about the value of many specific tests and treatments. The lack of scientific data or differing interpretations of existing data account for many, but not all, medical controversies.

In a *Wall Street Journal* opinion piece, two Harvard medical school professors (husband and wife), Jerome Groopman, MD and Pamela Hartzband, MD, insightfully related how pervasive controversies are in the practice of medicine.[9]

This is how doctors and patients make shared decisions—by considering expert guidelines, weighing why other experts may disagree with the guidelines, and then customizing the therapy to the individual. With respect to "best practices," prudent doctors think, not just follow, and informed patients consider and then choose, not just comply.

"No government bureaucrat will come between you and your doctor." The President (Obama) has repeatedly stated this in town-hall meetings. But his proposal to provide financial incentives to "allow doctors to do the right thing" could undermine this promise. If doctors and hospitals are rewarded for complying with government-mandated treatment measures or penalized if they do not comply, clearly federal bureaucrats are directing health decisions.

While making the point that excellent doctors often disagree with standard medical guidelines, Drs. Groopman and Hartzband criticized President Obama's proposal that strict adherence to government-sponsored treatment guidelines would protect physicians from malpractice lawsuits. Declaring "I was following standard guidelines" as a medicolegal defense means that deviating from (federally mandated) guidelines exposes doctors to risks of malpractice suits. With the threat of malpractice suits for deviating from guidelines, physicians might pressure their patients to comply with orthodox treatments despite their patients' preferences for alternative approaches. In the view of many, Congressional bills and state laws concerning medical "best practices" authorize treatments that infringe on physician and patient autonomy.

Despite the advent of evidence-based health care and tens of thousands of clinical practice guidelines drafted by experts, controversy abounds about the effectiveness and safety of many health care interventions, and it probably always will.

Tests and Treatments That Don't Work

In 1999, the Institute of Medicine estimated that errors in the delivery of medical treatment caused 44,000–98,000 deaths per year.[10] However, many more people also die from complications of medical tests and treatments that are not due to errors.

According to my analysis, 73,000 – 99,000 deaths occur each year in the U.S. due to complications of non beneficial, yet medical insurance covered, medical interventions. These are detailed in my book *Money Driven Medicine—Tests and Treatments That Don't Work*.[11] Using standard evidence-based medicine methods of analysis, I found that over 70 standard interventions are ineffective or that safer, equally effective alternatives exist. Table 1 (below), adapted from this book, details ineffective tests, their complications, and costs in 2007. Where the number of patients affected or the cost is in a range, the low estimate appears above the high estimate.

Adjusting for inflation,[12] in 2016 these medical interventions will cost Americans $1.1 billion – $1.4 trillion (36%–42% of all personal health care spending). In my view, if these tests and treatments did not exist, Americans would be healthier, live longer, and have more money. However, there would still be a crisis in health care because of the lack of sufficient preventive medicine strategies, excessive costs for many effective medical interventions, and too many administrators doing too much unnecessary paperwork.

Table 1. Consequences in 2007 of Tests and Treatments That Don't Work

Test or Treatment	Patients Treated Low High Estimate thousands	Deaths Low High Estimate	Serious Compli-cations Low High Estimate	Cost Low High Estimate $billions
Diet books, programs, and products	128,000	?	?	60.6
Drugs for obesity	2000 3000	?	?	2.5
Surgery for obesity	250	2500 5000	25,000 50,000	18.9 35.4
High cholesterol medications	14,000 17,000	15 ?	10,000 ?	29.5 32.1
High blood pressure medications	22,000	?	?	17.6 24.3
Tight blood sugar control in type 2 diabetes	5000 7000	?	?	25.2 37.8
Coronary artery bypass grafting	467	12,400	78,000 100,000	65.8
Angioplasties	1244	10,000	50,000	79.7
Coronary arteriography	1414	1400	1700 2600	59.0
Thrombolysis (clot busters)	210 350	2100 3500	26,000 44,000	0.6 0.9
Anticoagulants	13,100	24,400 51,400	232,000 458,000	18.5 31.2
Clopidogrel blood thin-ner for heart patients	4500	?	?	5.8
Antidepressant medications	18,000	170 ?	2,700,000 3,600,000	20.3
Excess cesareans	1280	?	?	18.9
Prematurity due to planned cesareans	250	?	?	15.1

Table 1. Consequences of Tests and Treatments That Don't Work (cont'd)

Test or Treatment	Patients Treated Low High Estimate thousands	Deaths Low High Estimate	Serious Complications Low High Estimate	Cost Low High Estimate billions
PSA tests	18,000	?		4.3
Prostate cancer surgery	66	180 600	23,000 79,000	4.3
Radiation therapy for prostate cancer	55	?	34,000 37,000	3.2
Screening mammograms	30,000	?	400,000	5.4
Arthroscopic knee surgery	350 425	?	11,000 26,000	2.4 3.2
Back pain tests and treatments	54,000	?	?	55.4
Cancer chemotherapy for non-responsive tumors	200 300	2,000 6,000	200,000 300,000	48.7 73.1
Futile treatments	500 1000	?	500,000 1,000,000	84 179
Other off-label prescribing of drugs	?	?	?	50.4 75.7
Hormone replacement therapy	5000	?	15,000	3.9
Routine medical checkups	64,000	?	?	15.1
Alzheimer's disease drugs	1000	?	?	1.9
Pap smears for women with no cervix	10,000	?	?	0.2 0.4
"War on drugs"	60,000	?	?	8.6
Antiviral drugs for hepatitis C	50 200	?	50,000 200,000	1.0 2.0
Unnecessary hysterectomies	420 456	250 500	100,000 200,000	13.7 14.5
Diet supplements	100,000 140,000	16 ?	260 ?	31.5
Total cost of ineffective tests and treatments		72,511 98,679	4,490,960 6,561,860	772 970

Changing Official Guidelines for Medical Interventions

Diagnosis and treatment guidelines change dramatically over time. Dr. Kaveh Shojania from Ottawa, Canada and colleagues tracked 100 recommendations for "best practices guidelines" published in prestigious medical journals. Within 5 1/2 years, half were considered no longer valid.[13]

Once medical establishment guidelines are in place and considered the "standard of care," clinical experiences with alternative approaches that may be superior become limited. Physicians may fear medical malpractice suits if adverse outcomes occur. For example, American Cancer Society and National Cancer Institute guidelines call for women to undergo screening mammography from age 40.[14, 15] In 2009, the U.S. Preventive Services Task Force issued a recommendation that screening mammograms begin at age 50.[16] What is a physician supposed to do?

A survey of physicians and other health experts found that about 44% thought that screening mammograms do not save lives.[17] However, if any PCPs do not order screening mammograms on women over 40 years old, they may be sued by patients developing breast cancer for failure to diagnose it earlier. Because of the existing mammogram screening guidelines, no randomized breast cancer screening trials are currently underway or have been initiated in the past two decades to scientifically settle the controversy.

A fallout of the conflict between the mammogram guidelines of the American Cancer Society and the National Cancer Institute versus the U.S. Preventive Services Task Force was that the National Committee for Quality Assurance had to change the way it grades health plans. Instead of measuring the percentage of women getting mammograms every one to two years starting at age 40, it began measuring the percentage getting mammograms beginning at age 50.[18] This illustrates the fallibility of top-down quality assessments of medical interventions by so called "unbiased experts." The data never supported screening mammograms as life saving in the first place, let alone beginning the screenings at age 40. This should make you question the results of standardized health care "quality measurements" in general.

Comparative Effectiveness Research

Patient-advocacy and health policy groups have hailed comparative-effectiveness research (CER) as a means of reducing health care costs without compromising the quality of care. The federal commitment of $1.1 billion under the American Recovery and Reinvestment Act (ARRA) ensured that the scientific community gives considerable attention to CER. Let us consider what CER is about.

CER may consist of systematic reviews of medical interventions, called meta-analyses, where all of the randomized trials published on an intervention are analyzed. It can also involve conducting new randomized clinical trials comparing old and new drugs or evaluating alternative treatments for a disease.

Major obstacles to obtaining accurate information from both these types of comparative effectiveness studies severely limits the conclusions and guidelines derived from these studies. For instance, reviews or meta-analyses may include favorable studies preferentially because drug companies neglect to publish studies with negative outcomes.

Setting up trials to compare two FDA-approved treatments for a condition, one expensive and one cheap, can be full of obstacles. A drug company selling the expensive drug has no reason to cooperate and waive the cost of the drug. Medicare may not cover the cost of the expensive drug, although another agency of the government may want to conduct the trial. For example, a comparative-effectiveness study, "Comparison of Age-Related Macular Degeneration Treatments Trials," proposed to evaluate the benefits of a drug called ranibizumab (Lucentis)—$5000 per year—with bevacizumab (Avastin)—$100 per year. Because of U.S. Government health agency roadblocks, the trial took nine years to initiate, during which time Medicare paid over $10 billion for recipients to receive Lucentis.[19] When finally completed, the trial showed no significant difference between the efficacies of the two drugs.[20-22]

Should CER be the Basis of Treatment Denials?

Regarding the $1.1 billion included in the federal stimulus bill, President Obama told the American Medical Association, "[We] . . . need to figure out what works, and encourage rapid implementation of what works into your practices. That's why we are making a major investment in research to identify the best treatments for a variety of ailments and conditions." President Obama wants a system, "where . . . doctors can pull up on a computer all the medical information and latest research they'd ever want to meet that patient's needs."[23]

In accordance with President Obama's statement, an Institute of Medicine (IOM) committee recommended "determining the most effective dissemination methods to ensure translation of comparative effectiveness research results into best practices."[6] This means enacting widespread changes in the practice of medicine from the top down, potentially including all the biases and special interest corruption of the data.

There are strong proponents and opponents of this approach to improving our medical system. Both have some valid points. Scientific evidence should guide any reform of our health care system. However, many argue against top-down determinations of which tests and treatments to cover with insurance. Because of the objections of many health care stakeholders, Congress promised that comparative effectiveness research will not become a basis for "cost-effectiveness research" that would lead to the denials of doctor-recommended treatments by insurers. Cost-effectiveness-based insurance company denials threaten to become a form of rationing.

An analysis by the RAND Corporation concluded that CER was of some value to provide information for doctors and patients about what works best in treating different health problems. However, they cautioned that reductions in wasteful medical interventions and improvements in patient health could not be guaranteed by an additional massive commitment to CER.[24]

"The Government Should Not Come Between Patients and Their Doctors"—President Obama

President Obama and most health policy makers agree in principle that the government should not come between patients and their doctors. However, government agency-endorsed medical treatment guidelines are increasingly driving practice patterns and treatment decisions of physicians. Private insurance companies usually follow the government's lead.

If government-endorsed guidelines were always right and improved patients' care, there would be justification for the government's intrusion into doctor-patient relationships. However, government insurance programs often pay for non-beneficial tests and treatments (Table 1 above) while denying coverage for health and safety-net interventions that would be very beneficial.

The financial clout of special interests unduly molds the opinions of government regulators, health care professionals, and the public about the value of medical products and services. Consequently, the determinations of government and private insurance industry policymakers regarding funding, or not paying for specific medical interventions and how much is paid, are often flawed. Political influences and economic factors, rather than evidence-based medicine or the true value of services to patients, often decide insurance reimbursement for health services.

A solution to the abuses of top-down regulation of medical care by the government and medical insurance companies will be discussed in Chapter 9.

Will Strict Regulation of Medical Research Make Evidence-Based Study Results Dependable?

For years, the medical media have reported on incidences of bias in conducting and interpreting the results of randomized trials and other studies in medicine. Results of industry-funded trials are notoriously more favorable to the products tested than the findings of National Institutes of Health-funded studies.[25] Trials with unfavorable findings regarding drugs or medical products may be reported in obscure journals or simply not published. Drug companies may commission several groups of researchers to test a drug for certain indications. They may then select the trials with favorable results to send for publication and bury the rest. If a researcher complains or publishes unfavorable trial results against the wishes of drug companies, the researcher risks losing support for their future research.

There have been many calls for regulating the process of conducting randomized clinical trials, including those for FDA approval of drugs and medical devices. Responding to the calls, a coalition of medical journal editors enacted a requirement in 2005 that researchers must register proposed clinical trials in a government database as a condition for publishing their results in medical journals. This may have stopped some of the most egregious special interest abuses in conducting research. However, the regulations imposed on industry-funded medical research so far have done little to correct the industry bias of reports published in medical journals. Many researchers and their special interest sponsors are ignoring the requirement, and journals are publishing the papers anyway.[26]

Diet and Lifestyle as Subjects for Evidence-Based Study

Overall, improved health outcomes depend on positive changes diet and lifestyles much more than on drugs or other medical interventions. Our health care system will not be reformed unless substantial resources are shifted from researching sickness treatment to evaluating preventive medicine and health-promotion strategies. However, because of the lack of financial incentives to special interests, relatively little research has been done on positive lifestyle changes or non-drug approaches to prevention and treatment of cancer, heart disease, and other chronic diseases.

Just like medical tests and treatments, preventive medicine interventions should be tested by rigorous research and shown effective to the satisfaction of practicing clinicians as a condition of acceptance and insurance funding. As with research into interventions for treating sick people, interpretations of preventive medicine research will often be controversial (Chapter 4). Although randomized controlled trials are not as suitable for lifestyle interventions (diet, exercise, etc.), rigorous observational studies may be conducted that qualify as evidence-based medicine. The future of this field, I believe, is with widened availability of online studies of diet, exercise, and other lifestyle interventions.

Outsourcing Medical Research to Other Countries

Currently, over 6000 new therapies, including drugs, procedures, and devices, are being tested in 80,000 locations in the U.S. However, the public has become increasingly suspicious of clinical research trials, and, consequently, not enough people volunteer to participate. In 2001, 86% of all clinical trials did not meet enrollment goals.[27, 28] Recruitment into randomized controlled clinical trials has not improved since then.

Consequently, many clinical trials are being outsourced to other countries. From 1990 to 2008, the outsourced trials for drugs intended for use in North America increased from 271 to 6485. Reasons to conduct clinical research in other countries include:[29]

1. Less expensive
2. Easier to recruit patients by paying them a small fee
3. Patients may believe that the medications are for treatment rather than experimentation.

4. Easier to find "drug-naïve" patients that have not previously taken other medications
5. Regulation in foreign countries may be less stringent than in the U.S.
6. Litigation risk is negligible
7. Human research subject protection by institutions may be lax.

This outsourcing of medical research raises ethical concerns. The application of results of trials in Russia, India, or China to patients in the U.S. should be questioned. This research outsourcing also costs American scientists many jobs.

An Alternative Format for Randomized Controlled Trials

In the typical randomized controlled clinical trial, participants must be recruited one by one by research doctors. Patients are told that they will be receiving an active experimental drug or a placebo. Neither the patient nor the physician will know whether a patient has the real drug or the placebo. Trials typically cost thousands of dollars per patient recruited. Extra time and clinic visits are often required of patients.

In order to greatly expand the number of people that will be able to participate in medical research in the U.S., consider an alternative to the usual randomized controlled clinical trial. Drug companies or medical device makers that need research subjects may recruit 10-20 or more ACCs to participate in a clinical trial. These trials would fit with ACC members' interests in improving care for an illness of personal concern. The ACCs might be randomly allocated to the active drug versus placebo or the real medical device versus no device. In all of the participating ACCs, all patients with the conditions under study would be carefully monitored for clinical outcomes.

All patients in ACCs randomized to receive the active treatment would then be offered the experimental treatment. For the particular medical conditions under study, the relevant clinical outcomes of the patients accepting the experimental treatments would be compared to the outcomes of patients in the same ACCs that declined the experimental treatments. Likewise, clinical outcomes of patients receiving the experimental treatments would be compared with patients with the condition under study in the ACCs that were randomized not to receive the experimental treatments. Statistical comparisons could then be made between groups to determine if the experimental treatments were effective.

The drug or medical device companies would pay the ACCs for participating in the trials. The experimental treatments would be free to the ACCs. The drug and device companies would recoup their investments in clinical research when/if their drugs/devices were shown to be beneficial, approved by the FDA, and became utilized by ACCs.

With this scientifically sound system of randomizing, plenty of patients would be available for clinical trials.

Summary and Conclusion

Disagreements about the efficacy of medical tests and treatments are the norm rather than the exception. Scientists have endorsed evidence-based medicine with the randomized controlled clinical trial as the gold-standard methodology for determining efficacy and basing standardized guidelines. However, moneyed special interests have often been able to corrupt the process of conducting and interpreting clinical research trials. Standard guidelines written by elite physician may later prove to be wrong.

We need a grand bargain that combines the best features of evidence-based medicine by individual clinicians and evidence-based health care guidelines by a consensus of experts. Both approaches have their strengths and weaknesses.

With ACC based reform, clinical research trials could be conducted by randomizing ACCs to receiving versus not receiving the experimental treatments. This will vastly increase the number of patients participating in clinical trials and the power of trials to answer important clinical research questions.

As a way to solve the problems with both evidence-based national guidelines and evidence-based medicine as practiced by individual clinicians, consider decentralizing health care guidelines and medical benefits packages to self-regulating ACCs. The next chapter will discuss shifting health care regulation from the government to private, competing, self-regulating ACCs.

Chapter 9
Self-regulation for ACCs

Virtually all health care policy wonks agree that at least one-third of medical expenditures go for useless or harmful tests and treatments[1] (over $1 trillion in 2016). However, they disagree on which tests and treatments are useless or harmful. Despite any increased money for randomized trials comparing effectiveness of different medical interventions, honest providers, patients, and payers will continue to disagree on the value of many tests and treatments.

Indeed, the inherently controversial nature of medical tests and treatments and rapid changes in standards of care should be factored into the recipe for reforming the health care system. I hope to convince you that the regulation of health care quality and costs can be reformed despite ongoing controversy about what works and what doesn't work in medicine.

For a look at the sorry state of status quo health care regulation by the government, let's see how Medicare performs as a regulator of medical quality and cost.

Medicare: Quality of Care versus Cost

The Dartmouth University Health Policy Institute published the "Dartmouth Atlas of Health Care" about variations in Medicare spending in 2009.[2] As mentioned in Chapter 5, Dartmouth data showed that Medicare recipients in McAllen, Texas had the highest per capita cost in the nation ($15,000 per enrollee in 2006) and received wasteful, mediocre health care. It found that Grand Junction, Colorado charged Medicare about one-third the McAllen rate per capita for high quality care provided by an integrated system of health care providers. Essentially, the medical care system in Grand Junction, CO functions as a cooperative with all the providers working together for the benefit of patients.

The Obama Administration promised to ask the Institute of Medicine, a non-governmental advisory group, to find formulas for putting the Dartmouth findings into action by setting payment rates that would punish inefficient hospitals, such as in McAllen, TX, and reward efficient ones, such as in Grand Junction, CO. This kind of top-down approach to cost control failed in this case, as have many top-down strategies in the past.

The Hobby Lobby Case

In what was, arguably, the most divisive legal case handed down in 2014, the U.S. Supreme Court ruled 5-4 in the Hobby Lobby case that corporations closely controlled by religious families cannot be required to pay for contraception coverage for their female workers. Justice Ruth Bader Ginsburg attacked the majority opinion as a "radical overhaul of corporate rights." She feared that it could apply to all corporations and to countless laws.[3] Clearly, conservatives won and liberals lost. The ruling further threatens the Affordable Care Act. It will spawn more anti-Obamacare litigation about what benefits must be covered to comply with the ACA.

While I personally favor a woman's right to contraception, I supported the Hobby Lobby decision. Like thousands of other medical interventions, contraception is *controversial*. In this case the controversy is religious rather than medical. Do we want the Supreme Court to rule on each case where people of different faiths or beliefs disagree about what should be covered by medical insurance?

The more logical approach would be to allow people to choose medical insurance plans that are in accordance with their religious, ethical, and, I would add, medical beliefs.

Personally, I don't want my medical insurance plan to cover PSA (prostate specific antigen) screening for prostate cancer or screening mammograms for breast cancer. I would rather my insurance money go elsewhere. I would be happy to purchase medical insurance that covered none of the 70+ tests and treatments in Table 1 from Chapter 8. However, I would like to see some currently non-covered medical interventions covered in the insurance plan that I buy. For instance, I would like insurance to pay $2800 for my hearing aids.

I don't expect everyone to agree with my choices of what I want and don't want covered in my policy. I don't mind at all if others make other choices and purchase other insurance. If we had this kind of choice in insurance, people would be happier and might have extra money. Ineffective and dangerous tests and treatments would be easier to discover. Medical costs for society would be able to be controlled.

Decentralizing Clinical Practice Guidelines

While evidence-based medicine as assessed by individual practicing doctors is essential to health care reform, evidence-based health care determined by elite academic physicians is arguably less important. Indeed, standardized, one-size-fits-all evidence-based health care may be an obstacle to some of the needed ingredients of true reform—patient choice, physician autonomy, and competition.

We know that top-down treatment guidelines are frequently corrupted by special interest money. Additionally, best practices guidelines rapidly become outdated. Therefore, we should consider abandoning attempts at requiring medical practitioners to rigidly adhere to government and industry sponsored medical guidelines as well as standardized health care benefit packages. Rather than suppressing controversial ideas about medical interventions and striving for guideline-dictated conformity, we can learn from medical controversies to practice better medicine.

How can we best learn from medical controversies?

The Grand Bargains' approach is to decentralize the medical practice guidelines and patient benefit packages offered by ACCs. Competing ACCs will have differing clinical practice guidelines and patient benefit packages.

Importantly, all ACCs will follow and document the medical interventions given to patients and the related clinical outcomes. This will give researchers lots of heretofore unavailable data relating to the efficacy and safety of thousands of medical interventions. This will give researchers new data on medical interventions because, unlike now, ACCs will differ in what medical interventions they do and do not offer. This will rapidly advance the practice of medicine.

For example, some ACCs may offer free screening mammograms and prostate-specific antigen (PSA) tests, and others may not. Over time ACCs can count deaths from breast cancer and prostate cancer and compare outcomes of different ACCs based on whether screening mammograms or PSAs were offered.

With decentralized clinical practice guidelines, benefit packages will be drafted by ACC staff in collaboration with health and social services experts and ACC members. Close monitoring and reporting of each ACC's services and the associated outcomes (health and social indicators as well as member financial security, educational attainments, employment, etc.) will drive ongoing enhancements of the benefits offered.

People will choose ACCs according to their preferences and priorities. People will be able to change ACCs at any time they think they will receive better services from a competing ACC. Transparency and competition in the ACC marketplace will foster continuous improvements in quality and encourage cost control.

When decentralized medical guidelines enable patients to forego expensive high-tech tests and treatments in favor of lower-tech, less costly approaches, the patients and providers should both reap the benefits. ACC members will receive lower premiums and/or access to additional therapies and health enhancement benefits. The providers will indirectly benefit when the guidelines and benefit packages their ACCs offer attract more patients. Patients will "vote with their feet" and choose health care providers based on the services covered (and not covered) and the cost of their premiums.

With no consensus about what medical tests and treatments must be eliminated, and with powerful vested interests supporting each component of the medical status quo, only deregulating medical guidelines will bring about quality improvements and cost savings. Competing ACCs will operate under different guidelines, offer different benefits to members, and keep track of the clinical outcomes. The resulting medical free market will result in non-beneficial tests and treatments being eliminated over time.

I will illustrate the potential of decentralizing the guidelines and benefits packages with an example.

Deregulation of Child Birth

Out of about 4 million births in the U.S. each year, fewer than 40,000 babies are delivered by midwives at home or in free-standing birthing centers.[4] Government insurance for the poor (e.g., Medicaid) does not cover home births. Few private insurance companies cover midwife or physician assisted home births for low-risk pregnancies.

A comprehensive registry of home births in North America by certified professional midwives published in the *BMJ* (formerly *British Medical Journal*) showed an excellent safety record.[5] None the less, if a home birth results in a bad outcome, even if it would have been unavoidable in hospital, midwives or physicians face possible malpractice suits or criminal prosecution. Standards of care and guidelines for births are written by obstetricians favoring hospital births. No consideration was given to the registry of home births when updating the obstetrical guidelines.

Clearly, access to back up hospital care is a requirement for safe home births. However, obstetrical guidelines mandating hospital births make hospital backup difficult to secure. Decentralizing birthing guidelines will allow women who want out-of-hospital births access to non-medicalized midwife care in birthing centers or homes with secure obstetrical care backup in hospitals. This is deemed optimal by many women. Besides medical freedom, at stake is tens of billions of dollars per year that could be saved by millions of low-risk pregnant women foregoing high-tech hospitals for certified professional midwife or nurse-midwife assisted births.

ACCs Drafting Reasonable Alternative Clinical Guidelines

Without a government role in health care regulation, how the ACCs provide services to members will be up to them. Without government regulation, ACCs will be largely self-regulated by the owners and em-ployees—enrollees and ACC professional staff.

Implementing a decentralized system of medical practice guidelines should be done with great care. Appropriate cautions should be taken with the drafting of any alternative clinical practice guidelines. In order for the ACCs to be accountable, they must keep accurate records on the health statuses of their patients, any alternative medical interventions utilized, and the clinical outcomes. These data should be available to outside researchers to audit the methodologies and results.

Practicing physicians that draft alternate guidelines for ACCs should be familiar with the relevant standard medical guidelines written by government regulators and special interest medical group affiliated experts (e.g., American Heart Association or American Cancer Soci-ety). These current medical establishment "standards of care" should be considered the default guidelines. Only if the leadership of an ACC, after input from all stakeholders, agrees to a different approach to a disease or health risk should a default guideline be discarded in favor of an alternative guideline. This assures caution and prudence.

It will be up to ACC committees working on alternative guidelines to consider input from the appropriate medical authorities, alternative care practitioners, and opinions of all interested ACC stakeholders. Before and after the alternative clinical practice guidelines are in place for medical conditions, the outcomes of patients receiving the alternative care for those conditions should be closely monitored. Each treatment guideline should be revisited periodically, whether standard care or an alternative approach, to reassess whether changes may be warranted.

Medical Research will Expand with Decentralized Guidelines

With decentralized medical practice guidelines and a diversity of medical intervention strategies available in different ACCs, medical research involving different intervention strategies will accelerate innovation and improve patient outcomes. With decentralized guidelines, more clinical questions can be studied more rapidly, with much less bias, and at lower costs. The universal implementation of electronic medical records will greatly facilitate the monitoring and reporting of medical interventions (whether conventional or alternative) and of patient outcomes.

Compared with medical interventions, relatively little research has been done on positive lifestyle changes or non-drug approaches to prevention and treatment. Improved health outcomes depend on positive changes of lifestyles much more than on drugs or other medical interventions. Our health care system will not be reformed unless substantial resources are shifted from researching sickness-treatment to evaluating preventive-medicine and health-promotion strategies. ACCs will be well situated and have financial incentives to collect data from members on different lifestyle change interventions to improve health.

Just like there should be robust evaluation of medical tests and treatments, preventive medicine interventions should be tested by rigorous research. As with research into interventions for treating sick people, interpretations of preventive medicine research will often be controversial. That's okay and to be expected. Further research studies will be needed. Yet more questions will arise. This is the nature of medical progress.

The decentralization of clinical practice guidelines will facilitate multiple innovative disease treatment and prevention approaches. Compared with relatively small, expensive, lengthy, and often biased randomized controlled trials; large observational studies of different ACCs with dissimilar clinical practice guidelines will give better quality research information faster and less expensively.

Cost Control Despite Ongoing Medical Controversies

Standards of care have been and will continue to be in constant evolution. Notwithstanding the inevitable controversies over the value of many tests and treatments, successful health care reform requires innovative efforts to reduce insurance funding for ineffective, dangerous medical interventions. While no amount of comparative-effectiveness-research or other medical studies will eliminate controversy about the value of many medical interventions, studies of costs of treatments and patient outcomes of competing ACCs will lead to cost control and better utilization of health care dollars.

ACCs will compete for members, in part, on how they deal with medical controversies. Regarding those controversies in clinical medicine, ACCs will also compete on the effectiveness of their research methodologies in finding practical and cost-effective guidelines and benefits packages that appeal to members.

Proposed New Research Methods in Determining Effectiveness of Health-Improvement Interventions

Randomized trials for testing drugs and other health interventions, funded privately and publicly, should continue. However, for many important treatment choices in medicine, conducting the necessary very large randomized trials to yield conclusive answers is impractical in terms of patients required, length of follow-up needed, and cost. In many of these situations, clinical decisions by practitioners about health interventions could be informed in part by online observational studies of health outcomes conducted by researchers in cooperation with ACCs.

Either of two alternative research approaches will give faster, more accurate, and less expensive findings and conclusions. One approach was described in Chapter 8 under "An Alternative Format for Randomized Controlled Trials." With this approach, a number of ACCs would be randomized to receive or not to receive an experimental drug or other medical intervention. This will work if doctors and patients do not have strong opinions about the likely efficacy of the treatment.

Where feelings are already strongly divided about a medical intervention among patients and physicians (e.g., contraception, midwife assisted birth, abortion, screening mammograms, drugs for mild hypertension, etc.), the other approach would be to conduct a study comparing outcomes and costs of ACCs that offer and don't offer the intervention.

For instance, clinical practice guidelines have recommended the treatment of mild (stage 1) hypertension with drugs for over 30 years. In 2012, the *Cochrane Database of Systematic Reviews* published a systematic review that I co-authored with three other doctors. It found no evidence supporting drug treatment for low-risk patients of any age with mild hypertension (systolic blood pressure: 140-159 mm/Hg and/or diastolic blood pressure 90-99 mm/Hg).[6] In addition, about 2 million low-cardiovascular-disease-risk Americans per year with stage 1 hypertension (about 9% of those taking drugs) suffer side effects from blood pressure-lowering drugs severe enough for them to stop treatment.

This also matters because the American Heart Association has projected that the cost for drugs and clinic visits for mild hypertension over the next 10 years will be almost $500 billion.[7] If blood pressure-lowering drugs do not benefit people with mild hypertension, this money can be used for helpful treatments or returned to ACC members in reduced premiums. A randomized controlled trial will never be done because it will require at least 50,000 patients, take over 10 years to complete, and cost at least $200 million.

With an online observational study, clinical outcomes in patients with mild hypertension in ACCs that offer drug treatment in addition lifestyle change programs might be compared with people in ACCs that offer diet, exercise, and stress management programs alone. With competing ACCs differing in their treatment approaches to mild hypertension (i.e., some continuing with drug treatment and others prescribing lifestyle change alone), millions of people might be enrolled in the observational study in a short time. Assuring the trustworthiness of an online study could be done by having the physicians of patients submit the data rather than the patients. Conclusive data might be generated within a few years at a much lower cost that with a randomized placebo controlled trial. If data remain inconclusive as often occurs even with randomized trials, medical scientists and patients can make up their own minds and act accordingly.

Online observational studies might help answer many clinical questions. Other examples would include the value of colonoscopy screening versus stool blood tests, and cholesterol-lowering statin drugs for coronary disease prevention versus a plant-based diet and rigorous exercise (Chapter 4).

For patients with various medical conditions, being involved with medical research will become as easy as logging onto one's computer periodically to input diet and exercise data, drugs taken, and other related information. As these studies evolve, statistical methods and other techniques will develop that more and more precisely assure the accuracy and honesty of the data. Low-cost, online, clinical observational studies will potentially involve tens of millions of patients and tens of thousands of research questions at any given time.

With this online system, studies will be completed much faster that with randomized controlled trials. ACC employed researchers, as opposed to drug company or other special interest funded researchers, will have no reason to be biased in interpreting their results. And ACCs, rather than academic medical institutions, will receive the clinical research funding from private industry and government agencies. ACCs will then pay the academic researchers for their work. Much more research will be conducted so the researchers and their academic institutions will not be unhappy.

With this methodology of conducting clinical trials, much of the approximately $70 billion projected to be invested by drug companies, private industry, charities, and research nonprofits[8] will flow to the ACCs. ACCs will also receive much of the $55 billion projected to be spent by the National Institutes of Health and other government agencies involved with medical research.[9]

Conclusion

Quality of care metrics currently rank physicians and hospitals according to their compliance of with top-down clinical practice guidelines. Pay-for-performance schemes similarly rely on conformity to medical-establishment-endorsed standards of care. However, since many medical guidelines are flawed and standards of care are in constant flux, we need other measures of quality of medical care. We must realize that quality of care means different things to different patients and physicians. For all these reasons, I recommend decentralizing the regulation of health care and making ACCs self-regulating.

Research studies are needed to improve quality of care. With decentralized regulation of health care, ACC involvement in medical research will greatly increase patient participation in randomized trials and observational studies. These studies will provide better quality data for analysis, improve the acceptability of findings, and, consequently, enhance the validity of the clinical research outcomes.

Vesting the medical practice guidelines with competing, self-regulated ACCs rather than government agencies or special-interest nonprofit organizations will be a major step forward in improving quality of care. Due to market-driven innovations that we can now only partially foresee, competition between ACCs for attracting patients will lead to a race to the top on quality simultaneously with a race to the bottom on costs.

Chapter 10
ACCs Can Best Deliver Social Services

As part of a *Los Angeles Times* series in 2009, "Innocents Betrayed," reporter Garret Therolf detailed the case of a 5-year-old South Los Angeles boy that almost died of malnutrition before a stranger delivered him to Los Angeles County child protective services. Before his dramatic rescue, eight separate LA County agencies had come into contact with the boy or his caregivers 108 times over four years without realizing the danger to the boy.[1] Although the responsibility for this tragedy lies as much or more with our dysfunctional social-safety-net system than the boy's mentally ill mother and her girlfriend, the Court gave the boy's caregivers long prison sentences.[2]

Los Angeles County child protective services investigators repeatedly found barriers to sharing information among social service agencies as contributing factors to inaction leading to deaths or injuries of LA County children. In 11 articles in this extensive year-long *Los Angeles Times* investigation, reporter Therolf never mentioned a pediatrician or family practitioner involved in any of the gruesome cases.[3] A child's doctor should be in the best position to coordinate social and medical services to best protect the child. While there are privacy issues with sharing information among social service agencies, social service personnel reporting information about health or safety risks of a child to the child's doctor does not breech anyone's privacy.

Unfortunately, low-income residents in the U.S. are likely to have no doctor, and this is even truer for impoverished children. The more primary care physicians for a population, the better the health outcomes.[4] Inner city poverty areas in Los Angeles and other cities have relatively few physicians.

From January 2008 through early August 2009, at least 268 children who had passed through the Los Angeles child welfare system died. Of those children, 213 were by unnatural or undetermined causes, including 76 homicides, 35 accidents, and 16 suicides.[3]

Agency spokespeople complained that they lacked adequate resources for their huge caseloads.[5] A friend of mine, who worked 25 years in this agency, told me that a previous study showed that adequately protecting the children of LA County required four times the number of social workers than had been allocated.

After the tragic stories of the abused and neglected children left unprotected by LA County social service agencies came to light, Richard Wexler, executive director of the National Coalition for Child Protection, wrote an opinion piece in the *Los Angeles Times* about a related problem—children needlessly put into foster care.[6] He wrote that overreaction to the failures of LA County Child Protective Services to remove endangered children from their families could make the system even more dangerous for children. In many instances case workers confuse parental poverty with parental neglect. Rather than helping poor but loving and competent parents with the financial resources to properly care for their children, they often move the children to foster homes.

He cited a study of 15,000 children put into foster care that showed that these children usually fared worse in later life than comparably maltreated children left in their own homes. Compared with children left with one or both parents, children placed in foster homes were more likely to commit crimes and become pregnant as teenagers. They were also less likely to be able to hold jobs as young adults.

Mr. Wexler wrote, "In fact, agencies like the Department of Children and Family Services can be arbitrary, capricious, and cruel. They do indeed leave some children in dangerous homes, even as they take more children from homes that are safe or could be made safe with the right kinds of help."

LA County's Social Services Mess: A Solution

In the case of protecting abused and neglected children in Los Angeles, the answer is a coordinated system with each child to have a primary care provider and for that PCP to be in charge. Pediatricians, family doctors, nurse practitioners, or physician's assistants should refer social workers, mental health professionals, and other welfare agency personnel to intervene to protect children as necessary. The social welfare personnel should report all relevant information to the PCP with their recommendations. PCPs for children should coordinate the relevant social service providers in responding to reports of child abuse or neglect. They should have all necessary resources to monitor high-risk families (e.g., homelessness, mental illness, crime, poverty, or substance abuse) to prevent harm to children.

Coordination of social and medical services is extremely important for children, substance abusers, the mentally ill, people with disabilities, and the elderly. In all these populations, PCPs should be in charge of managing the health care system's response to any abuse or neglect problems. Without this crucial coordination of all health care and social services providers by one PCP, the "social determinants of health" for patients will not be optimally addressed.

Social Determinants of Health

The Robert Wood Johnson Foundation Commission to Build a Healthier America issued a report titled, "Beyond Health Care: New Directions to a Healthier America." This report stated that the availability of quality medical care accounts for only 10% – 15% of good medical outcomes such as longevity.[6] With genetic conditions causing less than 5% of overall disease burden,[7] the "social determinants of health"—income, education, nutrition, social relationships, race, where someone lives, etc.—account for at least 80% of health outcomes. This fact dispenses with the fatalistic cop-out we've heard all too often—"It's all genetic."

Quality of life and longevity depend largely on these social determinants of health. Co-chair of the commission Alice M. Rivlin summed up the landmark report.

> Everyone must be involved in the effort to improve health because health is everyone's business. People should make healthy choices by eating better, getting enough physical activity and not smoking. Communities and employers should support those choices by creating healthy environments. And the federal government should make and enforce healthy policies, like ensuring that all subsidized food is healthy and junk food is eliminated from schools. . . . While each of us must make a commitment to our own health, society must improve opportunities for choosing health, especially for those of us facing the most challenging obstacles. We must acknowledge that some families and communities have a higher hill to climb than others. We cannot build a healthier America if we leave them behind.

Health care reform will fail if it addresses only medical interventions for sickness, long-term care, and preventive medicine. It must also address social factors. Attending to the social determinants of health should be done in an integrated fashion rather than depending on multiple fragmented government and nonprofit charity programs.

Social Isolation

While humans are naturally social, modern society's individualistic consumerism in the U.S. is often damaging to social relationships. We now have relatively few extended families living together. Young adults often delay getting married and having children. More of us are living alone, and becoming lonely. In the past 20 years, there has been a three-fold increase in the number of Americans who say they have no close confidants. Social isolation is on the rise.[7] Studies in Alameda County, California,[8] Tecumseh, Michigan,[9] and Evans County, Georgia,[9] all found that people with few social contacts were 2–3 times as likely to die than those with a good social network.[10]

In a scientific analysis of 148 studies of social isolation, researchers found that people with few social relationships were 50% more likely to die in a certain time period than those with stronger social relationships. This is about as strong a risk factor for death as smoking cigarettes or excess alcohol consumption.[7]

Government Policies versus Local Community Culture

In the book, *What Money Can't Buy*,[11] Susan E. Mayer, a social services researcher from the University of Chicago, showed that doubling the income of the poorest Americans would do little to reduce dropout rates of the children, decrease teen pregnancies, or improve child outcomes overall. Given existing cultural and social influences, government policies can easily hurt the social fabric, but top-down government programs and policies do relatively little to help the health and well-being consequences of poverty.

The influences of politics and government policies are usually trumped by the influences of culture, ethnicity, psychology, and other factors that operate at the local community level. The region you live in also makes a major difference in how you live and in what kind of environmental factors influence you. Also, where you live suggests the ways you would likely help people that are struggling.

There are certain high-trust regions where highly educated people congregate, producing positive feedback loops of close culture and good human capital programs. The different psychological, cultural, and social factors that determine good and bad health outcomes work together in ways that researchers don't entirely understand.[12] However, factors that seem to matter most are lifetime experiences, cultural attitudes, child-rearing practices, family formation patterns, expectations about the future, work ethics, and the quality of social bonds.

Therefore the cardinal rule of legislators trying to help the poor should be to adopt policies that support and strengthen local social bonds. In accordance with the common knowledge about social indicators of health and social services, decentralizing the authority and responsibility of local social-safety-net services via ACC alliances—the opposite of top-down social engineering—will improve our health and social outcomes.

Social Factors and Infant Mortality in Dane County, Wisconsin

The U.S. has a large racial gap in infant deaths, due primarily to a higher incidence of premature births among blacks. From the 1990s to the current decade, researchers noted that in Dane County, Wisconsin, which includes Madison, the rate of infant deaths among blacks dropped from an average of 19 deaths per thousand births to five deaths per thousand births, equaling the infant mortality rate for whites. While obstetrical services for low-income women in Dane County have not changed very much over the last two decades, researchers attributed the dramatic drop in infant mortality to a new federally supported clinic serving poor, uninsured people that cared for more black women in the 1990s using nurse-midwives. These midwives bonded with pregnant women, spending more time on appointments and staying with them through childbirth.[13] The improved social determinants of health for black women in Dane County represented by these midwives apparently accounted for the dramatically lower infant mortality.

This is a valuable example of *community* as the key to well-being, as opposed to the increasingly dominant concentration on *making money.* Money is of course important, but by itself it does not solve or offer much to the social human animal.

U.S. Social Services System Inadequacies

About 130 years ago, Dr. Rudolf Virchow, a famous German pathologist, anthropologist, and statesman (1821–1902), said,[14]

> Medicine is a social science, and politics is nothing else but medicine on a large scale. Medicine, as a social science, as the science of human beings, has the obligation to point out problems and to attempt their theoretical solution: the politician, the practical anthropologist, must find the means for their actual solution.... The physicians are the natural attorneys of the poor, and social problems fall to a large extent within their jurisdiction.

The close relationship between health and social problems remains today. Several European countries that spend about half what we spend for health care and yet spend much more than we do on social services have much better patient health outcomes than us.[15]

While welfare spending by our federal, state, and local governments has increased by over 200% since 2000[16] ($500 billion projected for 2016, Table 1), it is falling further and further behind in ameliorating the social determinants of health.

Table 1. U.S. Welfare Spending by Category Projected for 2016 (billions)[16]

Category	Federal	State and Local	Total
Housing	50	34	84
Family and Child	296	5	301
Unemployment[18]	45	70	115
Total	391	109	500

Social service programs for U.S. veterans of military service will cost about $104 billion in 2016.[17] The government bureaucracy administering these funds is separate from that administering other government social-safety-net funds. The VA disability system wastes resources and serves veterans poorly. Washington, D.C. politicians and insiders know full well that the highly dysfunctional VA disability system has gone far beyond the original purpose of compensating veterans for lost earning capacity. Disability payouts increased 18% in 2014 over the 2013 levels ($58 billion versus $49 billion). The system is arbitrary, out of date, and unfair. For instance, disability payments for sleep apnea, which is usually related to obesity rather than combat, total $1.5 billion a year. However, politicians decline to reform the system or even criticize the system publicly.[19] Reforming the VA disability system will require taking the system away from the control of politicians.

Workers' compensation is part of the social safety net. However, it is not included with welfare because employees pay for the insurance. Indemnity and medical payments to employees with work-related accidents or illnesses are on track to total about $40 billion in 2016, of which about 40% is for administration and legal costs (Chapter 11).[20] Many people are overpaid and many others are underpaid. It may depend more on your attorney than on your injury. This unfair state of affairs needs to be fixed.

In addition to the government's general fund spending on unemployment benefits, billions more in unemployment insurance will be collected from employers in 2016 by the federal and state governments.

These funds will be administered collaboratively by separate state and federal bureaucracies. Responding to economic pressures, especially during recessions, Congress politicizes the unemployment benefit payments in arbitrary and capricious ways. We need a better way of dealing with unemployment.

Lack of coordination of health and social services dilutes the benefits that social service professionals could otherwise be providing. As society is now configured, further increasing government spending on existing or new social-safety-net programs will do little or nothing to help the poor or to alleviate the adverse health consequences of poverty.

Any comprehensive health care reform proposal must have a mechanism to use existing government social-safety-net funds together with any available private funds for the poor, mentally ill, destitute, mentally ill, addicted, disabled, and unemployed. For instance, to best feed hungry people, we need better coordination to more efficiently utilize funds that come from the government and from local community sources—e.g., farmers' markets, local farms, community gardens, food banks, churches, soup kitchens, etc. If cost-efficiently allocated, safety-net funds can help prevent or alleviate the adverse effects of poverty—chronic illness, substance abuse, crime, lack of education, homelessness, etc.

Health care and social service providers now generally work under different bureaucracies, which are often competing with each other for funding from government agencies and charitable foundations. However, excellence in providing social services requires flexibility, a minimum of bureaucracy, and partnerships with PCPs that work well with local social services providers.

The optimal health care system will integrate evidence-based medical care, preventive medicine strategies, *and* social services.

Block Grants for Social-Safety-Net Services

Republicans have long sought to cap spending on welfare by having the federal government give social services block grants to the states to cover a wide range of human services for the poor, disabled, mentally ill, homeless, and otherwise down and out. Advocates of block grants claim that they increase government efficiency and program effectiveness by redistributing power and accountability through decentralization and partial devolution of decision-making authority from the federal government to state and local governments.[21]

However, critics of block grants—mostly Democrats—counter that block grants can erode the accomplishment of national objectives and can enable reduced government spending on domestic issues. Critics also fear that block grants may allow for reduced accountability of state government social-services administrators. Without the federal government's being able to hold state governments accountable for efficient and effective delivery of social services to the poor and disabled, states might race to the bottom in welfare benefits. State legislators might reason that meager welfare benefits might lead social-services recipients to move to other states.

Nevertheless, public sector social-services block grants to local authorities will have the effect of better integrating the public and private sector social services to the benefit of recipients and providers. Local authorities should be in charge of allocating and integrating all of the social-safety-net services.

But who should be those local authorities?

ACC-Based Reform of the U.S. Social-Services System

With Grand Bargains' reform, the federal, state, and local governments will ascertain their total spending on social services (i.e., Food Stamps, housing assistance, aid to families, etc.) and distribute it in risk-adjusted payments to ACCs. In the stalemate over block grants, the game-changer will be to shift responsibility for government-funded health care and other human services and entitlements to competing ACCs rather than to state and local governments. It will then be up to the ACCs to most effectively allocate these block grants for social services for their members.

Shifting social services to competing ACCs will foster the innovation, flexibility, and efficiency sought by the Republicans. The accountability sought by the Democrats will be provided by the ability of people to choose between competing ACCs rather than depending on governmental agencies operating as inflexible, bureaucratic, and inefficient, monopolies.

Consequently, the grand bargain for government-funded welfare reform includes shifting social-safety-net-services providers out of working for poorly coordinated government and private agencies. Instead, they will become integral components of patient-centered medical homes in ACCs.

If low-income people have trouble affording ACC insurance premiums, ACC social services resources could be tapped to provide assistance. However, instead of simply waiving medical insurance fees and doling out welfare stipends; providing jobs, healthy food, and housing should be strongly preferred as social service support. With flexible, innovative, coordinated management, welfare funds and appropriately utilized human resources will help people rise out of poverty to gainful employment. Public assistance will no longer become a route to dependence.

For homeless people, it will be the responsibility of ACCs to provide shelter. ACCs will fund and coordinate social services for abused or neglected children, substance abusers, domestic abuse victims, seniors, veterans, unemployed workers, incarcerated enrollees, parolees, and disabled people.

The ACC coordination of health and social-safety-net services will dramatically increase the positive impact of those services in peoples' lives. ACC-coordinated mutual self aid and volunteerism will supplement the professional services provided.

The cost control side of the welfare reform grand bargain is for the government social-safety-net budget to be indefinitely frozen at the 2016 level, which is $500 per year.

ACC Coordination of Fragmented Social Services

Despite a dramatic increase in spending,[16] our social safety net for the poor and disadvantaged is much more tenuous than at the turn of the 21st century. The health of Americans will deteriorate if our social safety net lags further behind in meeting the need.

To strengthen and coordinate social-safety-net services, the following grand bargains will be involved:

1. Grand Bargain #6: ACCs to Provide Long-Term Care
2. Grand Bargain #8: Government Welfare will be Administered by ACCs
3. Grand Bargain #12: ACCs to Administer Public Disability Benefits, Unemployment Insurance Benefits, and Workers' Compensation
4. Grand Bargain #13: ACCs to Provide Members Basic Prepaid Legal Services and Foster Legal and Prison Systems Reforms
5. Grand Bargain #14 and #15: ACCs to Assist Members Finding Jobs Paying at Least $15 Per Hour.
6. Grand Bargain #16: ACCs to Provide Members Financial Counseling
7. Grand Bargain #17: ACCs to Administer Social Security for Members
8. Grand Bargain #18: ACCs to Administer Public Sector Retirement Plans for Members
9. Grand Bargain #25: Veterans Health and Social Services to be Shifted from the Veterans Administration to ACCs
10. Grand Bargain #26: ACCs to Replace the Indian Health Service in Providing Health and Social Services

For all the services above, delivered by separate bureaucracies in a fragmented manner, government funding will be shifted to the ACCs for the delivery of and coordination of all health, social, and human services.

Instead of all these poorly coordinated government programs, with Grand Bargains-based reform an estimated $957 billion in social services funds will be administered by ACCs under this block grant plan.[a]

The redundancies, waste, administrative burdens, and failures to adequately help people in the current welfare system provide ample justification for shifting administration of government welfare spending and other social-safety-net benefits to ACCs. With intimate knowledge of both their patients and the local health and welfare services providers, direct practice PCPs with their patient-centered medical teams at the ACCs will provide and coordinate all health, welfare, and human services.

In a free market environment for health and welfare services, ACCs will efficiently and effectively employ social workers and other appropriate social-safety-net professionals to optimally benefit their patients. ACCs will have resources to employ or find employment for all who are capable of working (Chapter 12). The ACC system will enhance the positive impact of welfare spending while reducing the burden on the taxpayer.

While massive federal, state, and local social programs help many people, they tend to decrease the obligation each of us feels to assist unfortunate people in our own communities. ACCs will harness the efforts of individuals, religious and charitable groups, and social-services professionals to improve patient outcomes. The impacts of individual volunteers on overall social services will be magnified. Volunteers will become motivated to do more.

Possible examples of improved care with ACC coordination of funding for services ordered by direct practice PCPs will be the following:

- If a blind or disabled person requires a service dog,[22] the cost of training and caring for the dog should be covered by the combined health/social-safety-net insurance.

---

a $500 billion (Welfare) + $104 billion (Veterans social services) + $140 billion (federal and state unemployment benefits) + $40 billion (Workers' Compensation) + $173 billion (Disability benefits) = $957 billion

- A PCP trying to prevent or treat a patient's diet-related diseases (e.g., obesity, type 2 diabetes, coronary heart disease, cancer, etc.) faces the reality that poor people in the U.S. eat a lot of junk food. High calorie, low nutrient content food is cheap and all they can afford. That PCP should be able to prescribe fresh fruits and vegetables, whole grains, nuts, beans, and other nutritious foods and allocate social-safety-net funds to pay for those foods in an individually designed healthy diet (Chapter 13).
- When a homeless person sees his/her PCP, the PCP will be able to prescribe shelter along with medical treatment.
- When an elderly or disabled person requires assistance with activities of daily living, the PCP will be able to provide timely and uncomplicated funding for family and friends to provide care (Chapter 6).
- If a person is disabled, whether by a medical intervention, military combat, a sports injury, a car accident, an accident on the job, or other cause, a financial stipend could be provided to substitute for a paying job.
- Evidence-based intensive treatment for autistic children will be funded by insurance at the discretion of the PCP rather than based on the fine print of insurance policies or legal-system mandates.
- With ACCs in charge of health care and social services, provision of midwife services will depend on the demand of women. Midwife services are as much social as medical. Some ACCs will cover it and others will have exclusively hospital births. When choosing an ACC, women will be able to choose one that does or does not cover midwife services.

The Grand Bargain #26: ACCs to Replace the Indian Health Service in Providing Health and Social Services

Due to previous treaties with the U.S. government, Native Americans are entitled to their own health service and need not rely on Medicaid if they are poor. The federal Indian Health Service (IHS) provides free care to 1.9 million Native Americans, including indigenous people in Alaska and Hawaii, mostly living on tribal lands. An additional 8 million part- or full-blooded Native Americans, mostly living in urban areas, are not covered by IHS health care.[23, 24]

Unfortunately, the IHS is chronically underfunded and understaffed. A report to Congress by the U.S. Commission on Civil Rights concluded in 2004: "... our nation's lengthy history of failing to keep its promises to Native Americans includes the failure of Congress to provide the resources necessary to create and maintain an effective health care system for Native Americans."[23] Between bureaucratic hurdles, transportation issues, poverty, discrimination, lack of good jobs, and other social factors, Native Americans as a group receive substandard health care and have poor health outcomes. They have high infant mortality, low longevity, and high rates of alcoholism, obesity, and diabetes.

If not bound by treaties, Congress would probably get rid of the Indian Health Service (IHS) and force Native Americans to enroll in programs like subsidized private insurance or expanded Medicaid. However, most American Indians oppose abandoning the Indian Health Service. Switching from the IHS to Medicaid is not the answer. Obamacare will do little to help the health care of about 10 million Native Americans.

The answer is for ACCs to replace the IHS in providing health and social services. The IHS health care budget (projected to be about $4 billion in 2016[24]) as well as risk-adjusted government social service funds will be distributed to the ACCs chosen by the Native Americans.

Conclusion

The huge impact of the social determinants of health on individual and societal health outcomes justifies the integration of federal, state, and local social-safety-net funds with health care funds under the management of ACCs. With innovation, flexibility, and a minimum of bureaucracy, ACCs will be able to use the social-welfare funds along the lines of the 2016 federal budget to bring together local resources (charities, volunteer organizations, social services agencies, individuals, etc.) to better address the large number of serious social problems experienced by U.S. residents.

Methods of attending to homelessness, drug abuse, disability, mental illness, long-term care and other social challenges will differ between ACCs. Social services delivery methods and patient health and social outcomes will be monitored and reported by ACCs. The most successful approaches will be identified and copied by others.

ACCs will compete, in part, by the effectiveness of their programs to address the social determinants of health. To control long-term overall welfare spending, the government's allocation for social services will be frozen at the amount for 2016.

Chapter 11
Enterprise Medical Malpractice Liability and Legal System Reform

"The excesses of our legal system are harming society," according to Phillip K. Howard, an attorney and the founder of Common Good.[1] Howard asserts that we no longer have a legal system to protect individuals and society from wrongdoers. Instead, the law has become a weapon used by individuals and interest groups to advance their own interests over the common good. Because much litigation is harmful to the common good in many areas, Americans pay an ever-increasing amount of money on health care, education, government, and regulatory compliance costs. Despite paying more money, we get an ever-diminishing return in service, satisfaction, performance and safety.[2]

Whereas, in other developed countries, about 1% of the GDP goes to the legal system, in the U.S. over 2% of the GDP goes to litigation.[3] Returning our tort costs to 1% of GDP would reduce by half the litigation expenses of $350 billion projected for 2016.[4]

A poll commissioned by Common Good found that only 16% of Americans trust the legal system to protect them.[5] Lawyer jokes arise from this pervasive mistrust. Concerning this lack of confidence in the legal system, Howard makes the case that our excessively detailed laws and rigid and arcane government regulations leave no room for judgment or discretion. He argues that, without reform of America's legal and regulatory system, we will lose the freedom to take reasonable risks. He asserts that America is drowning in law, legality, and bureaucratic processes. He cites many examples of litigation or the fear of law suits constantly threatening not only doctors but educators, government workers, business people, and others.

In this chapter, I will begin with a proposal that addresses both reforming the medical malpractice system and reducing medical errors. Then I will address the wider scope of how Grand Bargains-based reform will facilitate a more functional overall legal system.

The Medical Malpractice Conundrum

In 1999, the Institute of Medicine estimated that 46,000–98,000 Americans die of medical errors per year.[6] Much attention has subsequently gone to efforts to improve patient safety. However, no overall improvement in patient safety has been documented.

In fact, a 2010 study showed that adverse events in hospitalized patients, including those caused by human errors (i.e., preventable), occur about 10 times as frequently as previously thought—at least 49 adverse events per 100 hospital admissions including about 20 errors.[7] Plugging this error rate estimate into the national estimates on hospitalizations for 2008 (last available year) translates into roughly 20 million patient injuries that year, of which about 8 million were caused by errors.

An unknown number of adverse events and errors were not documented in the hospital records. Additionally, almost half of all medical malpractice occurs in outpatient settings.[8, 9] Given the extent of medical errors, the track record of our medical malpractice system on reducing harm to patients has been questioned. Indeed, many analysts, including this author, think our malpractice system is responsible for *increasing* errors.

As mentioned in Chapter 1, the courts have a terrible record of distinguishing which injuries and illnesses are due to medical malpractice and which are just due to inherent risks of medical interventions and bad luck. Consequently we need to find a better way of dealing with bad outcomes for patients, including those due to medical malpractice.

Failed Government Strategies to Reduce Malpractice

To address the huge problem of errors by health care professionals causing injuries and deaths to hospitalized patients, Kathleen Sebelius, the former Secretary of the U.S. Department of Health and Human Services (HHS), unveiled the Partnership for Patients initiative in 2011.[10] This HHS patient safety plan targeted nine common types of errors in hospitals. The tools highlighted to reduce these errors included (1) checklists, (2) public reporting, (3) "evidence-based" guidelines, and (4) "pay for performance" (financial incentives). Except for checklists, these tools are quite problematic as detailed in Chapters 8 and 9.

According to a report issued by the Institute of Medicine (a branch of HHS),[11] not all "evidence-based" guidelines are valid. Furthermore, the report disclosed that the HHS has no mechanism to determine which guidelines are valid and which are not. Since financial incentives generally involve compliance with evidence-based guidelines, pay-for-performance bonuses won't improve care if the guidelines are not valid. Indeed, compliance with invalid guidelines may harm patients.

For example, venous thromboembolism (VTE: leg and lung vein clots) is one of the nine hospitalization-related adverse events targeted by the HHS' Partnership for Patients program. It occurs more commonly in patients with certain risk factors. The HHS refers to an "evidence-based" VTE guideline that recommends that physicians order anticoagulant drugs as prophylaxis (e.g., heparin injections) against the development of VTE for hospitalized patients with the risk factors.

I challenged the validity of that guideline in a peer-reviewed medical journal publication.[12] HHS leaders, drug companies, and anticoagulation experts have not rebutted my data and conclusions. Others have also questioned the evidence-basis for anticoagulation prophylaxis of hospitalized patients.[13, 14]

As of January 1, 2014, the American Academy of Orthopaedic Surgeons stopped mandating anticoagulant drugs as the only effective prophylaxis of patients undergoing joint replacement procedures, and endorsed aspirin (a much weaker blood thinner) as adequate venous thromboembolism prophylaxis.[15] A review of anticoagulant prophylaxis for patients in medical wards of hospitals found no benefit to this practice.[16] However, the HHS anticoagulant prophylaxis guideline linked to pay-for-performance evaluations remains.

We need to reduce preventable deaths and complications in hospitalized patients. However, forcing physicians to slavishly follow often flawed clinical treatment guidelines *is not the answer*. Nor will it make patients safe to capriciously expose to public scrutiny a relatively small subset of the estimated 8 million errors per year made by physicians and other health care professionals. In a very arbitrary fashion, this will damage the careers of some doctors without changing underlying problems leading to errors.

One component of how to make health care safer is for us to find strategies to address the underlying health care financing system that rewards excessive hospitalizations and unnecessary patient days in hospital (Chapter 20). Unnecessary days in hospital lead to avoidable errors and patient injuries. Inexplicably, the HHS Partnership for Patients program description makes no mention of strategies to reduce patient days in hospitals to improve care and decrease adverse events.

The Threat of Malpractice Suits Fails to Reduce Medical Errors

Studies show that there is no significant value of the threat of malpractice litigation in reducing errors or leading to systemic improvement in patient safety.[17] Indeed, our current malpractice tort system has presided over a high rate of preventable injuries for decades. Medical malpractice convictions have been falling steadily for the past decade and in 2012 were the lowest ever recorded.[18] However, this doesn't mean that the number of medical errors is going down.

In a large study conducted at Harvard, investigators found it is difficult to isolate individual failures from "system" failures.[19] While individual failures contribute to most errors, they are usually precipitated by or amplified by systems failures. Our tort system disproportionately focuses on individual failures.

For instance, a physician may order the wrong dose of a medication. The nurse sending the prescription should note the error and tell the doctor. If the nurse doesn't spot the error, the pharmacist should call the doctor and discuss the prescription. If the wrong dose of the medication isn't identified by the nurse or pharmacist and the wrong dose of the medication arrives on the ward, another nurse who distributes medications to patients might note the error and tell the doctor. If the patient takes the wrong dose of the medication because no one told the doctor of the error, the doctor is liable for medical malpractice.

Paradoxically, the threat of malpractice suits may perpetuate system faults that lead to errors. Due to the prospect of a devastating malpractice suit on the career of a doctor or other health care worker, the tort system itself contributes to hiding of errors by some or all members of medical teams. When errors are hidden, they are not openly discussed by the whole medical team. Consequently, opportunities to change the system to enhance patient safety may be lost.

Our Medico-Legal System Does Not Serve Patients Well

The medical malpractice system is capricious and arbitrary. It generally benefits affluent people who suffer serious adverse events—not moderate injuries affecting poor people. Seniors and disabled people are most often the victims of malpractice because they have more medical procedures than young healthy people. However, retired people and poor people with disabilities from adverse medical outcomes do not have as many economic damages as high-paid workers do. While obstetrician-gynecologists pay high insurance premiums because birth injuries are costly, gerontologists pay very low premiums.[20]

If a patient does win a malpractice judgment, it typically takes 5–10 years to receive the money. Seniors may die before compensation arrives. The courts, attorneys, administration, and insurance company overhead consume an average of 55% of medical malpractice insurance payments.[21]

Patients and taxpayers, not doctors and other health care workers, ultimately pay for medical malpractice with higher medical costs and with unnecessary medical procedures (defensive medicine—discussed later). Access to medical care may also be adversely affected by high medical malpractice premiums. Specialists might avoid practicing medicine in states with high malpractice premiums or unfavorable malpractice regulations. High-tech specialists utilizing risky procedures may also avoid high-liability-risk patients due to concerns about being sued.

Currently, patients injured and rendered disabled by medical interventions deemed to be not as a result of malpractice must suffer the economic losses without compensation. However, the courts are often wrong in attributing blame, and, in a civilized society, any people with disabilities need compensation for their lost capacity to work.

Patients, health care workers, and taxpayers are all victimized by the current medical malpractice system.

Problem Doctors Often Not Identified

Hospitals want to avoid alerting the government to potential dangers that might threaten the reputation of their medical institutions and practitioners. A Public Citizen Health Research Group report detailed how hospitals minimize the discipline of doctors for negligent or unethical behavior.[22] The report stems from analyzing independent studies and government reports from the National Practitioner Data Bank (NPDB). Congressional legislation requires hospitals and managed care organizations to submit reports to the NPDB about any disciplinary action that adversely affects a physician's hospital privileges for more than 30 days. However, in the first 20 years that the NPDB existed, 49% of U.S. hospitals never submitted a single report. Compared with predictions by the federal government and health care industry, only one-eighth to one-sixteenth of hospital disciplinary action reports have been filed.[23]

Due to the influence of the American Medical Association (AMA), the NPDB is not accessible by the public. Given that we have a capricious and error-prone medico-legal system and relatively few disciplined physicians are in the databank, public availability of the NPDB would not make us safer. Indeed, many practitioners not guilty of medical malpractice may well be in the NPDB. An unknown number of doctors convicted of malpractice in "sham peer-review" hearings (discussed later), appear in the NPDB.

Reducing medical errors, which is the purpose of medical malpractice litigation and much of government regulation of health care, needs to be approached very differently than with lengthy and expensive litigation in our error-prone court system.

Defensive Medicine

Policy experts define "defensive medicine" as ordering unnecessary or low-yield tests and treatments and referring patients to specialists out of concerns about malpractice suits. A study in Pennsylvania found that 9 of 10 specialists that performed high-risk procedures reported defensive practices.[24] These included over-ordering of diagnostic tests, unnecessary referrals, and avoidance of high-risk patients. Physicians more likely practiced defensive medicine if they faced tighter reimbursement rates, more assertive patients, greater administrative burdens, or increased likelihood of being dropped by liability insurers.

Defensive medicine reinforces itself. The more that physicians order low-predictive-value tests and give or prescribe aggressive treatments for low-risk conditions, the more likely such practices are to become the legal standard of care in court cases.[25]

Estimates of the cost of defensive medicine vary widely. Political leanings seem to color the figures. Table 1 shows some published estimates adjusted for inflation to 2016 dollars when personal health care is projected to cost about $3.3 trillion.[26]

Table 1. Estimated costs of defensive medicine in 2016

Authorities estimating the cost of defensive medicine	Cost estimate for defensive medicine
The Center for Medical Consumers[27]	Negligible cost[a]
U.S. Department of Health and Human Services[28]	$40 billion
Dr. Michelle Mello and colleagues from Harvard[29]	$60 billion
The American Medical Association[30]	$125–$225 billion
Former Secretary of Health and Human Services Tommy G. Thompson[31]	$133 billion
Drs. Daniel Kessler and Mark McClellan[32]	$164 - $295 billion
The libertarian/conservative Pacific Research Institute[33]	More than $260 billion

In addition to physician malpractice cases, suits over faulty medical devices and complications of drugs drive up medical costs with relatively little of the money going to the injured people. We need reforms also regarding suits against medical devices and drugs. These suits are expensive, they add to the cost of drugs and devices, and they do little or nothing to contribute to patient safety.

a   The Center for Medical Consumers and The New York Public Interest Research Group statement: "Liability concerns have a relatively small effect on practice patterns . . . some so-called 'defensive medicine' may be good medicine—averting unnecessary patients' injuries."[27]

Following Guidelines as Protection from Lawsuits

In a speech to the American Medical Association in June 2009, President Obama noted that too many doctors order unnecessary tests and treatments only because they believe it will protect them from a lawsuit. His solution: "We need to explore a range of ideas about how to put patient safety first, let doctors focus on practicing medicine and encourage broader use of evidence-based guidelines."[34] President Obama's answer to the medical malpractice issue is to provide a safe harbor for doctors that follow evidence-based guidelines. Anyone who could demonstrate that he has followed the recommended course for treating a specific illness or condition could not be held liable.

However, as noted in Chapter 8, the benefits to patients of many tests and treatments in medical practice are *controversial*. Universally recognized "evidence-based medicine guidelines" do not exist for the majority of medical interventions in common use today.

Where evidence-based clinical guidelines exist, research suggests that doctors follow them only about half of the time.[35] In one study, about half of best practices recommendations published in elite peer-reviewed medical journals were found to be invalid within 5-1/2 years.[36]

To put it mildly, clinical guidelines applicable to all U.S. practitioners offer no panacea to prevent unjust lawsuits.

Sham Peer Reviews

As mentioned in the introduction, my former employer, the L.A. County Department of Health Services administration, targeted me as a whistleblower and retaliated with an unfounded malpractice allegation. They fired me in 1998 and I lost my medical license permanently because of one medical malpractice conviction by an administrative law judge—the price of whistleblowing.

I'll briefly tell the back story, which was alluded to in the Introduction. The hospital administration closed my highly successful Pain and

Palliative Care Service in 1995 amid a financial crisis in which L.A. County + USC Medical Center faced possible closure. At that time, patients writhing in pain in acute-care hospital beds because of poor palliative treatment were a cash cow for the hospital.

Excellent home hospice treatment for the pain and distressing symptoms of cancer and AIDS patients cost the hospital an estimated $9 million in lost Medicaid revenue per year. The hospital financial bottom line won out over pain relief for cancer and AIDS patients.

After the closure of the Service, I submitted over 80 incident reports detailing cases with poor pain and symptom management to my hospital's quality-assurance committee. None were ever investigated.

My op-ed piece in the *L.A. Times* on the dysfunctional Medicaid reimbursement system that overpaid for inpatients and underpaid for outpatients marked me as a clear whistleblower.[37] My letter to the Chief of the Health Care Financing Administration threatening a *qui tam* (whistleblower's) law suit over wasted taxpayer money and patient harm from the Medicaid reimbursement system was ignored by the U.S. Department of Health and Human Services and the 11 legislators that I carbon-copied.[38] Meanwhile, the administration almost immediately retaliated by placing me on administrative leave and subsequently dismissing me.

The hospital administration accused me of malpractice in a single clinical case: My team of medical residents admitted a man to my internal medicine inpatient service with alcoholism, liver failure, advanced tuberculosis, and a deep venous thrombosis (leg vein clot). I assessed that his risk of dying of lung emboli (thromboses or clots from the leg travelling to the lungs) to be less than the danger of dying from bleeding from the blood thinners heparin and warfarin (Coumadin, the active ingredient in rat poison). Accordingly, I stopped the anticoagulant drugs. Unfortunately, he died of emboli in his lungs about a week later.

I said that I was sorry that the man died, but maintained that his high risk of bleeding justified my decision to stop the anticoagulants. The details of the case can be found in my book, *Whistleblower Doctor—The Politics and Economics of Pain and Dying*.[39]

My case falls into the category of "sham peer review." According to the Alliance for Patient Safety, "Sham peer review is the use of the peer review system to discredit, harass, discipline, or otherwise negatively affect a physician's ability to practice medicine or exercise professional judgment for a non-medical or patient safety related reason."[40]

Partially in recognition of sham peer-reviews, the California State Legislature called the medical peer-review system "broken." A report on the peer review system commissioned by the California State Legislature observed in 2009,[41]

> The present peer review system is broken for various reasons and is in need of a major fix, if the process is to truly serve the citizens of California... This report cites the inconsistencies in the way entities conduct peer review, select and apply criteria (e.g., implicit vs. explicit review), and interpret the law... One major recommendation is to re-design the peer review process, including establishing a separate, independent peer review organization that has no vested interest in the review outcome, except the protection of the public.

My petition to the California Medical Board for license reinstatement in 2009 was denied because I refused to admit that I made a medical error in stopping the blood thinner in the venous thrombosis case. If I had made that admission as recommended by the prosecuting Deputy Attorney General and my own attorney as well as the Superior Court Judge, I would have committed perjury. My appeals of the decision to the California Supreme Court were denied.

This personal experience with the medical malpractice system has helped me understand the problems with the tort-based legal process of compensating patients harmed by medical interventions. Both physicians and patients are unfairly treated while lawyers and legal system bureaucrats profit handsomely. Legislators remain clueless.

Comprehensive medical malpractice system reform must fix this injustice to physicians and other health care workers.

Malpractice Reform Should Promote Patient Safety

Physician groups, hospital administrators, insurance companies, the AMA, and conservative politicians talk about a "malpractice insurance crisis," highlighting excessive payments for non-economic damages, frivolous lawsuits, high malpractice premiums, and defensive medicine. These are all issues of concern. However, the bigger crisis is about a medical culture that allows too many iatrogenic (doctor and health care system caused) injuries to patients. Uncapping medical damages lawsuit awards and safeguards against frivolous lawsuits will not reduce medical errors. Reforms should go beyond improving the accuracy of liability determinations and cost control. Clinical practice changes designed to prevent risk of injury and improve patient safety need to be the focuses of malpractice reform.[42]

Since physicians largely control patient care, they can play a critical role in developing systematic approaches to reduce patient injuries. For physicians, better communication with patients and others requires individual effort. However, physicians also need the support of a system that fosters good communication. Reforms must encourage the cooperation of doctors and allied health workers to act collectively to find ways of making care safer.

I agree with patient safety experts who believe that effective malpractice system improvement requires fixing medical organizational systems rather than solely blaming individuals for adverse events.[6, 43] Since medical systems, as much or more than individuals, tend to be at fault in medical errors, it makes sense to shift liability from individuals to medical systems.

Grand Bargain #11: ACCs to Adopt an "Enterprise Liability" Malpractice System to Reduce Medical Errors

As discussed in Chapter 1, enterprise liability will be the legal system to handle medical malpractice allegations with ACC-based care.

Enterprise liability means the responsibility for patient safety lies with the enterprise (e.g., ACC) and not solely with the individual physician or allied health care worker. [44]

Each error or unfortunate patient outcome will become an opportunity to help spur the needed corrections in the system of health care delivery. In most cases, ACCs will consider medical errors "system problems" rather than errors caused solely by an individual practitioner. ACC physicians and other health care providers will need no malpractice insurance for services authorized by ACCs. All payments for medical malpractice occurrences will be the responsibility of the ACCs.

Enterprise liability will give each staff member of each ACC a stake in ensuring that all its PCPs, specialist consultants, and other ACC care providers are competent and diligent. It will assure that entire ACC organizations work collaboratively to reduce risks of harm to patients. Medical errors will be deterred because all ACC health care providers and other ACC stakeholders will have the analysis procedures in place to find and correct clinical practice system errors.

For physicians and other health care workers that willfully harm patients or are deemed hopelessly incompetent or negligent by coworkers, ACC staff will have every reason to fire them and report them to legal authorities.

To take enterprise liability a step further, economic damages will be allocated for adverse outcomes causing disability without adjudicating whether the problem was due simply to the risk of the intervention or due to malpractice. Ascertaining blame takes a lengthy, expensive, and error-prone litigation process that Grand Bargains-based enterprise liability avoids.

ACCs will hire legal teams to mediate prompt and fair compensation to patients for serious harm from medical interventions. Enterprise liability will eliminate individual malpractice insurance, allowing about $11 billion projected to be paid by health care workers in 2016[21] to be used instead by the ACCs to compensate injured patients.

Currently, about 65% of malpractice payouts go toward the cost of future medical care.[45, 46] With ACC-based malpractice system reform, compensation to patients for future medical costs will be unnecessary. ACCs will continue to provide health and safety-net care after any adverse event.

Indemnity payments for economic losses for the disabled comprise the remaining roughly 35% of malpractice payouts. For justice in determining indemnity payments, it will be less expensive and more beneficial for patients to rely on the judgment of the PCPs of injured patients and ACC-appointed expert advisors in this area rather than engaging the expensive, highly fallible, bureaucratic legal system. Lawyers specializing in health law employed by ACCs will have much more gratifying careers helping injured people than litigating cases in the courts.

Of the approximately 8 million patients in 2016 that will be affected by medical errors,[7] less than 15,000 are projected to receive payouts through malpractice litigation (0.2%). In 2012, total malpractice payouts totaled $3.1 billion. This indicates that we are grossly under compensating people that are injured by medical interventions, whether the injuries are due to malpractice or bad luck.

With ACC-based enterprise liability reform, I estimate that ACCs will be compensating injured patients for financial losses (excluding non-economic and punitive damages and the future cost of health care) with roughly $40 billion in 2016,[19, 21, 45] [b] almost 40 times the amount now paid to patients awarded malpractice judgments.[c] With enterprise liability combined with ACC administration of public disability benefits

b   Estimated economic cost of adverse events from medical interventions: $3.1 billion (i.e., payouts due to malpractice in 2012[18]) x 0.35 (about 65% of payouts for future health care and 35% are for economic costs[45, 46])/0.002 (about 0.2% of malpractice victims receive payouts[9, 47, 48]) / 0.4 (about 40% of adverse events are cause by medical malpractice[7]) x 0.03 (cases not litigated generally involve less severe injuries: estimating 1/30th as severe) = $40.7 billion
c   Current payouts to patients that win malpractice judgments: $1.09 billion ($3.1 billion total malpractice payouts x 0.35 (35% goes for patient indemnity payments) = $1.09 billion). $40.7 billion (total economic cost of medical adverse events) / $1.09 billion (current indemnity payments) = 37.7 (i.e., we should be compensating malpractice victims more by about a factor of 40).

(Chapter 19), this compensation for economic losses of ACC members will be equitably allocated to patients who suffer serious adverse events due to medical interventions whether caused by malpractice or not.

For ACC-authorized drugs and medical devices, the responsibility for product liability will be shifted from pharmaceutical companies and medical device makers to the ACCs. Class action settlements in the billions of dollars against drug companies (e.g., Merck for Vioxx, a pain pill that caused heart attacks) will be eliminated.

Concerns about losing prescriptions from ACCs will serve better than fear of product liability suits to reduce the marketing of drugs and devices that do more harm than good to patients. The savings to pharmaceutical companies and medical device providers will also be passed along in lower drug and device costs.

ACCs will select mediators (likely attorneys specializing in health care) to recommend payments to patients for economic losses. Performance of these mediators will be documented by the ACC-affiliated financial services companies and scrutinized by patients, providers, and any other interested health care stakeholders. Unsatisfied patients could appeal the decisions to civil courts of law.

As part of the selection process of choosing ACCs, patients could evaluate the records on allocations of funds for economic losses due to adverse medical events.

For additional protection against economic losses from accidents and illnesses, people with high incomes and high-spending patterns could protect their incomes with additional private disability insurance as they do now.

With enterprise liability-based malpractice reform and the decentralization of clinical practice guidelines (Chapter 9), wasting money and resources on defensive medicine will not serve ACCs, their staffs, or patients. In ACCs, cultures will develop fostering the avoidance of the ordering of unnecessary medical interventions as defensive medicine. This will improve patient care and save lots of money.

The elimination of both provider malpractice premiums ($\approx$ \$11 billion/year) and defensive medicine (> \$50 billion/year) will be more than enough to compensate all people for economic losses due to medi-cal malpractice ($\approx$ \$40 billion). With the integration of unemployment and workers' compensation benefits and public disability insurance funds (Chapter 19) together with enterprise liability, social-safety-net funds will be allocated much more efficiently.

Practicing medicine through patient-centered medical homes within ACCs under a system of enterprise liability will also remove the financial incentives for sham peer-reviews. Whistleblowers that expose poor-quality care will not be targeted for retaliation by other health care workers or ACC managers. Nor will exceptionally competent doctors be targeted in sham peer reviews by mediocre competing physicians.

Enterprise Liability will Help ACCs Reduce Patient-Days in Hospital and Reduce Errors

As a hospital-based practicing physician for 25 years, I can attest that hospitals are life-saving for many patients with major trauma, high-risk pregnancies, and many other conditions. However, hospitals are also dangerous places. To prevent adverse events and errors in hos-pitals, we must hospitalize fewer people and for shorter periods of time.

The current hospital bed utilization rate per capita is about half that of 40 years ago. Consequently, the hospital error and injury rate is down. Reducing hospital bed utilization by half again would pre-dictably reduce hospital-related adverse events and errors significantly while decreasing overall health care costs.

Why do patients spend unnecessary days in hospitals?

With the current business model of hospitals, physician "pay-for-performance" means filling as many beds as possible with insurance-reimbursable patients. While no hospital administrator wishes harm on patients, adverse events occurring to unnecessarily hospitalized patients increase hospital revenues. In the hospital business, more er-rors injuring patients is a side effect of financial incentives to maximize profits by filling beds.

Financial incentives drive the pattern of excessive patient days in hospital. Hospitals compete to fill beds. About 200 million acute care days in hospital in 2016 are projected to cost over $1 trillion ($5000/day on average).[26, 49] Hospitals that fill fewer beds than their competitors will go out of business.

For example, medical treatments in hospital in the last year of life for patients with advanced chronic illnesses (e.g., cancer and heart failure) will consume about 30% of Medicare spending (about $200 billion projected for 2016[26, 50]). Much of this "care" in a hospital is unnecessarily burdensome for patients. In many of those cases, hospitalizations could be avoided by earlier access to palliative care/hospice programs (Chapter 5). In addition, managing acute exacerbations of chronic medical problems with "home hospital care" has been shown to be safe, effective, and less expensive (Chapter 20). Patients and family members often prefer it over hospitalization.[49]

With member-owned ACCs responsible for hospitalization policies, there will be incentives for more judicious use of days in hospitals and for the development of alternatives to hospitalization. This will markedly decrease acute care patient days in hospital, improve quality of care, reduce errors, and save money.

Grand Bargain #13 Part 1: ACCs to Provide Members Basic Prepaid Legal Services

ACC-based overall legal system reform will begin by providing prepaid basic legal services for ACC enrollees funded by risk-adjusted government welfare money and savings from administrative efficiencies. ACCs will hire lawyers, paralegals, and others charged with advising clients about legal matters. At the discretion of the ACC legal experts, ACCs may represent members in filing or responding to legal suits.

Whenever possible, disputes will be kept out of the courts. The emphasis for ACC legal teams will be on mediation, fairness, justice, and minimizing legal costs.

Organically restructuring of the overly intrusive legal system will be made much more possible in conjunction with other Grand Bargains-based reforms. These include health care enterprise liability, social services, disability allocations through ACCs, ACC facilitated employment (Chapter 12), and financial counseling (Chapter 24). Reforms in each of these bureaucratic, dysfunctional sectors of society will lead to the reduction of the associated legal system ramifications.

With Grand Bargains-based reform, the proposed prepaid legal services provided by ACCs will reduce the responsibilities now assumed by the U.S. Department of Justice (DOJ) and avoid the need for much DOJ work. For example, prepaid financial counseling services by ACCs will reduce the incidence of financial and mortgage fraud, which the DOJ prosecutes.

These basic ACC legal services will magnify the benefits of comprehensive health system reform, integrated social services, expanded job opportunities, and ACC financial counseling services. These ACC legal services integrated with other human services will decrease overall litigation. Consequently, the overall litigation costs in the U.S. can be expected to drop over a few years from 2% of GDP currently to about 1% of the GDP as in other developed countries. Tens of thousands of redundant legal system workers will be assisted to find other jobs by their ACCs (Chapter 12).

ACCs will compete with each other, in part, on the performances of their legal services departments.

Prison Overpopulation Crisis

Being "tough on crime" has aided politicians in getting elected fairly consistently over the past three decades. Consequently, the prison population in the U.S. has gone from about 460,000 inmates in 1980 to 2.2 million in 2012.[51] The overall cost of incarceration has skyrocketed from about $5 billion in 1980 to $84 billion projected for 2016.[52] The U.S. now leads the world in the proportion of the population in jail.

Nonviolent drug offenders account for about half of convicts.[53] Financial crimes, such as writing bad checks, have also landed more people in jail in recent years.

Because mental illness treatment is difficult to access for many, about 40% of mentally ill U.S. residents have been in jail at some time in their lives. About 16% of currently incarcerated people have been diagnosed with major mental illnesses. About three times as many mentally ill people are in jail than in psychiatric hospitals.[54]

An Urban Institute study found that almost 70% of males released from prison will return to prison.[55] The factors leading to such a high recidivism rate include the individual's social environment of peers, family, and community as well as the state-level policies toward felons. Poor educational achievement, abuse in childhood, substance abuse, and mental illness increase the risk.

Even in non-recessionary times, ex-convicts face tremendous challenges in returning to society. People can legally discriminate against ex-cons in housing, employment, and education. Felons are not eligible for college Pell Grants from the government.

In California, the cost of incarcerating people now exceeds the funding for higher education and impedes the state's properly funding education. It also detracts from dealing with health and social-safety-net services for the poor. Prison guard unions exert considerable power over state legislators—longer sentences increase their pay and job security.

Grand Bargain #13, Part 2: ACCs to Foster Prison System Reform

To break the cycle of incarceration, parole, and re-imprisonment, the ACC legal teams will monitor and intervene with their clients that get in trouble with the law. For people without financial resources, the ACC legal teams will represent clients in court. For this purpose, public defender funds (federal: about $1 billion[56] and state and local: about

$2.2 billion[57]) will be shifted to the ACCs. Public defenders and affiliated staff members will move to employment with the ACC legal teams. Should their clients be convicted of crimes and go to jail, the ACC legal teams will, if appropriate, advocate for their early release.

Once an ACC enrollee convicted of a crime is released from prison, the ACC teams for social-safety-net services, education, and legal and financial services will assist him/her in reintegrating back into society. As with other ACC enrollees, ex-convicts will be offered shelter, food, employment, educational opportunities, substance abuse treatment, and mental health therapy as required.

ACCs need financial incentives to prevent their members from committing crimes and to decrease the recidivism rate of members released from jail or prison. Sometime after the ideal roll out of Grand Bargains' reform in 2016 (if we are quick), I propose that ACCs administer the funding for the jails and prisons of the country. The projected cost of jails and prisons should be transferred from the federal, state, and local government in a risk-adjusted manner to the ACCs. Then ACCs will then be responsible for funding the cost of incarceration of all of their members in jail. This will give ACCs an immediate interest in working with the 12 million people that churn through the jail and prison system each year. It will be particularly important for the ACCs to help prevent re-incarceration for the approximately 700,000 people released from prison each year. Jails and prisons will bill ACCs for the time that each ACC member spends in jail or prison.

Even in the short run, it will cost more for the ACCs not to provide comprehensive crime prevention services. ACCs will compete on preventing crimes of members and on successfully reintegrating ex-convicts back into society. Consequently, they will focus on legal defense and crime prevention strategies. Over time, a lot fewer people will be locked up.

With comprehensive and integrated assistance for those convicted of misdemeanors and felonies, ACC-based reform will lead to major decreases in the prison recidivism rates. I conservatively estimate that the cost of prisons will fall by half over the next decade.

Redundant prison system workers will be assisted to find other jobs by their ACCs.

Summary and Conclusions

The tort system for medical malpractice is unfair, costly, slow, and error-prone. Shifting from Obamacare ACOs to ACCs with enterprise-liability medical-malpractice reform will foster the medical culture's changes needed to reduce medical errors and improve patient safety. Errors will be less likely to be hidden and more likely to be analyzed by ACC personnel to find the system-changes needed to prevent recurrences.

Enterprise malpractice liability reform will enhance the benefits of social services, workers' compensation, unemployment, and disability compensation. Consequently, ACC's will compensate an order of magnitude more injured people. It will also reduce litigation costs, speed the process of compensating the injured, and eliminate the perceived need for defensive medicine.

Administration of disability insurance by ACCs will ameliorate the economic impact of disabling injuries and illnesses however they are caused. This will make injured patients much less litigious. Rarely will they take advantage of the availability of appealing the ACC mediators' economic loss compensation decisions to civil courts. Payments will be prompt rather than delayed and uncertain. In addition to severe injuries, moderate injuries also will be more likely to be compensated. Access to physicians will not be compromised by high medical malpractice premiums. Indeed, no malpractice insurance will be needed by individual doctors.

Within ACCs, PCPs and disability-compensation mediators, rather than the courts, will determine the payments of economic damages for adverse events associated with medical interventions. Consequently, health system problems will be spotted and corrected to reduce future errors. Physicians and other health care workers with patterns of repeatedly hurting patients with medical errors will more easily be exposed. Those doctors and allied health workers that do not improve their quality of care will lose referrals and go out of business.

With ACCs being self-insured with enterprise liability, defensive medicine practices of physicians and other health care workers will plummet. Due to competition between ACCs, the overriding incentive will be to provide the needed care most efficiently. Tens of billions of dollars will be diverted from wasted services driven by malpractice fears. Instead, people will be given appropriate compensation for disabilities without respect to the cause. ACCs will compete in part on fairness and promptness of compensating people disabled by medical interventions or by other causes.

For civil and criminal law issues, prepaid legal services by ACC legal teams will help restore the integrity of our legal system while promoting economic justice. This will reduce current litigation expenses significantly. A reduced burden of litigation will increase freedom and stimulate private enterprise.

ACC services (health, social, financial, legal, educational, and employment) will be coordinated to reduce the risk of members committing crimes and becoming incarcerated. Imprisoned members will be supported with legal services by ACCs during incarceration and will be helped to reintegrate into society upon release.

A centerpiece of prison system reform will be for ACCs to take over the administration of financing the jails and prisons of the country. Once this is instituted, it will become in the economic best interests of all ACC members to support crime prevention and ex-convict rehabilitation.

ACCs will compete in part on quality of legal counseling and representation services. Legal, law enforcement, and prison system workers made redundant by legal system reforms will be assisted to find other jobs through their ACCs.

Chapter 12
Jobs, Jobs, Jobs

Thirty-one separately budgeted offices with almost 18,000 employees comprise the Employment and Training Administration of the Department of Labor. President Obama's projected budget request to Congress for the Department of Labor in 2016 request is $68 billion.[1] About 94% of the budget will go for aid to states, individuals, and businesses.[2] States also have employment development departments with big bureaucracies and budgets.

What has resulted from all these human resources and funds? Are all these programs going to help us reach full employment anytime soon?

No.

Government employment policy prescriptions have failed American workers, and the government itself predicts these policies will lead to unqualified disaster on the future employment front.[3a]

The Unsatisfactory Status of American Workers

Worker productivity in the U.S. has increased significantly because the same work now requires fewer workers and no increase in wages. Since the low point of the Great Recession in the second quarter of

---

a   The Bureau of Labor Statistics projects an employment increase of 15.1 million jobs from 2012 -2022.[3] If this estimate is correct, these 15.1 million new jobs over a decade will do nothing more than keep up with the 125,000 new workers reaching employment age and being added to the labor force each month. 125,000 new workers/ month x 120 months = 15.0 million new jobs

2009, the U.S. "economic recovery" has consisted of 85% corporate profits and 15% new hires and wage increases. Despite the fact that U.S. corporations now hold almost $2 trillion in cash, they have decreased contributions to employee health plans.[4]

During the Great Recession, a *New York Times*/CBS News poll found that more than half of the nation's unemployed workers cut back on doctor visits or medical treatments because they were out of work. While depression and/or anxiety affected almost half of the unemployed, only about one-quarter of jobless people sought help from mental health professionals. Children of unemployed patients had high rates of behavioral problems. Working-class people especially felt at risk of permanently falling out of their social class. The formal and informal safety nets have been overwhelmed. Of those receiving unemployment benefits, most said the amount did not cover basic necessities.[5] For many, the situation will not be better in 2016.

Absent borrowing money from future generations, the government is only able to increase public sector jobs when businesses are prosperous, hire more workers, and pay more taxes. After the $800 billion economic stimulus did not nearly enough to boost employment, future Franklin Delanor Roosevelt-style public sector jobs programs seem unlikely to work.

As before the Great Recession, tens of millions of able bodied people are out of the work force because they care for their children or their disabled parents or friends. In these especially hard times, should these workers be financially compensated? We need to have a better system of compensating people for caring work, without which society would crumble. As will be detailed, the Grand Bargains' jobs plan will pay these people.

Despite the bleak situation for many workers, there are ever more products and services needed throughout the economy. We need more farmers, construction workers, educators, health care professionals, information technology experts, entrepreneurs, and innovators. Thankfully, plenty of people remain ready to work.

The Business Climate for American Entrepreneurs Sucks

Increasingly, business owners perceive the government as burdensome. They object to government attempts to drive businesses to support the larger interests of society (e.g., increasing employment, minimum wage laws, worker safety protections, limitations on working hours, environmental safeguards, paid family leave, the employer mandate for health care, decent pensions, social insurance, etc). They understandably feel that, if businesses don't make money, they don't promote anyone's agenda.

The larger and more powerful corporations become, the more leverage they have to invest some of their profits to eliminate or weaken the intrusions of government into their operations. These investments generally take the form of lobbyists and political campaign contributions. The prizes they seek are subsidies, tax breaks, favorable regulations, government contracts, etc. Conservatives call these benefits to businesses by the government, "crony capitalism." Liberals call it, "corporate welfare."

Moving corporate operations to foreign countries to avoid the U.S. corporate income tax is another common strategy to enhance the financial bottom line (Chapter 21). Hiring low-wage undocumented immigrants gives a company an advantage. Guiding their low-wage employees to seek government welfare rather than to militate for higher wages may also help businesses to compete in the domestic and global markets.

We live in a globalized consumer economy with 70% of the U.S. GDP coming from sales of products and services. Until we all decide to radically reduce our personal consuming patterns, we need policies that allow businesses to grow and compete internationally for economic growth. Businesspeople don't feel that politicians understand this reality. Apart from subsidized energy consumption for growth, which is not recommended, businesses would be helped most to grow and compete by less taxation and fewer government regulations. Fewer obligations to provide employee benefits would also entice more business owners to invest in their companies and to hire more employees.

Despite businesses' having many obstacles, 70% of jobs created in our economy have been in small businesses.[6] U.S. businesspeople, entrepreneurs, inventors, and investors are among the best in the world and are eager to compete with anyone on a fair playing field. Naturally, they seek to foster and protect that fair playing field.

Grand Bargain #14: ACCs to Provide Members Jobs

Currently, only 72% of men and 58% of women over 20 years old participate in the labor force.[7] Grand Bargains' reform will greatly expand the number of workers in the labor force.

Each ACC will have a "department of employment." The task of members of ACC departments of employment will be to provide every work-ready ACC member the opportunity for a job. Realistically, 100% employment will never be achieved. However, an achievable goal will be 98% of a much expanded labor force[b] to be employed.

Financial resources that will be available to ACC jobs-departments to keep members employed will include the budget of the Employment and Training Administration and federal and state welfare budgets. Federal and state employment enhancement funds will be sent in risk-adjusted[c] block grants to ACCs (Chapters 10 and 19).

ACCs will also tap savings from reducing waste and inefficiency in health care and social services to create tens of millions of jobs and to stoke economic activity.

Grand Bargain #15: Raise Minimum Wage to $15/Hour

As mentioned in Chapter 1, a game-changing grand bargain to help workers and the economy will be to raise the minimum wage to $15

---

b   The civilian labor force consists of employed and unemployed people actively seeking work, but does not include any Armed Forces personnel. It also excludes people in institutions, retired people, and full-time students.
c   Risk-adjusted: more funding for poor people that wealthier people.

per hour (about \$33,000 in 2016). For employed people, supplemental welfare will no longer be needed.

To help businesses afford the increase in labor costs, the corporate income tax will be eliminated and employee benefits greatly reduced (Chapter 21). Instead, ACCs will provide the employee benefits.

In utilizing ACC funds to foster employment, ACC job-placement managers will need to consider the best interests of all stakeholders. These interests include enrollees needing jobs, businesses requiring workers, ACC members that consume the products and services of local businesses, taxpayers, and the local environment. As a source of labor and financial investment, ACCs managers will also have leverage with local businesses to incentivize them to produce health-promoting products and services. For instance, to attract workers and financial support from ACCs, fast food restaurants may need to shift to a more plant-based, less processed, more healthful cuisine.

To fulfill their mandates to assist all work-ready members to find employment, ACCs will begin by paying members for valuable and necessary work now being done for free. Long-term care providers of up to 10 million disabled and/or elderly people will receive income from their ACCs for the care they are already delivering on a voluntary basis for their relatives and friends (about \$330 billion in 2016, Chapter 6).[8]

Given the challenges with child care in the U.S., we should also consider helping parents cope financially.

The Status of Child Care in the U.S.

When my three daughters were young, my then wife stayed home to care for them. She continually searched for educational enrichment opportunities for the kids. The children went to piano lessons, soccer practice, children's theater, ballet classes, and many other activities. We joined a child care cooperative of about 25 families in our neighborhood. Many of the families also had a stay-at-home mother. We never paid for a baby sitter that I can remember, and our kids enjoyed visiting their young friends while we were gone. Our children benefited greatly by my then-wife's being able to stay home to care for them. Unfortunately for the current generation of children, few parents are able to afford to put child care ahead of a paying occupation.

For families with both parents working full-time, and for single-parent families, the challenge of child care is much more difficult than with families having one middle-class income and two parents. This can strain the budgets of young families and reduce funds for enriching children's educational and recreational activities. In an increasing number of families, the needs of children can take money from necessities like food, housing, and medical care.

Care of children is seriously undervalued in the U.S. The average wage for child care workers is $8.78 an hour.[9] A preschool teacher with a postgraduate degree and years of experience may earn only about $30,000 a year.

Paying parents has been suggested as a way to help low-income families meet living expenses and to recognize the importance, social worth, and value of child rearing.[10] It is also a way to stimulate the economy. Parents will have money for products and services, and they will tend to spend available money immediately.

A Grand Bargain for Kids: ACCs to Finance Child Care

As part of ACC-based health care and social services reforms, ACCs will administer funding for parents to care for their children. This will be a popular benefit with ACC members, and will improve health and social outcomes of children and their parents.

There are approximately 60 million children under 14 years old in the U.S.[11] I propose beginning with funding for 10 million full-time equivalent parenting jobs, costing about $330 billion in 2016.[d] Funding will come in part from risk-adjusted allocation of social services

---

d $33,000 per minimum wage job (including employer and employee Social Security taxes) x 10 million parenting jobs = $330 billion in 2016.

funds from the government to the ACCs, and part from health care cost savings.

ACCs of families with children could figure out the most efficient way of allocating the child care funds. Priority will probably be given to parents of children under 5 years old. Some families might form cooperatives like my family did and provide child care for each other. This would spread the child care income to more families.

With the funding for child care, ACCs will also have leverage to incentivize parents to provide healthful and high quality educational and recreational experiences for their children. ACCs could contract children's health experts to guide and monitor parents toward more healthful diets and exercise activities for children.

ACCs will compete, in part, on their innovativeness and fairness in allocating the funds for child care and the outcomes of the children and parents.

20 Million New Jobs in Energy, Agriculture, and Beyond

Shifting from income taxes to consumption taxes, particularly the taxes on freshwater (Chapter 21) and non-renewable energy (Chapter 22), will require the creation of millions of new jobs. More workers will be needed in the sectors of energy, agriculture (Chapter 13), infrastructure construction (Chapter 15), national security (Chapter 17), and business. The income generated and spent from these new jobs will foster additional secondary jobs in a virtuous cycle throughout the economy.

The National Technical Assistance and Research Leadership Center at the John J. Heldrich Center for Workforce Development at Rutgers University, together with the U.S. Department of Labor, estimated that nearly 4 million new jobs could be created in energy efficiency and alternative energy production in the U.S.[12] With the consumption tax on non-renewable energy (Chapter 22), renewable energy (solar, wind, biomass, etc.) will become cost competitive with fossil fuels and nuclear energy, spawning a new gold rush of business activity and employment.

With food production having to become much less energy-and water-intensive, more people will be needed to produce what we eat. Prompted by the taxes on freshwater and non-renewable energy, moving to a post-carbon sustainable future will require as many as 4 million more U.S. agricultural workers (Chapter 13).[13]

As will be discussed in Chapter 21, tax reform will provide $50 billion in 2016 to be invested in long-deferred infrastructure projects. This will employ at least 1 million construction workers (Chapter 15). Over the next decade, the goal will be to spend $3.6 trillion on bringing our infrastructure to 21st Century standards, in accordance with the analysis of the American Society of Civil Engineering.[14]

ACC members enhancing national security will require an initial investment of $50 billion to train and deploy development workers in Third World countries. This will employ at least 500,000 professional development workers from the U.S. in engineering, sanitation, public health, agriculture, education, and other professions in 2016. By the end of the next decade, foreign development aid should total at least $500 billion per year and employ 5 million U.S. workers (Chapter 17).

With the elimination of corporate income taxes and employee benefits other than Social Security, businesses will net over $800 billion more profit in 2016 to devote in part to hiring new employees (Chapter 21). Businesses already have about $2 trillion in reserves that could be invested in jobs that will increase profits. Considering that 60% of the retail costs of goods and services go to the wages of company employees, businesses will be positioned to launch a net hiring of about 20 million new workers, earning from the minimum wage to millions of dollars per year, averaging the mean U.S. wage of $47,000.[15e] The projected 2 million high earners in that group (10% of 20 million) will contribute substantially to income tax collections. The personal income

e   ($800 billion additional net profits in 2016 + $700 billion (half of repatriated corporate offshore tax sheltered assets (Chapter 21)) x 0.6 (60% of company income going to wages) / $47,000 per added worker (projected from Social Security's National Average Wage Index[15]) = 19.2 million new jobs

tax and Social Security payroll tax dividends of the new jobs created, and the added taxes from repatriating offshore tax sheltered funds, will be detailed in Chapter 21.

Disruptive Process of Moving to Full Employment

Using ACCs to facilitate full employment will involve shifting about one-third of the economy to ACCs (i.e., about $6 trillion in 2016, Chapter 21). This will potentially disrupt most businesses and workers in the country. At least 40 million existing jobs will be subject to moving from the government or corporate sectors to ACCs or being made redundant. Millions more workers will move to more satisfying new jobs paying more money. Some workers with the highest incomes may see drops in earnings due to less crony capitalism/corporate welfare and more competition in the marketplace. In the end, there will be a net increase of at least 40 million well-paying jobs.

Of about 21 million people projected to be employed in the $3.5 trillion health care industry in 2016,[16] perhaps 7 million will work in the approximately $1 trillion administrative and clerical areas of medicine. With Grand Bargains' market-based health care reform, many of these administrators will become redundant. However, they could be retrained by their ACCs to take other positions in health care and other fields.

These people should receive fair treatment and opportunities to train for other positions. Likewise, Grand Bargain-related downsizing of jobs in some economic sectors (e.g., finance, law, prisons, non-renewable energy, etc.) and increasing jobs in others (e.g., alternative energy, agriculture, infrastructure, national defense/foreign development assistance, child care, elder care, etc.) will cause disruptions. Many public sector workers (e.g., government agency administrators in health care and social services) will move to ACCs to do more satisfying work in similar fields that is more efficient and beneficial to clients.

Any health care and economic-reform proposal will face opposition. First, it must be clear to most people that the status quo is fast becoming not an option. People must understand that Grand Bargain-based reform will greatly help individual people, poor and rich, as well as the country. The transition won't be easy. To succeed, we will need diverse ACC leaders with innovative ideas that attract supporters and ACC members. People with markedly different ideas about the best way forward about health and human services will have "laboratories" of ACCs to try out their ideas.

One common sense way of creating jobs is for workers to work fewer hours per week. This will improve worker quality of life as well as increasing employment.[17, 18]

Reducing Annual Hours Worked per Worker

Government mandated shorter work weeks (i.e., 32–37 hours) have been successfully used in Europe to combat unemployment. Relative to Europeans, Americans are workaholics. In 2002, the average American worker spent 1815 hours on the job compared with less than 1500 hours in France and Germany.[19] If the average work week for the 146 million U.S. workers dropped from 1815 hours to 1650 hours with almost the same kind of work and quantity of work done (i.e., about halfway between the hours/working in Europe versus the U.S.), over 14 million jobs would be created.[f]

One obstacle to transitioning to a shorter work week is the high cost of health insurance to employers. It costs more than the minimum wage for a full-time worker to pay the average family's private health insurance premium.[20][g] But with ACC-based health care, this will no longer be an obstacle.

---

f   1815 hours/year/worker x 146 million workers/1650 hours/year/worker = 160.6 million workers: 160.6 million – 146 million = 14.6 million additional workers

g $19,584 projected for the average annual family premium in 2016[20, 21]/1815 hours per year = $10.16 per hour for health insurance. People earning the federal minimum wage ($7.25) can never afford private health insurance.

Some studies show that a four-day work week increases consumption and dynamizes the economy. It improves education of workers due to usage of the extra time to take classes and courses. Also, workers' health improves from less work-related stress and usage of the extra time for exercise. A shorter work week saves fuel used in transportation, reduces carbon-related emissions, uses less office lighting, and helps the environment. Studies have found that overall, productivity on per-hour basis increases with a shorter work week.[22]

Job sharing is another effective way for spreading the wealth while improving lifestyles of workers. Germany and the Netherlands have aggressively used job sharing in the Great Recession to avoid layoffs. In California, furloughs of government workers, although traumatic for many affected, have saved jobs while lowering the huge state government budget deficit.[23]

Moving the minimum wage to $15 per hour will make it possible for a minimum-wage worker to still live on $28,000 per year with a 36 hour work week.[h] ACCs, employers, and workers will be able to experiment with shorter work weeks.

Part-time Community Service Work for High School and College Students and Retired People

Families with high school age students have been under increased financial stress especially since the Great Recession.[i] Many high school students drop out of school to take low-wage jobs, out of real or perceived necessity. Poor, idle teenagers are more likely to get into drugs and gangs and have unintended pregnancies.

With Grand Bargain-based reform, ACCs will have an additional $50 billion from the new consumption taxes in 2016 to provide for

h   36 hours/week x 52 weeks/year x $15 /hour = $28,080 /year
i   In 2013, about 40% of high school aged children (about 6 million students) were eligible for food assistance at school, indicating that their families earned less than 185% above the poverty line ($38,200 for a family of four).[24, 25]

students wanting a college education without going into debt (Chapter 16). Partly with those funds, ACCs may:

- present teens with part-time paying work to help them remain in high school until graduation,
- offer motivated teens money towards tuition for college
- give young students alternatives to gangs and crime,
- ease the financial stresses of many poor families, and
- provide communities with an additional workforce for public service projects.

Public service projects for high school and college students might include:

- tutoring school children and/or adults,
- providing elder-care assistance,
- coaching children in athletics,
- planting trees,
- working on environmental restoration projects, and
- growing fruits and vegetables in urban community gardens.

Similarly, financial incentives at ACCs could allow retired seniors to work part-time on community service projects or in other employment.

Financial Processing Services for Part-time Workers to be Provided by ACCs

Just as is now the case, many people will have a number of part-time jobs. Currently, these are often in the informal economy, without Social Security deductions or employee benefits. With Grand Bargains' reform, ACC financial services departments will process the payroll for people with part-time jobs. This way Social Security, health care premiums, and pension deductions may be easily and accurately processed from all employers.

Whether part-time workers are ACC-employed or employed by private businesses, ACC financial services companies will be available to collect wages and withhold deductions. This will help members integrate their ACC health, social, and other human services into coherent long-term financial plans. With this ACC financial service, people will become cost conscious and frugal savers rather than over-consumers (Chapter 24).

Health Care Jobs with Grand Bargains-Based Reform

The physician workforce will increase by at least 30% with Grand Bargains reform (Chapter 19). Direct practice PCPs will have much more time to spend with each patient compared with now (Chapter 3). Consequently, PCPs will need to send fewer referrals to specialists. Specialists will probably perform fewer high-tech procedures. Fees of specialists will drop along with the hours of administrative work required (Chapter 20). The distribution of the physician workforce to the inner city and rural areas will be much improved because funding for health care will not depend on the patients' income.

ACC-based reforms will significantly alleviate our current nursing shortage. Reducing the administrative burden of nurses dealing with insurance companies alone will free up many nurses to care for patients. With ACCs having the resources to play roles in health care provider training, more slots in schools of nursing will also be created (Chapter 19). Public funding for PCP nurse practitioner training will enable more nurses to become PCPs.

Health care providers will have increased cost-consciousness about ordering expensive and possibly unnecessary "imaging studies." Consequently, some laboratory and imaging technicians (x-ray, MRI, ultrasound, etc.) may need to retrain for other work.

The medical insurance industry will undergo a major transformation involving retraining for most of its employees (Chapter 18). This will not involve a significant gain or loss of workers. The new roles for insurance company workers in ACC-affiliated financial services companies will leave these people more secure and with a much-improved public image. However, insurance company executives will likely see downsized salaries because of free-market pressures of competing to work for ACCs. Investments in ACC-affiliated financial services companies will not be needed. These financial services companies will not be traded on the stock markets.

ACC-affiliated financial services companies will not be underwriting and assuming risk but rather distributing funds as prescribed by ACC physicians and managers. The ACC-affiliated financial services companies will be doing processing of requests for payments for products and services. Bookkeepers and accountants will be needed to keep track of funds being received from government block grants and from patient premiums as well as money going out to health and human services providers.

For example, say Ms. Brown works for a medical insurance company, determining which medical treatment claims to approve and which to deny based on the terms of the policies. Ms. Brown might move to a job with an ACC-affiliated financial services company handling the distribution of payments to health care vendors as directed by ACC physicians and managers. Rather than deciding whether and how much to pay health care providers, she would implement payment of the amount designated by the ACC decision maker.

Say Mr. Smith works for a medical insurance company as an actuary,[j] determining how to structure medical plans in terms of premiums, co-payments, deductibles, etc. Mr. Smith might move to work as an actuary for ACCs. His job would then be to determine the estimated costs of implementing different options for benefit packages of medical and

---

j   An actuary analyzes the financial consequences of risk. Actuaries, working in the medical field, use mathematics, statistics, and financial theory to study risks of future events such as injuries, disease, and death. Actuaries may work for insurance companies or other businesses that need to manage financial risk.[26]

social services. The analyses of Mr. Smith would be considered by the ACC members, staff, and other stakeholders in deciding the medical guidelines and benefits packages.

Within the constraints of new incentives for cost-effectiveness in health care, the pharmaceutical industry will be encouraged to innovate in the new ACC-centered health care environment. The increased emphasis on health promotion and palliative care (Chapters 4) and better approaches to evidence-based medicine (Chapter 8) will likely reduce the overall volume of medication consumed. However, randomized trial evidence of efficacy certified by the Food and Drug Administration (FDA) will be easier to accomplish since ACCs can be randomized to receive or not receive experimental drugs to offer patients (Chapter 6). Determinations of efficacy of experimental drugs will be faster than now because of more trial data and the collection of data on all health interventions and health outcomes (Chapter 8). Jobs in the pharmaceutical sector will depend ultimately on the value of their products to patients. With ACC-diet and exercise coaching and more health promotion options leading to better health and more personal responsibility, fewer drugs will be taken by the average person.

Millions of new health-related jobs will be created in the areas of health promotion (Chapters 4), palliative care/hospice (Chapter 5), alternative therapies (Chapter 6), and medical social services (Chapters 10). Because of the current shortages, training slots for physicians, nurse practitioners, and physician assistants will rapidly increase in number as will be discussed in Chapter 19. Especially considering the paid employment of 10 million caregivers for seniors and the disabled at home (Chapters 6 and 25), the health care workforce will grow substantially.

Grand Bargains' Reform Synergisms Will Reduce Poverty

More than half of personal bankruptcies in the U.S. are related to health care costs.[27] With universal ACC-based health insurance and much lower out-of-pocket health care expenses, health problems will no longer lead to bankruptcies.

People with adverse health outcomes due to any cause may lose the ability to work. Whether their injuries stem from medical malpractice or just bad luck, these people risk becoming financially destitute. The enterprise liability portion of Grand Bargains' legal system reform will support disabled people (Chapter 11). ACCs will have incentives to use their creativity and ingenuity to most effectively provide funds and services to those affected by disabling medical problems (temporary or permanent).

With the multiple integrated health, social, legal, and financial services provided by the ACCs to seniors and disabled people (Chapters 23-25), they will be much less likely to fall into poverty. If desired, seniors and disabled people will be provided part-time or full-time jobs by their ACCs. Consequently, retirements will be much more financially secure with ACC reforms.

Over 40% of children now meet family income requirements for government subsidized meals at school.[25] With ACCs able to pay parents for caring for their children, we will no longer have so many children in poverty who depend on school meals. ACCs will have financial incentives to assure that families can pay for healthy nutritious meals for their children at their schools and at home.

Permanent Homes for the Homeless

People with schizophrenia, post-traumatic stress (e.g., war veterans), and those affected with other severe psychiatric disorders are at increased risk of becoming homeless and ending up on suicide-watch hospital wards. Increasingly, social problems are at the root of homelessness—substance abuse, prolonged unemployment or sudden loss of a job, lack of affordable housing, domestic violence, frustration over sexual expectations, etc.[28]

Homelessness in the U.S. is a huge problem.[k]

A United Way study in Los Angeles followed four chronically homeless people for four years as they lived on the streets, and were monitored after social service agencies provided them with permanent housing. According to the study, emergency room visits went from 19 among all four homeless people to one, and drug/alcohol rehabilitation stints went from six to none. Incarcerations were eliminated.[32] [l] Based on this study, the authors calculated that providing permanent housing to a homeless person could save taxpayers $20,000 a year.

ACCs will find it not only the humanitarian thing to do, but it will be to the financial advantage of all their members to provide housing to those in need. Once homeless people are given shelter, ACCs will offer opportunities for job training, jobs, and educational enhancement, as well as counseling and rehabilitation related to substance abuse and mental illness.

Summary and Conclusion

Since the beginning of the Great Recession in December 2007, levels of unemployment worsened and then, if you believe Department of Labor statistics, substantially improved. However, income inequality and underemployment dramatically increased. Trillions of dollars in savings and investments have been lost from pensions and the portfolios of individuals. Millions more people are in poverty—many of whom are food-insecure.

Massive deficit spending to stimulate the economy and other government attempts to boost employment have been woefully ineffective. The federal government's own projections of future U.S. employment

---

k   Homelessness affects 840,000 people on any given night,[29] 2.5 to 3.5 million people each year and 7 million people at some time over a five year period,[30] and 12 million people at some point in their lives.[31]

l   Based on the 840,000 homeless people in the U.S. on a given night, taxpayers will save at least $17 billion per year by ACCs providing permanent homes to the homeless: 840,000 homeless people each night x $20,000 per year = $16.8 billion.

are dismal. All the while, corporate news coverage tends to celebrate any small employment gains, not taking into account larger structural unemployment.

Despite over $2 trillion in cash reserves, large corporations have not substantially increased hiring. The all-time highs in the stock market are not trickling down to workers. Small businesses struggle with government regulations, high business taxes, the employer mandate for employee health care, and uncertain demands for their products and services.

Neither government programs nor trickledown economics in the private sector has worked to generate sufficient jobs. A fundamentally different approach to job creation is needed.

Prime functions of ACCs will be to assure the productive employment of enrolled members, thereby preventing the health and social consequences of poverty. Flexibility and innovation in accomplishing these goals by the ACCs will be a great asset in adapting to current and future economic and environmental developments.

ACCs will pay for parents to care for their children. For frail elderly or disabled people, ACCs will employ 10 million family or friends as caretakers. The $3.6 trillion investment in infrastructure projects over the next decade (Chapter 15) will provide additional resources for construction businesses to hire millions of well paid workers. Employment in agriculture, energy, health care, and national defense/foreign aid will grow substantially. These jobs will transform lives, improve health and education outcomes, and stimulate the economy. With member input, ACC managers will be tasked with efficiently utilizing their financial and human resources to optimize employment while assisting members in obtaining the products and services that they consider essential.

Pluralism will prevail in ACC approaches to creating good, sustainable jobs. No two ACCs will do it the same way. Many tradeoffs, compromises, and employment strategy reassessments will occur. The reduction in the use of products and services subject to the new consumption taxes will displace workers. However, new jobs will be needed to provide additional products and services that contribute to health, environmental sustainability, and national security.

Disagreements between employers, employees, and consumers will occur. Some people may change ACCs over employment related disagreements. Grand Bargains-based reforms with the central role of ACCs will be a continual work in process.

To help businesses thrive and thereby hire workers, ACCs and their members will assume the cost of most employee benefits. ACCs will be responsible for health insurance, workers' compensation, unemployment insurance, retirement planning (i.e., Social Security and public sector pensions, Chapters 18, 19, and 23), and other human services. Employees will find it easier to move to more fulfilling jobs, since their benefits will be with their ACCs rather than with employers. For workers with multiple employers or part-time workers, ACC financial services companies will provide payroll processing services to assure the proper deductions for Social Security, health care premiums, and pensions. This will facilitate financial literacy education and coaching people to develop viable overall financial plans (Chapter 24).

The $15/hour minimum wage together with at least 40 million new jobs will assure economic sustainably and eliminate deficit spending. The $15/hour minimum wage will also provide an opening gambit in the strategy to break the impasse on immigration reform (Chapter 14).

ACC members dissatisfied with jobs provided by their ACCs could switch to other ACCs. ACCs that do not maximize the employment potential of enrollees will lose market share and risk going out of business.

ACCs will employ people to perform all necessary medical, social and other services for their enrollees. When there are demands for new products or services, ACCs will partner with employers and entrepreneurs to facilitate the creation of necessary jobs. ACC investments in businesses that employ their enrollees could go to potential employers in private businesses or nonprofit organizations. Innovation and experimentation will be encouraged.

Chapter 13
Food and Agriculture Policy Reform

Regarding our government's dysfunctional food policies in relationship to the health care reform debate, University of California Berkeley Journalism Professor Michael Pollan says it best: [1]

> Even the most efficient health care system that the administration could hope to devise would still confront a rising tide of chronic disease linked to diet. That's why our success in bringing health care costs under control ultimately depends on whether Washington can summon the political will to take on and reform a second, even more powerful industry: the food industry.

Food system problems are highly linked to health care system failures, increasing welfare spending, high unemployment, wealth inequality, and unsustainable consumption of energy and freshwater. Our corporate-agriculture, factory-farm system of food production utilizes cheap fossil fuels and unrestricted water to replace the jobs of millions of farm workers. This has been dressed up as progress.

Without food system reform, there will be no:

1. health care system reform,
2. reductions in chronic disease rates,
3. full employment,

4. energy independence, or

5. lasting improvement in the economy.

Optimizing the health of people depends on what foods we produce and eat, how we process those foods, and what agricultural methods we employ. We need interconnected, mutually-reinforcing reforms to improve the American diet.

The U.S. Government's "Healthy Diet": Bad Medicine

U.S. government nutrition experts from the National Institutes of Health (NIH) officially recommend the "Therapeutic Lifestyle Change Diet" (Table 1 below) for people at risk for developing coronary artery disease (i.e., everyone).[2] They claim that it reduces chances of chronic vascular disease and early death.

Table 1. The National Heart, Lung, and Blood Institute's
Therapeutic Lifestyle Change Diet[2]

Component	Recommendation
Calories (energy)	Adjust total caloric intake to maintain desirable body weight
Polyunsaturated fat	Up to 10% of calories
Monounsaturated fat	Up to 20% of calories
Saturated fat	Up to 7% of calories
Total Fat	25%–35% of calories
Cholesterol	Up to 200 mg per day
Carbohydrates	50%–60% of calories
Dietary fiber	20–30 grams per day
Protein	Approximately 15% of calories
Physical Activity	Include enough moderate exercise to expend at least 200 kcal per day

What is the evidence concerning the effectiveness of this Therapeutic Lifestyle Change Diet?

None.

The American Heart Association (AHA) diets conform to the Therapeutic Lifestyle Change Diet recommendations (i.e., 30% of calories as fat). The AHA step 1 diet calls for saturated fatty acids < 10% of calories and the AHA step 2 diet requires saturated fatty acids < 7% of calories. A pooling of all published reports of trials comparing regular American diets with AHA diets showed very small cholesterol-lowering patient-benefit with the AHA diets.[a] With data from the same studies pooled, these very small reductions in serum cholesterol were completely worthless in reducing morbidity or mortality of subjects on AHA diets versus those on regular diets.[4]

As part of the "Women's Health Initiative,"[5] a diet trial compared a more ambitious 20% fat, omnivorous[b] diet with a regular American diet. At the beginning of the trial, 74% of the women (ages 50–69) were overweight or obese and that changed negligibly after eight years in both groups.[6] Related to this finding, a review article in the journal *Current Opinion in Cardiology* about the Women's Health Study concluded: "Although the dietary modification trials did not show any significant reduction in the incidence of coronary heart disease, it is currently recommended to continue using a heart-healthy diet."[7]

Related to this conclusion is an adage attributed to Benjamin Franklin: "The definition of insanity is doing the same thing over and over and expecting different results."

In the prevention of degenerative chronic diseases of diet and lifestyle, the government has been more often the problem rather than the solution. As detailed in the documentary film, *Fed Up*, Big Food has repeatedly pushed the government to give out compromised health information.[8] The documentary makes the case that the U.S. Department of Agriculture (USDA) has a stronger allegiance to farmers than

a   27 studies involving 30,902 person-years of observation showed that the AHA Step 1 diet lowers total cholesterol by only 3% on average and the AHA Step 2 diet lowers it by 6%.[3]
b   Omnivorous diet: a diet that includes plants, meat, dairy, and eggs.

to the health of the public. USDA employees, probably with the best of intensions for improving public health, have been co-opted by food politics, government bureaucracy, and agribusiness money.

From a public health standpoint, the government-endorsed Therapeutic Lifestyle Change Diet and the diets that conform to its guidelines like AHA diets are worse than ineffective. They cause harm, because they keep many people from receiving potentially worthwhile dietary advice.

Even if government nutrition experts knew exactly what diet would be optimal to prevent diet-related chronic diseases, politics and food industry money would surely prevent them from leading Americans to adopt healthful diets. Too many powerful food related corporations would suffer financially.

For example, in the late 1970s, politics trumped food and nutrition experts assembled by the U.S. Senate Select Committee on Nutrition and Human Needs. After much deliberation, the Committee, led by Senator George McGovern, recommended that Americans adopt nutrient-rich diets that:[9]

- Increase consumption of complex carbohydrates and "naturally occurring sugars;" and
- Reduce consumption of refined and processed sugars, total fat, saturated fat, cholesterol, and sodium.

In order to achieve the above dietary recommendations for nutrient intakes, the Committee recommended that Americans:

- Increase consumption of fruits, vegetables, and whole grains;
- Decrease consumption of:
  o refined and processed sugars and foods high in such sugars;
  o foods high in total fat and animal fat, and partially replace saturated fats with polyunsaturated fats;
  o eggs, butterfat, and other high-cholesterol foods;
  o salt and foods high in salt; and

- Choose low-fat and non-fat dairy products instead of high-fat dairy products (except for young children).

Due to lobbying by agribusiness and the corporate food industry, these guidelines were never enacted by the government and politicians that endorsed them were discredited by a corporate food industry campaign.

Government Food Assistance for the Poor: Subsidizing Obesity and Chronic Diseases

In 2015 (and probably in 2016), the federal government is projected to distribute about $107 billion worth of food assistance for the poor (Food Stamps now called the Supplemental Nutrition Assistance Program, the School Lunch Program, the Women, Infant and Children Program, and others).[10] Food stamp recipients, with only about $3–$4 per day with which to eat, can only afford cheap, government subsidized junk foods. Instead, this money for those needing assistance should be used for healthful nutrition. However, food stamps will not pay for much of what the federal government or many independent food scientists recommend that Americans should be eating.

While the USDA funds a small program recommending that Americans eat five or more servings per day of fresh fruits and vegetables,[11] the government does not subsidize farms growing the fresh fruits, vegetables, beans (other than soy), nuts, and seeds needed for a healthful diet. Instead, it subsidizes sodas, processed flours, meats, dairy products, and extracted oils (canola, corn, soy, etc., for deep frying).

In 2004, Consumer Reports reported that the advertising budgets for the food, beverage, candy, and restaurant industry exceeded the communications budget for the USDA's "5 A Day" campaign (i.e., recommending eating at least five servings of fresh fruits and vegetables per day) by over 1000 to 1 ($11.3 billion versus $9.6 million).[12] Consequently, frugality with food purchases leads consumers to government subsidized, low-nutrient, high-calorie food choices rather than a healthful variety of fresh unprocessed plant-based foods. Pervasive media messages by food corporations reinforce those unhealthful but cheap choices.

Diet-related Diseases Linked to Government Food Commodities Subsidies to Farmers

The most common diet-related chronic diseases are type 2 diabetes, heart disease, stroke, obesity, and certain cancers (breast, prostate, ovary, colon, rectum, and pancreas). Nationally, we spend about three-fourths of the personal health care budget treating these and other preventable chronic diseases that are related to diet (about $2.5 trillion projected for 2016).[13]

For instance, over a lifetime, an average case of type 2 diabetes will cost more than $400,000 in medical products and services.[1] Every third person born since 2000 is projected to eventually come down with type 2 diabetes. Poor people receiving government food assistance bear the greatest risk. Sugar, salt, and saturated fat laden government food aid promotes type 2 diabetes. So Food Stamps appear to be as much an assault as a gift.

In the farm bill of 2013, the federal government allocated up to $30 billion per year for farm subsidies.[10] Topping the subsidy list were corn, wheat, and soy. When highly processed by big food corporations, these foods promote the common diet-related diseases. Corn is processed into high fructose corn syrup to sweeten sodas, pastries, candies, and other low nutrient, high calorie foods. Most corn harvested goes to feed animals like cows and pigs. The meats of these animals contain lots of artery-clogging saturated fat and cholesterol. While whole wheat and sprouted wheat baked foods have lots of fiber and vitamins, consumers buy mostly the cheaper refined white flour products with high calories and low fiber. Soy beans are processed into, among other things, hydrogenated oil used for deep frying potatoes and onions to make them into junk foods.

Fast food restaurants can offer cheap food (e.g., cheeseburgers, fries, and sodas) largely because of massive government subsidies to agribusiness for the ingredients. The minimum-wage laborers employed in these restaurants are also government subsidized by welfare programs that disproportionately support low-wage fast food employees.[14]

I'm giving my biased side of the great food debate. There are other views.

No Consensus on what Constitutes a Healthful Diet

The consensus among independent nutrition experts of all persuasions is that the USDA and HHS dietary guidelines for Americans are wrong. However, which specific errors exist in the guidelines remains highly debatable. For instance, Steven Malanga, a senior fellow at the libertarian-conservative Manhattan Institute, contends that the guidelines should never have recommended a reduction in the amount of meat and dairy products. He argues that medical breakthroughs—statin drugs, blood pressure pills, and bypass surgery—account for the decrease in heart disease in the last 40 years, not less meat and dairy food consumption. He attributes the guidelines' recommendation to replace fats with carbohydrates with causing our current epidemics of obesity and type 2 diabetes.[15]

I agree with his conclusion about refined carbohydrates (e.g., sugar and white wheat flour) causing obesity and type 2 diabetes. However, I disagree with his endorsement of meat and dairy products as heart healthy foods.

On the other hand, Vegetarian Resource Group nutrition experts, while praising the new guidelines' shift toward a more plant-based diet, complain that:

1. the emphasis on combining plant proteins should be eliminated since this is not a practical problem;
2. the guidelines err in implying that vegan diets increase the risk of fractures due to reduced calcium uptake; and
3. the guidelines do not recommend expanded vegetarian and vegan choices in the USDA "School Meals Program."[16]

These are but two examples of a wide spectrum of views about the optimal diet.

In order to reverse the massive epidemics of diet-related chronic diseases, we need a consensus on a way forward to improve the diets of Americans. We cannot depend on the USDA and HHS for guidance since they contributed to the diet-related epidemics. However, we don't all necessarily need to agree on what are the most healthful diets. So the necessary consensus about a way forward on preventing diet-related chronic diseases doesn't mean we all agree on the optimal diet.

How to Find the Most Healthful Diets Despite Strongly-Held, Diverse, Dietary Opinions

Pluralism in our opinions about optimal diets and dietary patterns can be used to help us to scientifically discover what really are the most healthful diets. However, we need to agree to employ evidence-based mechanisms to monitor and analyze the effects of various diets on the nutrition-related health outcomes of us all.

With Grand Bargains' reform, ACCs will promote different diets. Through our choices of ACCs, families should plan to adopt the most healthful diets according to their own interpretations dietary information. In essence, we will be setting up a huge ongoing observational study of our own diets and related health consequences (e.g., rates of obesity, diabetes, cancer, heart disease, etc).

Currently, USDA crop subsidies and food assistance to the poor foster the adoption of diets that are high in processed foods, heavy in saturated fat, salt, and sugar. The government's role should be to enact policies that level the financial playing field between differing dietary choices (i.e., plants, meat, dairy, refined sugar, processed or unprocessed food, etc).

Shift Governmental Agricultural and Food Subsidies Distribution Role to ACCs

The Grand Bargains' game-changer that can level the financial playing field is shifting the responsibility for administering the government subsidies to farmers and to poor people. Instead of the USDA issuing the subsidies, individual ACCs should do it. This way, each ACC can use its share of the food subsidies to encourage members to adopt the diets that they consider the most healthful (Chapter 19, Table 1).

ACCs controlling all food subsidies will greatly reduce economic disincentives to more healthful diets for U.S. residents. However, what exactly is the optimal diet will remain controversial. Given widespread disagreement about what constitutes a healthful diet, decision makers of individual ACCs should determine the diets to promote with educational campaigns, economic incentives, availability of urban farming cooperatives, farmers markets, etc.

With ACCs' assuming the responsibility and accountability for helping people avoid diet-related chronic diseases, many healthy diet promoting strategies will be tried. Compliance with the various recommended diets and the resulting health outcomes will be monitored. People will choose ACCs partly based on the diets and health-promotion strategies recommended along with the diet-related health outcomes of members.

ACCs will receive up to $30 billion per year now directed for farm commodity subsidies.[17] ACCs will also collect the USDA food assistance funds ($107 billion projected for 2015 for Food Stamps, school lunches, etc).[10] Possible ways that this money, together with health care insurance funds from ACC members, may empower ACCs to help members to improve their diets include:

1. boosting the availability of fresh produce from farmers' markets,
2. organizing food buyers' clubs to buy staples and other foods in bulk to save money,
3. contracting with local farms to provide food for their clients (i.e., Community Supported Agriculture);
4. assisting some of their unemployed enrollees to find jobs in food production and distribution;
5. facilitating the hiring of enrollees to grow fruits and vegetables in vacant lots in cities; and
6. creating innovative strategies to provide food security and healthful, affordable diets for all, while fostering fair wages for food production and service workers.

To help people eat high quality food for better health, ACCs will need all possible tools to improve the diets of their patients. Educating their patients about selecting good foods and monitoring what patients eat will be the places to start.

Scientists and lay people will compare healthy food assistance strategies and overall health outcomes of the competing ACCs. Aided by the published results of diet-composition analyses related to health outcomes of patients in ACCs, the best food assistance strategies of the ACCs will be copied by others. Better diets will also reduce ACC sickness costs.

Widespread Opposition to USDA Farm Subsidy Programs

Numerous health-related groups have criticized (1) the disease-promoting USDA commodity subsidies for junk foods, and (2) Department of Health and Human Services (HHS) welfare payments for the impoverished workers that serve them.[18, 19] In addition, agriculture subsidies have been criticized by the United Nations and the World Trade Organization because USDA financial assistance prevents fair competition for sustainable food systems in developing nations. In essence, the government is facilitating U.S. farmers to export our highly processed, freshwater- and fossil-fuel-intensive foods, rather than to help farmers in developing countries to grow healthful, unprocessed local foods for their people. Organizations opposing the U.S. farm subsidy policies are wide ranging and include the libertarian Cato Institute's Center for Trade Policy Studies,[10] the European Commission,[20] Union of Concerned Scientists, the Center for Rural Affairs, and Oxfam America.[21]

Exporting over $100 billion of U.S. grown food per year[22] greatly enriches a few corporate farmers but harms many other stakeholders. The competitive advantage of U.S. farmers in exporting food to foreign countries lies largely from direct government farm subsidies (i.e., crony capitalism) and in our relatively cheap water, fossil fuel, and labor. Developing countries would benefit much more from our aid in helping their farmers produce their own food and from the U.S.'s stopping the subsidies to competitors of their native farmers.

Subsidies for Energy, Water, and Agribusiness

Each year, governments of countries around the world spend over $1 trillion in subsidizing agriculture, energy, water, fisheries and transport. These unsustainable subsidies harm the environment, damage human health, are socially regressive, and distort trade interactions.[23] The U.S. government provides an estimated 25% of those damaging subsidies—about $250 billion.

Grand Bargains' tax reform should counteract these subsidies that harm the public health, the economy, and the environment (Chapter 21 and 22).

The highly interrelated crises in health, agriculture, energy, and the economy all have many causes. However, subsidies leading to misallocation of government *and private funds* underlie them all. Improving health care, health, the economy, and the environment all depend on subsidy reform and removing perverse incentives that undermine a "green" economy.

Non-Renewable Energy Subsidies

In the U.S., the biggest government subsidies are for energy. Fossil fuel and nuclear energy subsidies stimulate demand, have hidden costs in all products, and prevent the development of alternative technologies that may reduce pollution, including greenhouse gas emissions (Chapter 22).

In a 2007 interview with *Time* magazine reporter Joe Klein, Presidential nomination contender Barack Obama said:[24]

> I was just reading an article in the *New York Times* by Michael Pollan about food and the fact that our entire agricultural system is built on cheap oil. As a consequence, our agriculture sector actually is contributing more greenhouse gases than our transportation sector. And in the mean time, it's creating monocultures that are vulnerable to national security threats, are now vulnerable to sky-high food prices or crashes in food prices, huge swings in commodity prices, and are partly responsible for the explosion in our health care costs because they're contributing to type 2 diabetes, stroke and heart disease, obesity, all the things that are driving our huge explosion in health care costs.

It appears that President Obama understands the health consequences of agriculture being dependent on cheap oil. Yet federal government taxation, spending policies, and subsidies continue to favor agriculture's unsustainable reliance on fossil fuel. Obama needs to translate his understanding into new agriculture and food policies.

The fossil fuel inputs to agriculture (heating, chemicals, etc.) and food processing (packaging, heavy machinery, processing chemicals, etc.) are such that 10 calories of energy are used to produce 1 calorie of food on average.[25] However, variation in the carbon footprint of food is wide with animal products having a much heavier carbon footprint than plant-based products. [c]

The grand bargain of a consumption tax on nonrenewable energy will change this (Chapter 22). The tax will also reduce the vulnerability of relying on long-distance transport for food. The average serving of food in the U.S. has traveled 1500-2500 miles from farm to plate.[25] This requires petroleum, mainly diesel fuels for trucking.

Water Subsidies

According to the U.S. Geologic Survey, the percentage of freshwater going to the domestic sector (households) is only about 2% of all freshwater drawn from public reserves. Of the freshwater consumed, about 70% goes for the production of food (agricultural irrigation, aquaculture, livestock, etc.) at highly government-subsidized rates.[26] Most of the rest goes to industries and businesses.

Unfortunately, we have been using freshwater in the U.S. at unsustainable rates.[27] It is widely recognized that we need to reduce our consumption of freshwater for all purposes.

Ocean fish stocks are low and continuing to decline. Yet governments subsidize the fishing industry directly and with little or no cost of water. Rationales for fish subsidies include subsidies help fight poverty, or that the subsidies enhance development, that other countries do it, and that fish eating is required for a healthy diet.[28] These reasons do not

c   Calories In / Calories Out for Various Common Foods

Food Type (Animal Product)	Energy In/ Energy Out	Food Type (Plant-Product)	Energy In/ Energy Out
Lamb	83.3	Tomatoes	1.67
Pork	27.0	Apples	0.91
Salmon (farmed)	17.5	Potatoes	0.83
Tuna	17.2	Peanuts	0.71
Beef (grain fed)	15.6	Dry Beans	0.56
Eggs	8.93	Rice	0.48
Chicken	5.52	Wheat	0.45
Milk	4.85	Corn	0.40

make sense. Along with two co-authors, I wrote an article published in the *American Journal of Cardiology* that challenged the alleged cardiovascular benefits of eating fish.[29]

According to the American Farm Bureau,[22]

- One in three U.S. farm acres is planted for export.
- Thirty-one percent of U.S. gross farm income comes directly from exports.
- About 23 percent of raw U.S. farm products are exported each year.

In 2010, U.S. farms produced food valued at $370 billion. Of that food, about $255 billion was sold domestically and $115 billion worth was exported to other countries.[22] Since food production accounts for 70% of our freshwater consumption, this means that we are exporting about 23% of our freshwater in the form or highly subsidized food to other countries.[d]

For example, in 2012, during a severe drought in the western U.S., California farmers in the Central Valley and other regions exported more than 50 billion gallons of water to China in the form of alfalfa to feed Chinese cattle. Alfalfa is a particularly water thirsty crop. Due to antiquated water right laws in California, the water cost little or nothing to the farmers who exported it.[30]

To determine how we can best conserve freshwater, we need to understand the concept of the "freshwater footprint" on various food products. The amount of freshwater drawn from public reserves required to produce a quantity of food can be expressed as gallons of freshwater per pound of food produced (gal/lb) or gallons of freshwater per kilocalorie (gal/kcal) of energy in the food. Plant-based food products have much lower freshwater footprints than animal foods. The wide variation in water footprint estimates for beef depend on whether

---

d   0.70 (70% of freshwater consumption goes for exported food) x 0.33 (33% of U.S. farm acres are planted for export) = 0.23 (23% of U.S. freshwater is exported in the form of food).

animals are raised in a dry or wet climate, whether they are fattened in feedlots, whether the studies are cattle industry funded versus non-profit organization funded, and other variables.[31-34]

Plant-based food products have much lower freshwater footprints than animal foods.[e] With Grand Bargains reform, freshwater excise taxes will significantly raise the cost of food, depending on the water footprint of the food (Chapter 21).[f]

The proposed excise taxes will counteract these counterproductive, economy distorting subsidies, encouraging us to reduce consumption of commodities that harm health and/or the environment (Chapters 21 and 22). We can't afford overconsumption of water and energy, and neither can the fish, our bodies, or the climate.

Our Reliance on Unsustainable Industrial Agriculture

America's industrial agriculture system consumes fossil fuel, water, and topsoil at unsustainable rates. The International Food Policy Research Institute and World Resources Institute jointly published a "Millennium Ecosystem Assessment." It concluded that agriculture is the "largest threat to biodiversity and ecosystem function of any single human activity."[35] Up to 40% of global croplands are experiencing soil erosion, reduced fertility, or overgrazing.[36] We are threatening our agricultural capital to an unprecedented degree.

e   Water Footprint of Plant-based Foods and Animal Products[32]

Plant-based food	Gallons / pound	Gallons / kcal	Animal product	Gallons / pound	Gallons/ kcal
Sugar crops	24	0.18	Milk	122	0.48
Vegetables	39	0.35	Eggs	392	0.64
Roots/ tubers	46	0.12	Chicken meat	519	0.79
Fruits	115	0.55	Butter	666	0.19
Cereals	197	0.13	Pig meat	719	0.57
Oil crops	284	0.21	Sheep/goat meat	1052	1.12
			Beef	1800 (441-12,008)	2.69

f   Excise taxes are taxes paid when purchases are made on a specific good, such as water.

The heavy use of petrochemical pesticides in industrial agriculture is associated with elevated cancer risks for farm workers and possibly consumers. Several pesticides are coming under greater scrutiny for their links to endocrine disruption and reproductive dysfunction.[37] Obesity, type 2 diabetes, and some cancers are among the health consequences.

In a *Solutions* magazine article, legendary farmer, writer, and philosopher Wes Jackson detailed a long list of the components of the interconnected ecological and cultural crises caused by our unsustainable agricultural practices:[38]

- soil erosion,
- loss of wild biodiversity,
- poisoned land and water,
- salinization (poisoning with salt),
- expanding dead zones, and
- the demise of rural communities.

Mr. Jackson concluded that the same thing that drives climate change helps drive the agricultural crisis—cheap fossil fuel. Compounding the problem, big agriculture depends on lucrative exports of our fossil fuel and water intensive crops. Food exports from the U.S. hurt farmers in poor countries while consuming petroleum and water and degrading our agricultural land.

Meat production contributes disproportionately to ecological damage, in part because feeding grain to livestock to produce meat—instead of feeding it directly to humans—requires huge amounts of water and energy. This makes animal agriculture more resource intensive than other forms of food production.

More efficient practices of livestock production will have a favorable environmental impact. According to the Food and Agriculture Organization (FAO), "Environmental problems created by industrial production systems derive not from their large scale, nor their production intensity, but rather from their geographical location and concentration."[39] The FAO recommends reintegration of crop and livestock activities. In other words, sustainability requires getting rid of feed lots, greatly decreasing growing crops for animal feed, and raising livestock near to crops.

The proliferation of factory-style animal agriculture creates environmental and public health concerns. These include pollution from the high concentration of animal wastes and drug-resistant infections in humans due to the extensive use of antibiotics for animals subject to close confinement conditions.

Antibiotic Use on Factory Farms

On factory farms, antibiotics used in healthy animals to prevent infections and to promote growth modestly reduce the cost of the meat to the consumer. However, the short-term advantages of antibiotics are offset by the emergence of drug-resistant bacteria such as salmonella and E. coli. Antibiotic-resistant strains of microbes evolving on factory farms may be passed along in meat sold to consumers. Among many medical groups that have called for a ban on giving antibiotics to healthy animals to prevent infections and promote growth are the American Medical Association and the Infectious Diseases Society of America.

Studies show that drug-resistant E. coli strains found on poultry and beef in grocery stores have genetic markers that match those of the same bacteria in sick patients. Microbes can infect people as they handle uncooked meat products or, if cooking is not thorough, when eating meat. The drug-resistant strains can also enter the environment by contact with manure or the clothes of farm workers.[40]

Because of concerns about promoting antibiotic resistance, the European Union barred most non-treatment uses of antibiotics in 2006. Farmers in Europe have adapted without major increases in costs. The U.S. Food and Drug Administration is considering following suit[40] and should do so.

Wasted Food

While government-subsidized food sales at home and abroad continue, our market incentives do almost nothing to discourage food waste. From 40%-50% of all food produced in the United States goes uneaten—left in fields, spoiled in transport, thrown out at the grocery store, scraped into the garbage, or forgotten until it spoils.[41, 42] The cost of wasted food in the U.S. exceeds the cost of food assistance to the poor.[g] For the average household, wasted food translates into almost $1400 value in food per year. Wasted food also hurts the environment by accounting for about 19% of the waste dumped in landfills, where it ends up rotting and producing methane, a greenhouse gas.[40] Food waste accounts for at least 25% of all the freshwater used in the country.[42]

Composting, both on the household and municipal levels, offsets food waste and helps to grow more food (without petrochemicals).

With Grand Bargains-based health and economic reform, competing ACCs will find it very important to address wasted food. Due to higher food costs because of consumption taxes on non-renewable energy (Chapter 22) and fresh water (Chapter 21) and higher wages for food production and service workers (Chapter 12), food will nominally cost much more than now (Details on food price rise with Grand Bargains-reforms follows in this chapter). Consequently, ACC staff and members will find it mutually beneficial to work together to limit food waste.

By informing members about food waste, monitoring waste by conservation coaches, and innovating in food distribution methods; waste can be greatly reduced. The savings will benefit ACC enrollees, the environment, and the country. Local gardening for raising food, including on apartment balconies and growing sprouts in kitchens, will help to not only save money but contribute to better health, food security, and lessening petrochemical inputs to raise food. Additional space for growing food will come from converting lawns to vegetable gardens and fruit tree orchards.

---

g   Cost of food wasted in the U.S. per year: at least $165 billion per year[42]
Cost of U.S. government food assistance: $107 billion in 2015[43]

Changing Agricultural Methods to Abate Climate Change

According to the Intergovernmental Panel on Climate Change, about one-third of global greenhouse gas emissions come from food systems—the ways we produce, process, distribute, and consume the food.[44] In the U.S. about 18% of greenhouse gas emissions relate to agriculture and the transportation, storage, preparation, and decomposition of food.[39, 45, 46] This is a bigger share than that of transportation.[39]

Higher greenhouse gas estimates for agriculture come from the international nonprofit organization "Grain," a group that supports small farmers and social movements in their struggles for community-controlled and biodiversity-based food systems.[h] Considering ways of mitigating the major components of climate change that are related to agriculture, Grain scientists suggest several strategies:

- using agroecological practices to rebuild soil organic matter lost from industrial agriculture,
- decentralizing livestock farming and integrating it with crop production,
- distributing food mainly through local markets instead of transnational food chains, and
- stopping land clearing and deforestation for plantations.[48]

According to the Food and Agricultural Organization of the United Nations, livestock production occupies 70% of worldwide agricultural land used and 30% of the land surface of the Earth.[49] To avoid the consequences of catastrophic climate change, industrial-scale livestock production must decrease significantly. Both human and environmen-

---

h   Grain estimates that worldwide, industrialized, fossil-fuel intensive agricultural methods account for between 44% and 57% of total global greenhouse gas emissions. In Grain's estimate of greenhouse gas emissions from industrialized agriculture, the components of agriculture-related greenhouse emissions are the following: agricultural activities: 11%–15%, land clearing and deforestation: 15%–18%, food processing, packing, and transportation: 15%–20%, and decomposition of organic waste: 3%–4%.[47]

tal health will benefit from people shifting towards a more plant-based diet and eschewing the chewing of factory farm animal products.

Food Prices will Rise with Agricultural Reforms

The USDA estimates that the cost of food will be about $1670 billion in 2016, about $5200 per person.[50] With Grand Bargains-based economic reform, food prices on average will increase due to higher costs of water (Chapter 21), increased energy costs (Chapter 22), and higher pay for agricultural and food service workers (Chapter 12). However, the increases in food prices will be concentrated in water- and fossil fuel-intensive foods and in labor-intensive food services (processed foods and food away from home). The costs at the grocery store, farmers' market, or direct from the farmer of fresh fruits, vegetables, whole grains, beans, and nuts will go up relatively little.

About 18% of energy goes to food production and services in the U.S.[45] Consequently, about 18% of the $700 billion revenue from the non-renewable energy tax will relate to food. The non-renewable energy tax will increase the cost of food to consumers by about $126 billion.[i] Similarly, 70% of the freshwater consumption in the U.S. goes for the production and consumption of food. Therefore, 70% of the freshwater excise tax will be passed onto food, depending on the water footprints of the various food products, raising about $210 billion in 2016.[j]

The third component of the increase in the cost of food will be with higher wages for labor (Chapter 12). Whereas, farm laborers and food services workers constitute about 15% of the workforce (21 million workers),[22, 43] they are disproportionately poorly compensated and make up about 30% of the lowest paid workers. In addition to the estimated 3 million full-time, migrant, and seasonal farm laborers in the

---

i $700 billion (nonrenewable energy tax, Chapter 22) x 0.18 (18% of energy goes to food production) = $126 billion
j $300 billion (freshwater tax, Chapter 21) x 0.70 (70% of freshwater goes to food production) = $210 billion

U.S.,[51] about 2 million more farm laborers will be needed to produce the food on smaller, more decentralized, less fossil fuel intensive farms with better labor conditions. This will translate into approximately $260 billion additional labor cost of food in 2016.[k]

Consequently, combining the tax on freshwater (70% of freshwater relates to food production), the tax on fossil fuels and nuclear energy (18% going to food production), an increase in the minimum wage to $15 per hour, and 2 million additional required farm laborers would be expected to raise the cost of food by about $600 billion.[l] However, with this great an increase in the cost of food, our profligate waste of 40% – 50% of our food will be in the spotlight. Out of about $165 billion in food waste per year,[42] let's conservatively estimate that individual and ACC conservation coach efforts will reduce food wasted and save consumers at least $50 billion.

Also, the fossil fuel footprint of food production will decrease because of the shift from large, agribusiness, fossil-fuel intensive, monocrop farms and ranches to more decentralized, local, labor-intensive, organic farms. Less petroleum products will be needed for transportation, storage, packaging, storage, refrigeration, pesticides, chemical fertilizers, and food processing. ACCs will find it economically advantageous and healthful for members to help farmers and the food industry reduce the food-miles traveled by food products. ACCs will also help in the shift from fossil-fuel-intensive monocropping on mega-farms to diversified organic agriculture on smaller farms closer to population centers. We can estimate that the $126 billion of fossil fuels projected to be going into agriculture in 2016 will be reduced by 30% (about $40 billion).

---

k   Additional pay for the 21 million current farm laborers and food service workers = $264 billion (($660 billion total increase in wages due to raising the minimum wage to $15 per hour) x 0.3 (food workers constitute about 30% of all low wage workers) = $198 billion + $66 billion (from 2 million additional farm laborers @ $33,000 per year due to decreased fossil fuel intensity of farming and better labor conditions) = $264 billion).

l   Total additional food related consumption taxes and labor costs: $210 (freshwater taxes) + $126 billion (nonrenewable energy taxes) + $198 billion (increased pay for current food and agriculture workers) + $66 billion (additional farm laborers) = $600 billion.

At the disposal of ACCs to help the farmers and the food industry make this huge transition, will be the administration of USDA food assistance to the poor ($107 billion, Chapter 10), USDA farm subsidies ($25 billion, Chapter 19), and mortgages for farms administered by ACC-affiliated credit unions and savings and loan banks (Chapter 24).

Accounting for the savings in food waste and non-renewable energy with food system reform, an overall increase in food costs of about 30% will be expected. The average individual's food and beverage bill, including eating out, will rise from about $5200 to about $6900 in 2016.[m] We can expect food cost reductions as health-promoting shifts in food-consumption patterns (e.g., less processed food, more fresh fruits and vegetables, etc.) occur.

With the consumption taxes on freshwater alone, the retail price of one pound of factory farmed beef will be increased by about $7.00.[n] Grass-fed beef would have dramatically lower water and fossil fuel footprints and therefore cost to the customer.

Families will save money by consuming a more healthful diet with more plant-based foods, smaller portions of meat, pasture-raised rather than feedlot raised livestock, growing vegetables and fruit at home or in community gardens, and less food wasted. ACCs will be responsible that their members do not suffer food insecurity despite the increased prices. The increase in food costs for the poor will also be ameliorated by the minimum wage hike to $15 per hour and increased employment (Chapter 12).

ACCs will be able to use educational programs and financial incentive programs to assure that members consume what they consider to be the most healthful possible diet.

---

m $600 billion (projected additional fuel, water, and labor costs for food) – $50 billion (less food waste) – $40 billion (less non-renewable energy) = $510 billion. $510 billion / $1670 billion = 0.305 (≈30% higher cost of food). Food and food services costs per capita in 2016, status quo: $5200 ($1670 billion (total cost of food and food services in 2016) / 321 million U.S. residents ≈ $5200. With Grand Bargains food system reform, food and food services projected costs in 2016: $2210 billion / 321 million U.S. residents ≈ $6900

n   1800 gallons of freshwater per pound of beef x $0.004 / gallon (tax on freshwater) = $7.20 (freshwater tax per pound of beef).

Incentives for Changing to a More Plant-Based Diet

The average American animal-product-centered diet consumes up to seven times the energy and generates up to seven times the greenhouse gases as a completely plant-based diet.[34] Since animal products require much more fossil fuel to produce than plants, transforming to agricultural and food processing systems with less energy consumption and greenhouse gas emissions will require transitioning to a more plant-based diet. Fortunately, the disproportionately higher cost of animal products due to the greater inputs of freshwater and fossil fuels will help incentivize this transition to more plant-based food.

Individuals and ACCs will have stakes—not steaks; pardon the pun—in increasing plant-based foods in diets that reduce the health impacts and costs of chronic diseases. Any increase in plant foods relative to animal products will have positive health, environmental, and economic effects.

As will be detailed in Chapter 22, the $2.40 per gallon tax on gasoline and comparable taxes on other non-renewable energy will lead to more decentralization of the production of food to smaller, more diversified, mostly organic, less energy-intensive farms situated much closer to population centers. Urban agriculture will also be financially incentivized because it requires relatively little fossil fuel and provides recreation, social contacts, and exercise for city-dwellers.

Downsizing Agricultural Exports and Imports While Strengthening U.S. Farms and Farm Communities

Domestic and foreign farmers ship a tremendous amount of food into and out of the U.S. each year. However, Grand Bargains-based transitioning to a post-carbon economy will require the vast majority of food to be produced and consumed locally. This calls for some major changes in farm policies to assure that farmers prosper throughout the disruptions of the transition.

Among the many factors listed by the USDA as affecting global agricultural trade are (1) global supplies and prices of farm commodities, (2) government support for agriculture, and (3) trade protection policies. Things that are not listed by the USDA as affecting the importing and exporting of farm crops are the cost of energy, water, and labor.[52] The USDA assumes that farm labor will remain about the lowest paying of occupations. In part to stem the unsustainable and environmentally damaging volume of imports and exports of farm products, Grand Bargains' reform will markedly increase the cost of fossil fuel, freshwater, and labor.

According to the USDA, the "productivity" of U.S. agriculture is growing faster than domestic food and fiber demand. The USDA has responded with policies to expand global trade in farm commodities. U.S. farmers and agricultural firms rely heavily on exports to sustain prices and revenues ($144 billion in farm products exported in 2013). These exports depend on cheap fossil fuel, water, and labor. If U.S. residents suddenly reduced food waste from 40%- 50% of all food produced to 0% and inputs of energy, water, and labor increased 30% according to Grand Bargains-based reform, farmers would suffer an economic disaster. This must be averted.

For agricultural products in 2013, there was a $40 billion net positive trade balance (U.S. farm product and processed food exports: $144 billion versus exports: $104 billion imports). Since export income comprises over 30% of all farm sales, farm state legislators doggedly seek to protect and expand farm exports with each version of the farm bill. They have been largely successful.[21]

Since global free trade underpins U.S. government economic policies including those in agriculture, one price for expanding U.S. agricultural exports is to allow a free flow of imports. To justify our economic interests in sustaining and expanding the positive trade balance of agriculture in keeping with our overall global free-trade stance, the USDA encourages agricultural imports. The USDA officially endorses imports saying that they:[52]

- expand food variety,
- provide year-round supplies of fresh fruits and vegetables, and
- control increases in food prices.

I don't buy any of the reasons for shipping food around the world in tankers powered by bunker fuel. This is not part of transitioning to a post-carbon global economy for several reasons:

- Food variety in the U.S. is already arguably second to none in the world without food imports.
- Since fresh fruits and vegetables are perishable, eating them in season from local sources is preferable to buying imports from agribusiness corporations.
- By "controlling increases in food prices," the USDA must be referring to using the exploitation of very low-wage workers from Third World countries to keep a lid on the low wages paid to U.S. farm workers. However, social justice requires that we increase U.S. worker wages.

We need an alternative to the well-meaning but dysfunctional U.S. trade policies that seek to double-down on subsidizing the exports of our fossil fuel- and water-intensive agricultural products. At the same time, we need to make sure that U.S. farmers not only survive but thrive in what will be a highly disruptive transition to food production with lower carbon- and freshwater-imprints and with well-paid farm and food service workers.

Assuming that in 2016 Grand Bargains' reforms result in U.S. farm product imports and exports both decreasing by 30% due to the marked increase in food prices, farmers will have $44 billion worth of reduced exports.[o] Farmers will also have $32 billion worth of increased domestic sales due to the 30% reduction in food imports.[p] U.S. farm

---

o $144 billion (U.S. farm exports estimated for 2016) x 0.30 (30% reduction in farm product exports) ≈ $44 billion
p $104 billion (U.S. farm imports estimated for 2016) x 0.3 (30% reduction in farm product exports) ≈ $32 billion

product imports and exports will be expected to decrease progressively in future years as we transition into a global post-carbon economy.

In 2016, part of the Grand Bargains' agricultural strategy is for the USDA to shift about $133 billion in subsidies for farmers and poor people to the ACCs for administration. Consequently, ACCs will have the resources and the mandate to help the agricultural community make up for the loss of USDA crop subsidies and other agricultural assistance and for the decrease of an estimated $12 billion in net sales due to reductions in farm products imports and exports.[q]

This will be a huge transition for agriculture that will take up to a decade to reduce non-renewable energy use in agriculture and food services by over 80%. President Obama pledged to reduce overall greenhouse gas emissions 83% by 2050.[53] Grand Bargains' reforms will accomplish this in agriculture by 2025.

Further ACC financial assistance in the transition will come from opportunities for farmers to enlist to do national security work as teachers of the latest organic farming methods to farmers in developing countries (Chapter 17). ACC-affiliated financial services companies will also be available to provide loans and crop insurance to farmers (Chapter 24).

Summary and Conclusion

Food subsidies include cheap water, cheap fossil fuel, underpaid workers, USDA food assistance for the poor, and USDA crop subsidy payments to farmers. Unfortunately, these subsidies tend to make junk food cheaper relative to wholesome food. USDA subsidies are unsustainable due to adverse health impacts and strains on non-renewable resources as well as topsoil.

Our unsustainable agricultural practices, resulting in a chronic-disease-promoting diet, contribute to our failures in health care,

---

q   Net decrease in farm sales due to decreases in exports and imports of farm products: $44 billion – $32 billion = $12 billion

energy, the environment, climate change, the economy, and national security. These diverse crises all call for integrated solutions to inter-related problems.

Our food system is now dominated by large-scale agribusinesses using monocropping and intensive petrochemical fertilizers and pesticides. An essential component of abating climate change is for us to transition to smaller-scale, mostly organic, locally produced food. This was strongly endorsed by the United Nations in a report entitled, "Wake Up Before It's Too Late: Make Agriculture Truly Sustainable Now For Food Security in a Changing Climate."[54]

Even with minimal subsidies, organic food successfully competes with USDA subsidized corporate food for a growing niche market. Additionally, because less fossil-fuel-intensive organic methods are more labor-intensive, they can help us put more people to work in highly meaningful jobs.

To improve health of individuals and the public at large, Americans must change the diet that contributes to $2.5 trillion per year in medical bills for preventable chronic diseases. With Grand Bargains' economic reforms in place in the food system, ACCs could compete with each other in part by contracting with local farms and urban agriculture entrepreneurs to provide healthy food while increasing employment in farming and food distribution.

In part because of the advertising clout of special interests, and in part because of the limitations of our nutritional science studies to date, no consensus exists about how Americans should change their diets. This leads to political paralysis in the areas of governmental policies regarding food and agriculture.

After throwing out the unscientific USDA/HHS national dietary guidelines, Grand Bargains' health and economic reforms will empower competing ACCs to each develop their own recommended dietary guidelines and strategies to encourage compliance of members. This pluralistic approach to food policies will allow ACC members and staff at the local level to use their own strategies to reduce diet-related morbidity and mortality. Nutrition scientists will study the varying dietary intakes of people from different ACCs and relate them to health outcomes. Then ACC health professionals and the public will be able to use the information to determine what dietary changes to promote. Based on this information, ACCs will develop innovative and effective strategies to incentivize members to adopt healthful eating habits.

Methods to test as potential aids to improve members' diets may include (1) social networking, (2) financial incentives, (3) educational media, (4) support groups, (5) health lectures, and (6) feedback from physicians on diet diaries. The process of improving diet-related health outcomes will be ongoing. ACCs that inspire members to adopt truly evidence-based healthy diets will save money on sickness care. This money may be returned to ACC members in health promotion programs, better paying job opportunities, social services, and lower health care insurance premiums.

The taxes on freshwater (Chapter 21) and non-renewable energy (Chapter 22) will make local, sustainable, largely plant-based agriculture a "win-win-win-win-win" situation. It will benefit U.S. residents enrolling in ACCs, ACC staff, taxpayers, the government, and the environment. Aided by consumption taxes that incentivize healthful food and wise agriculture policies, ACC nutrition and public health experts will incentivize healthful eating and will replace the USDA policies that have inadvertently contributed to spawning diet-related disease epidemics and the degradation of our environment.

The environmental and economic consequences of our unsustainable agricultural methods (pollution, climate change, fossil fuel dependence, chemically tainted food, topsoil depletion, food insecurity, etc.) are just as serious as diet-related chronic diseases. ACCs that succeed in facilitating diets that improve health outcomes and environmental sustainability will succeed financially and will attract more members.

Chapter 14
Immigration Reform: A Foundation For Zero Population Growth

I practiced medicine for 17 years at the LA County + USC Medical Center where at least 20% of the patients were undocumented (illegal) immigrants. For me, health care for undocumented immigrants is not a matter of abstract statistics and cost figures. It's about the Hippocratic Oath. The "Pain and Palliative Care Service" that I directed provided hundreds of undocumented immigrants with morphine and other medicines for severe pain from terminal cancer or AIDS. For certain, few of them would have been able to obtain relief of pain in their own countries.

At the LA County + USC Medical Center, I worked with hundreds of intern- and resident-physicians who emigrated from their homelands to the U.S. for their post graduate medical training. I found them to be highly intelligent, hard working, dedicated, and compassionate. If all immigrant physicians in the U.S. were deported, we would lose over a quarter of our doctors. Of course, the U.S. needs to dramatically increase the physicians trained in this country to reduce the need for immigrant physicians over the long term (Chapter 19). However, immigrant physicians will remain vital to the excellence of American medicine.

Likewise, a large proportion of nurses come to the U.S. from other countries. Many engineers that develop our innovative technologies were born elsewhere. The field of education in the U.S. depends heavily on immigrants. If all the undocumented farm workers were deported tomorrow, we would starve.

Benefits of Legal and Illegal Immigrants to the U.S.

Michael Bloomberg, former Mayor of New York City, testified to a U.S. Senate committee that the economy of his city, and that of the entire nation, would collapse if undocumented immigrants were deported en masse.[1] He told the Senators that New York is home to 3 million immigrants, including a half-million that are undocumented. Bloomberg said, "Although they broke the law by illegally crossing our borders . . . our city's economy would be a shell of itself had they not, and it would collapse if they were deported. The same holds true for the nation."

Mr. Bloomberg and many others recognize that the U.S. is a country of immigrants, including innovative entrepreneurs and highly educated leaders. He recommended that immigrants completing advanced degrees in U.S. universities should automatically receive green cards on graduation.

In the formation of a coalition advocating for immigration reform, Mayor Bloomberg was joined by other big city mayors and the chief executives of Hewlett-Packard, Boeing, Disney, News Corp., and other large corporations. They all strongly recommend a path to legal status for all undocumented immigrants now in the United States. The coalition calls itself the "Partnership for a New American Economy." The goal is to reframe immigration reform as the solution to repairing and stimulating the economy.[2]

Referring to immigrants, Walt Disney Company Chairman and CEO Robert Iger, a member of the partnership, said, "It's our great strength as a nation, and it's also critical for continued economic growth. To remain competitive in the 21st Century, we need effective immigration reform that invites people to contribute to our shared success by building their own American dream."

Statistics on Undocumented Immigrants and Health Care

According to the Center for Immigration Studies, about 62% of un-documented immigrants are medically uninsured.[3a] Undocumented immigrants tend to be younger and healthier than the average legal U.S. resident, so their unreimbursed medical care (e.g., treatments that they receive in emergency rooms but for which they cannot pay the bills) is proportionately less costly than other uninsured people. Projecting from Medical Expenditure Panel Survey data for the period 2000-09,[4] the cost of publicly funded health care for undocumented immigrants in 2016 will be about $3 billion (less than 0.1% of all personal health care costs).[5, 6]

Balancing Health Care Concerns for Immigrants

While Obamacare excludes undocumented immigrants as recipients of public funding of medical treatment besides emergency care,[7] the enforcement of this provision has been questioned. Conservatives fear that proof of citizenship may not be required to access Medicaid benefits.[8] Even though only a small fraction of undocumented immigrants, if any, would likely receive public funding with the proposed Medicaid expansion, the issue has been a major obstacle to Obamacare's goal to insure as many as possible of the uninsured.

President Obama has indicated that he would oppose using public funds to medically insure undocumented immigrants, with the exception of children.[9] Mr. Obama also promised that his immigration reform proposal would include a path to citizenship. His proposals await the new Congress in 2015.

Public health programs to control infectious diseases (e.g., Ebola, tuberculosis, HIV/AIDS, etc.) will not be effective if they fail to control infections in immigrants like everyone else. As long as legal and illegal

---

a   About 6.9 million out of an estimated 11.1 million illegal immigrants are not medically insured.

immigrants reside in the U.S., they will have pregnancies, injuries, and diseases that require medical attention. For humanitarian and public health reasons (i.e., prevent the spread of infectious diseases), we need to care for these people.

Economic considerations arise in discussions of undocumented and legal immigrants. A Rasmussen Report Poll found that 83% of voters nationwide do not want taxpayers to foot the bill for medical treatment of undocumented immigrants.[8] An effective health reform plan must ensure that medical providers are not forced to provide un-compensated treatment to uninsured people, including legal or illegal immigrants.

By all accounts, unlimited illegal immigration into the U.S. would have adverse economic, social, and environmental consequences. The North American continent's population is already way beyond ecological carrying capacity without a major decrease in percapita consumption. As part of resolving the immigration morass, we need policies regarding health care for undocumented immigrants that address humanitarian and public health concerns without increasing taxpayers' costs. Consequently, health care reform and immigration reform should both incorporate a mechanism providing that immigrants pay the full cost of their own health care. This will satisfy the concerns of many conservatives about the economic impact of immigration.

We also need policies that allow us to control immigration into the U.S. in a way that is fair to U.S. citizens and legal immigrants and, as much as possible, to undocumented immigrants. Regarding the control of immigration, we need to consider not only the numbers of new immigrants each year, but also the long-term population growth rate due to immigration.

A Brief History of U.S. Immigration Policy

The present U.S. immigration law, enacted in 1965, replaced the national-origin quota system. "Family reunification" became the visa "preference category" most utilized. After subsequent modifications of preference categories, 90% of immigration visas became based on family reunification of immigrants. Skills-based immigration has received less than 10% of the available slots. Consequently, we may turn away foreign born visa applicants who have completed advanced degrees in U.S. universities while permitting the immigration of children, parents, or spouses of citizens who themselves previously immigrated legally or illegally.

Overpopulation and limited economic opportunities in developing countries and relatively high-paying jobs in the U.S. maintain a steady stream of legal and illegal immigrants. Remittances from U.S. immigrants to their homeland relatives and friends constitute a major component of the economies of many developing countries.[10] This increases the pressures for people to immigrate to the U.S. These factors should be considered in designing immigration policy.

Zero Population Growth Essential for the Sustainability of Human Life as We Know It

Environmentalists, economists, policy makers, and the public cannot afford to ignore unsustainable population growth.[10-12] Poverty, climate change, civil strife, wars, environmental pollution, inadequate access to education, and depletion of resources are all exacerbated by overpopulation.[10, 13] Without controlling the worldwide population, we will not be able to achieve any of our important goals regarding health, welfare, environmental sustainability, prosperity, or security. Immigration policy should be seen in this context. In designing immigration policy, the upmost aim should be zero population growth in the U.S. and, to the extent possible, worldwide.

Due to the poor economic conditions during the Great Recession, the lifetime average number of babies per woman (total fertility rate[b])

---

b   The total fertility rate of a population is the average number of children that would be born to a woman over her lifetime if: (1) She were to experience the exact

in the U.S. hit an all-time low of about 1.9 babies per woman in 2010.[15] This is slightly below the rate to just replace the population (2.1 babies per woman on average for developed countries[14]). This means that all of our population growth comes from immigration. Additionally, immigrant women within the U.S. have more babies than native born women. In 2010, with the immigrant population comprising 13% of the U.S. population, 23% of all U.S. births were to foreign-born women that immigrated to the U.S.[15]

Research shows that the most important factor in determining average family sizes is not necessarily the availability of family planning, sterilization, or abortion services. Family size is a response to the perceived costs and benefits associated with children. Some conditions raise family-size targets and others lower them. Motivation of parents or potential parents is the key to family size. Individual women or their mates and families make decisions regarding family size. Over the longer term, culture adapts in ways that facilitate, or not, (1) early and universal marriage, (2) spacing between children, and (3) non-reproductive roles for women. These individual and cultural processes form the basis of purposeful, adaptive behavior regarding family size.[10]

Motivated by high rates of teen pregnancy and sexually transmitted diseases in the U.S., public schools took on the responsibility of sex education. During the 1980s, 17 states mandated that schools teach "comprehensive sex education," and 30 more states supported it. Educators define comprehensive sex education as a curriculum that begins in kindergarten and continues into high school, covering reproductive biology, the psychology of relationships, the sociology of the family, the sexology of masturbation and massage, and many other topics.

This approach has the appeal of inexpensively reaching the vast majority of American schoolchildren. It reassures parents that their children will learn ways to protect them from AIDS and other sexually transmitted diseases. Exploring the relationship of young people hav-

---

current age-specific fertility rate through her lifetime, and (2) She were to survive from birth through the end of her reproductive life.[14]

ing sex, getting pregnant, and bearing children with overpopulation of the planet is not a goal of these comprehensive sex education classes. However, unless sex education taught in schools can be effective in preventing unwanted pregnancies and sexually transmitted diseases, it will be ineffective in limiting the sizes of families.

What is the evidence that comprehensive sex education can prevent pregnancies and sexually transmitted diseases?

The evidence is very weak.

New Jersey has been the leading state in implementing comprehensive sex education. New Jersey students average 24 hours a year of sex education from primary school through high school. Teachers are well trained and experienced in presenting the family-life curriculum. Opinion polls show wide support among parents of sex education in schools.

Sex education is offered as the alternative to failed attempts to control teenage sexuality through social norms and religious values. Comprehensive sex education classes present information about the technical aspects of sexuality along with exercises to build communication skills in sexual situations. The thesis is that, once teenagers learn the scientific information about sex, pregnancy, and sexually transmitted disease and they develop the skills of communicating about their feelings about sex, they will be prepared to be sexually responsible. The effectiveness of comprehensive sex education depends on the power of knowledge to change behavior. However, the available evidence suggests that sexual knowledge only weakly relates to teenage sexual behavior.

Donald Kirby, PhD, a leading researcher in the field of sex education, reviewed the medical literature on approaches to reduce adolescent sexual risk-taking, unintended pregnancy, childbearing, and sexually transmitted disease, including HIV. Surprisingly, he found that only a few sex education programs actually delay the initiation of sex, increase condom or contraceptive use, and reduce unprotected sex among youth. He found that, in addition to high quality sex education, three other programs components were especially effective in preventing unprotected sex:[16]

1. one-on-one clinician-patient protocols in health settings,
2. service learning programs, and
3. a particular intensive youth development program with multiple components.

To have better results in preventing unwanted pregnancies, perhaps we need sex education in schools (or homes) and more effective contraceptives. However, we need to go beyond these strategies to include programs with these more holistic and intensive approaches to reducing unprotected sex and unwanted pregnancies.

Patient-Centered Medical Homes in ACCs to Lead Efforts to Prevent Unprotected Sex and Unwanted Pregnancies

If Dr. Kirby's research findings are correct, a key to moving toward zero population growth nationally and worldwide is to create settings for one to one human relationships to form between mature mentors and young people in the reproductive age range. In addition, service learning programs and youth development programs should be readily available.

Patient-centered medical homes in ACCs will be ideal settings for health care and social services providers to help children and adolescents develop the knowledge, skills, and behaviors necessary to prevent unprotected sex and unwanted pregnancies. Under the direction of pediatricians, family medicine doctors, nurse practitioners, or physician assistants, primary care team members will lead children and adolescents in service learning activities and youth development projects. As stakeholders, parents and other relatives of the children and adolescents will collaboratively work with PCPs and their team members to design the most effective programs and activities to facilitate the coming of age of youth in their relationships with others.

There will not be a one-size-fits-all set of activities and experiences designed for and by young people within ACCs or even in patient-centered medical homes within ACCs. ACCs will have the flexibility to use whatever educational methods they want to use to help young people develop mutually beneficial and affirming relationships and to delay having babies. ACCs will be able to experiment with strategies to help couples limit the sizes of their families. For instance, educational opportunities, employment opportunities, and mentoring will be essential ingredients in a campaign for zero population growth.

The approaches to sex education, activities in youth groups, service learning experiences, and other programs for children and adolescents will be collaboratively determined. The intention will be for the programs and activities for youth to foster cultures that lead to low rates of unprotected sex, unintentional pregnancies, and abortions. Delaying childbirth until after college or trade school and small family sizes should be encouraged. Activities to build self esteem and prevent sexual abuse should be worked into the curriculum. The utilization of family planning services, contraception, and abortion and the format of sex education will be at the discretion of the ACCs with input from stakeholders. Some ACCs may support some celibacy-based pregnancy- and STD-prevention strategies for some or all of their families.

High birth rates will be costly for ACC members. Health care premiums for children will not be subsidized. Wages will replace welfare for feeding, clothing, sheltering, and educating children. Consumption taxes will not favor people with many children. For these reasons and for the general well-being of ACC members, their communities, the country, and the world, ACCs will compete to achieve low birth rates consistent with overall zero population growth in the U.S.

Birth rate-lowering strategies learned in ACCs will be exported to other countries. As will be detailed in Chapter 17, the main Grand Bargains' strategy for helping people in developing countries control population growth will be through a major national security program to provide wide-ranging development assistance. Funded by federal revenue, ACCs will be able to send their members trained as development professionals to, among many other things, help people in other countries achieve control of population growth. Rather than just focusing on sterilizing women and men or disseminating birth control devices, strategies should be in alignment with Dr. Kirby's research on holistic methods of preventing unwanted pregnancies and unprotected sex. As pertaining to his research, service learning projects and youth development programs will be encouraged.

The Conundrum of Better Economic Opportunities Associated with Higher Immigrant Birth Rates

The usual reasons listed to account for large families include (1) poverty, (2) retirement security, (3) cheap child labor, (4) lack of education, particularly of women, (5) high infant mortality, and (6) lack of access to family planning services. However, another major reason has been shown to be increasing economic opportunity and optimism about the future. Paradoxically for poor people emigrating from Third World countries to the U.S., a windfall of resources may fuel population growth. For instance, the birth rate of foreign-born women in the U.S. in 1990 was 70% higher than U.S. born women.[15]

Since the 1930s, overpopulation researchers have noted that fertility and prosperity are inversely related.[17] Given the finite carrying capacity of regions of the world where cheap fossil fuel, water, and other resources are not readily available, an increase in the birth rate could mean that the entire village or community would endure harsher economic conditions. Some argue that, in poorer countries with abundances of the usual reasons for rapid population growth, the momentum for growth may only be constrained when dire economic conditions cause people to reduce the sizes of families.

For instance, between the end of World War II and 1970, Africa's economic progress was associated with an increased birth rate—averaging about six children per woman. Even as the high illiteracy and infant mortality rates were decreasing, the birth rates rose. In Africa, researchers reported that perceived large increases in basic resources as well as opportunities to emigrate tended to fuel excess population growth. On the other hand, deteriorating expectations for economic opportunities and the absence of emigration options was apt to be associated with decreased fertility.

Some would use the observations from Africa to argue that fostering development (health care, education, agriculture irrigation systems and technologies, etc.) only leads to increased fertility and unsustainable population growth. Basically, they are saying that helping people develop is futile, because, with the fruits of economic development, they over-reproduce and return to poverty.

I disagree that this is needs to be the case.

Cuba represents a counter-example to the thesis that evolving from a Third World country with high rates of poverty, illiteracy, and infant mortality to a country with a prominent middle class will lead to an explosion of population growth. In the 1950s before the Communist Revolution, the Cuban crude birth rate per year averaged about 27 per 1000 population. In the early 1960s, the birth rate increased to 35 per 1000 people and then gradually declined to 14 per 1000 people by 1980, where it has remained. In association with the marked decline in the Cuban birth rate were the advents of food rationing giving universal food security, universal health care, universal education through high school, the highest literacy rate in the Americas, Social Security for the elderly, and the fall of infant mortality to as low as or lower than that of the U.S.

On my trip to Cuba, I spoke with many young men and women. Almost all were actively pursuing careers and few had children. Many Cubans I talked to envied people in the U.S. because of our material possessions. They strongly aspired to have more consumer items. One of their personal strategies to acquire more of what they wanted seemed to be to delay having children and limit the size of their families. When

I asked them about it, they generally told me that they were waiting until they could afford children.

The Cuban government makes the funding of children's programs a high priority. Children under six years old receive more from the food ration than others. Child care and education are free as are many athletic, artistic, and musical extra-curricular activities. However, young Cuban families must struggle harder with each child they bring into the world. Birth control and abortion are free in Cuba and do not carry a major stigma. The Cuban government does not directly or indirectly pay families to have more children that I could see. A friend, who is a Cuban native, confirmed my impression.

On the other hand, U.S. tax policies facilitate poor people to have more babies:[18]

1. The Child Tax Credit provides up to $1000 for every child under 17.
2. The Earned Income Tax Credit applies to low-income people as long as they have some wages. With each child, the amount of the credit increases.
3. Child and Dependent Care Credit covers up to 35% of child care expenses, or up to $3000 for a child under 13.
4. Additionally, employers of low-income people may exclude up to $5000 from their taxable wages for child-care expenses.
5. For many states, tax write-offs benefit parents paying for parochial-school tuition and supplies for children in kindergarten through high school.
6. The American Opportunity Credit allows for up to $2500 for tuition and related expenses.
7. The Lifetime Learning Credit for higher education has a maximum benefit of $2000 per year.
8. If you don't claim either of the education tax credits, you may deduct up to $4000 of tuition and fees.
9. A 529 college savings plan shelters savings from taxes.

U.S. welfare policies have a similar effect in facilitating more births:[19]

1. Temporary Assistance for Needy Families (TANF) provides cash assistance for low-income families with children.
2. Medicaid funds about 40% of births in the U.S.
3. The Women, Infant, and Child Program helps low-income mothers with expenses for infants and children.
4. Food Stamps and school nutrition programs feed low-income families.

Congress created all of these programs with the best of intentions to help poor people who have children. Undoubtedly, they have helped many poor families escape hunger, homelessness, and adverse health consequences of poverty. However, some adverse consequences have included (1) perverse financial incentives to have more babies than families can afford without welfare, (2) encouraging the break-up of low-income families[c], (3) disincentives to work, and (4) welfare dependency.

Cuba offers lessons about fostering strategic economic development while limiting population growth:

1. Economic gains need to be carefully administered to promote local agriculture, public health (adequate housing, sanitation, family planning, etc.), health care, education, retirement security, and infrastructure. Higher worker pay by itself may tend to increase population growth.
2. As opposed to developing societies with wide wealth inequalities, economic gains that are equitably distributed throughout the society will better tend to constrain population growth.

The bottom line is that we need to help people in Third World countries develop in ways that that will constrain the tendency of economic

---

c   It is easier for a single-mother to live on welfare than for a couple with children to live on one or even two minimum wage salaries.

progress to spur a population explosion. This will be discussed in more detail in Chapter 17.

Requirements for Immigration Policy Reform

The immigration policy challenge is to design strategies that simultaneously accomplish the following:

1. utilize the skills and talents of immigrants
2. avoid allowing undocumented or legal immigrants to access taxpayers' funds for health care and social-safety-net services or to take jobs from citizens
3. design a policy for immigrant workers that adds to the federal treasury
4. offer fairness to immigrants willing to work hard and play by the rules
5. provide a legal path to citizenship
6. allow for a mechanism for the government to be in control of the flow of immigrants into the U.S.
7. deport immigrants that commit felonies
8. structure immigration reform so that it leads the U.S. to achieve zero population growth
9. maintain support to people in Third World countries receiving remittances from U.S. immigrants, ideally by training development assistance professionals who immigrated from those countries and sending them back to their native lands (Chapter 17)
10. change from a legal immigration system that is predominantly family-reunification based to a largely skills-based system
11. favor legal immigration over illegal immigration
12. expand the number of legal immigration slots available to accommodate the need for more farm workers in a post-carbon economy and more construction workers (Chapters 13, 15, and 22)

13. require a minimum of cost to administer immigration programs and to police the flow of immigrants

Immigration reform has become politicized. There may be grains of truth in the talking points of people on all sides of the issue. We need a game changer that addresses all 13 of the above considerations.

A tax on the labor of undocumented immigrants should be considered as a policy option that will be in accordance with all these requirements. Both undocumented immigrants and citizens will be advantaged. It will appeal to liberals and conservatives. It won't be easy. However, it will be much less brutal, more socially just, and better for the economy than now.

Grand Bargain #20: Undocumented Immigrants will Remain Working in the U.S. with Their Employers Paying a $3 per Hour Labor Tax

As mentioned in Chapter 1, a $3 per hour tax on the labor of undocumented immigrants will be deducted by employers from the hourly wage (minimum $15/hour, Chapter 12). Employers of legal immigrants will not need to pay this labor tax. This tax is designed to:

(1) provide an economic disincentive to illegal immigration compared with legal immigration,
(2) advantage citizens and legal immigrants over undocumented immigrants in earning money,
(3) generate federal revenue, and
(4) allow hardworking, law-abiding, undocumented immigrants a path to citizenship.

About $60 billion in 2016 from a new undocumented-immigrant labor tax will thus go into the U.S. treasury.[d]

This undocumented-immigrant employment tax will address economic concerns of conservatives as to the financial impacts of undocumented immigrants, while raising the effective minimum wages of illegal immigrants to $12 per hour. Highly trained immigrants with advanced degrees and unique technological skills will have little trouble affording the undocumented immigrant tax.

This grand bargain addresses both immigration reform and widening economic inequality. It will provide all workers enough in wages, so they don't need to rely on social-safety-net services (e.g., Food Stamps and Medicaid). It will advantage the employment of citizens and legal immigrants over undocumented immigrants. With a predominantly skills-based immigration system, highly educated professionals will be able to immigrate to the U.S. much more readily.

Better than costly high-tech fences along our southern borders and repressive deportation campaigns, this undocumented-immigrant employment tax will put economic pressure on undocumented immigrants, making it less likely for excessive numbers to immigrate to the U.S.

Provisional Documentation of Workers and Dependents

Proper and effective implementation of this labor tax on work of illegal immigrants will be important. It will require instituting a completely new category of immigrant with "provisional documentation." An undocumented immigrant working in the U.S. and his/her dependents could qualify for and receive "provisional documentation" status, by the following:

1. demonstrating that his/her employer(s) has/have paid the $3 per hour tax to the federal government on all labor for a minimum of a three months

---

d   7 million working undocumented immigrants[20] x $3/hour x 2080 hours/year = $62 billion

2. joining an ACC and documenting that the premiums for the worker and all dependents have been paid for three months

3. showing that his/her employer(s) has/have sent Social Security taxes (12.4% of earnings) for three months to the employee's ACC to be held in a separate account

4. documenting that they received no safety-net assistance from their ACC.

Provisional documentation status will not mean that the worker and his/her dependents will receive Social Security cards. Achieving legal immigrant status (Green card, etc.) will require the worker to adhere to the above three conditions for two full years. If during this two year process of becoming documented, the worker is unable to maintain employment or does not adhere to the three above requirements, he/she may withdraw the Social Security funds from the ACC for him/her and any dependents to return to their native country. For undocumented workers with two or more employers, the chosen ACC may serve to manage the income and taxes from multiple employers.

These conditions are not meant to be easy for undocumented immigrants or their employers. If undocumented immigrants do not join ACCs and have their employers pay the undocumented workers' taxes and the Social Security taxes, they will not receive provisional documentation or be on a path to citizenship. In helping people find jobs, ACCs will favor citizens, legal immigrants, and provisionally documented immigrants over undocumented immigrants.

Employers will not be able to profit by paying undocumented people substandard wages. Paying less than minimum wages or paying under-the-table and not withholding taxes will be unlawful and will get employers into trouble.

This Grand Bargains' immigration policy will be fair to immigrants, employers, other workers, and taxpayers. Undoubtedly, not all currently undocumented immigrants will be able to succeed on the path to eventual citizenship. Many may use their accumulated Social

Security funds and any other savings to return to their native homes with skills and resources that will help them and their communities.

With this immigration policy in place, the tens of billions of dollars that we now pay to patrol our southern border and for Immigration and Customs Enforcement (ICE) officers to deport record numbers of immigrants may be redirected more constructively. Undocumented immigrant communities will no longer be terrorized by the fear of deportation for petty offenses or simply for being undocumented.

Undocumented Immigrant Health Care without Taxpayer Funding

For humanitarian and public health reasons, medical services for uninsured legal and undocumented immigrants will be available with Grand Bargains-based health care reform. However, as noted above, the immigrants themselves will foot the bill. Like everyone else, all immigrants enrolled in ACCs will have to pay their health care premiums—$2960 per year per child ($247/month) and ranging from $3490-$7820 per year ($291-$652/month) per adult. Depending on the medical benefit package offered by the chosen ACC, these prices could be much lower (Chapter 18).

Uninsured immigrants will be treated for emergencies, as will other uninsured people, funded by the federal government. Once entering the health care system through having emergency care, uninsured immigrants will be encouraged to enroll in an ACC and pay current and back insurance premiums. If they cannot afford the back premiums, they can still be enrolled in an ACC by paying current premiums but will forfeit their chance for eventual citizenship until they have paid all outstanding premiums. Undocumented or provisionally documented immigrants will not be eligible to receive social-safety-net services through ACCs.

If all of the currently undocumented immigrants paid the health insurance premiums, it would generate about $60 billion per year.[e] Consequently, no taxpayer funds will be needed for health care of these people.

Grand Bargains Reform will Reduce Illegal Immigration

Initially, all undocumented immigrants may not comply with these fair but challenging new rules. All of the employers of undocumented immigrants may not initially choose to obey the new law. However, the disadvantages of noncompliance for both undocumented employees (e.g., no provisional documentation, no path to citizenship, etc.) and their employers (misdemeanors, fines, business disruptions, etc.) will lead the vast majority to abide by the new law.

People emigrate from their homelands to the U.S. seeking political asylum or economic opportunity. They generally have the best of intentions. Most undocumented people find employment in low-paying jobs in agriculture, food services, landscaping, and construction. With Grand Bargains-based health care and economic reform, the economic incentives for undocumented people to emigrate from their home countries without the required legal status to the U.S. will be reduced in the following ways:

- Pursuing a path to citizenship will require paying for ACC-based health insurance for the immigrant and all his/her dependents.
- Among undocumented people, competition for jobs will be increased because legal residents and provisionally documented immigrants—but not undocumented people—will be assisted by ACCs to find employment.
- A $3 per hour labor tax will be levied on undocumented workers, coming out of the income of the workers.
- The cost of living will be higher due to the consumption taxes.

---

e   9.6 million adults x $5930 per year on average ($56.9 billion) + 1.5 million children x $2960 per year ($4.4 billion)[3, 21] = $60.3 billion total health care insurance bill for undocumented immigrants

- Safety-net assistance will not be available to undocumented people.

Despite these hurdles, people from other countries will continue to come to the U.S., seeking opportunities for a new life. With this Grand Bargain-based predominantly skills-based immigration policy, it will be much easier for highly educated professionals to immigrate here and make their contributions in business, medicine, engineering, or education.

For less well educated but hard working people from Mexico, other parts of Latin America, and other countries, Grand Bargains-based reforms will create opportunities for new jobs. Construction will be booming because of the investments in repairing and replacing infrastructure (Chapter 15). Agriculture will be shifting away from fossil-fuel-based farming to more decentralized, organic, labor-intensive methods of food production with better working conditions (Chapter 13).

These will present openings for immigration. The Grand Bargains-based incentives are stacked to be strongly favoring legal immigration.

Summary and Conclusion

The U.S. is a nation of immigrants and continues to benefit greatly from the hard work, innovations, and leadership of many foreign born residents. Most undocumented immigrants come to the U.S. to work hard and to make their contributions to building a great society. However, the population growth of undocumented immigrants has been unsustainable environmentally and economically. We are not in a position to allow undocumented or legal immigrants to access taxpayers' funds for health care and social-safety-net services or to displace citizens from employment. We also need to be able to count on the ACC environments changing the culture that leads to large families among immigrants that will be finding new economic opportunities. The dysfunctions throughout our systems of health care, welfare, taxation, and immigration have created a quagmire, victimizing all of us—immigrants, employers, politicians, and citizens.

A way forward is needed—a multifaceted solution for a complex set of problems.

Grand Bargains-based health care and economic reform offers a solution to this conundrum. We need to (1) tax the labor of undocu-mented immigrants (i.e., taxing both employer and employee), (2) shift legal immigration from primarily family-reunification-based to predominantly skills-based immigration, and (3) increase the quota for legal immigration based upon our needs for workers with certain skills (e.g., highly educated, highly skilled workers). With these re-forms, skills-based, legal immigration will be preferred by would be immigrants.

Zero population growth in the U.S. needs to be a part of the overall solution to the immigration conundrum. Grand Bargains' reform will constrain the birth rates among immigrants from developing countries by requiring that all immigrants join ACCs and pay premiums for themselves and their dependents. The Grand Bargains' reformed tax code (Chapter 21) will not offer subsidies to parents with dependent children. ACC administration of social-safety-net and social insurance services will foster the development and education of all children. How-ever, ACCs will not have incentives to encourage immigrants or others to have more children than they can afford over the long term. Within ethical boundaries, ACCs will be free to innovate and experiment in how to best achieve small families that are well-educated, prosperous, and community minded. The availability of family planning through patient-centered medical homes is only one of many modalities to prevent unwanted pregnancies. These efforts will moderate population growth to sustainable levels in the U.S. and provide a foundation for spreading zero population growth around the globe through world-wide sustainable development work (Chapter 17).

Thus, requiring undocumented immigrants to join ACCs, pay premiums, pay the undocumented labor tax, and to begin to pay into Social Security, will result in undocumented residents subsidizing legal residents by tens of billions of dollars per year.[f] At the same time, ACC care will provide all U.S. residents, including immigrants, the benefits of prompt diagnosis, treatment, and prevention of health problems. And Grand Bargains-based reform will grant undocumented immigrants the all-important path to citizenship.

---

f   The tax on labor of undocumented immigrants ($\approx$\$60 billion/year) and ACC premiums for 11 million relatively healthy people ($\approx$\$60 billion/year) will subsidize legal residents.

Chapter 15
Public Infrastructure Investments

As a member of a local community gardening organization, I mentored some students from a local high school. They wanted to work with us vegetable gardeners to fulfill their required community service obligations for graduation. They called their student club, the "Youth Environmental Leaders." Richard (not his real name), one of my mentees, an Asian boy in his sophomore year, was an honor student in math and sciences. At the garden, he enjoyed socializing with the other students and with mentors. Richard worked hard on vegetable gardening, planting trees, and in a wetlands restoration project. He more than fulfilled the learning hours under the community service required for graduation. He went off to an excellent college to major in civil engineering.

About five years later, Richard and some other students came back to visit with me at the same garden. I asked them all what they had been doing with their lives. Richard had graduated in civil engineering but had not been able to find work in his major. Instead, he had been working as a cashier at a local auto parts store and lived with his parents. He said that he continued to send out his resume but that jobs were scarce. With all the bridges that need repair or replacement, road maintenance work, and other infrastructure projects urgently required for safety and functioning of the economy, I wondered why Richard couldn't get a job.

Why Enhance American Infrastructure?

America's infrastructure connects businesses, communities, and people. Our economy and quality of life depend on it. We need good transport systems by land, water, and air; energy transmission systems that deliver reliable power from a wide range of energy sources; and water systems that drive industrial processes as well as provide clean water to our homes.

Our communications infrastructure has changed drastically in the last two decades. Instead of cables and wires for landlines that were independent of the electric grid and required almost no electric power, we now have a vast system of microwave towers for cellular phones. Instead of talking on the phone or writing letters that depend on a postal system, we have internet that is increasingly wireless. These electricity-consuming systems can suffer more kinds of massive breakdowns than telephone polls, cables and postal delivery trucks.

Apart from building cell phone towers and installing Wi-Fi radio frequency systems almost everywhere, we have not invested adequately in maintaining our infrastructure systems let alone expanded it sufficiently to meet our future population and economic needs.

In 2013, the American Society of Civil Engineers estimated that the U.S. has a backlog of needed infrastructure projects that will cost about $3.6 trillion.[1] The more those projects are delayed, the higher will be the costs to complete them and the more citizens and the economy will suffer in the mean time.

In this globalized economy, we are competing with China and other countries that invest more in maintaining and expanding their infrastructures. Not only is infrastructure essential to support healthy, vibrant communities, it is critical for long-term *qualitative* economic growth, jobs, household income, and exports.

The challenge to maintain today's infrastructure lies in availability of cheap energy and petroleum materials (Chapter 22). The U.S. built its high oil-consuming infrastructure when oil was a fraction of today's true, unsubsidized cost. Fortunately, there is much employment opportunity to rebuild for a less energy-wasteful infrastructure. In the process the urban landscape will be beautified, more healthful, and safer for all travelers.

The advent of unconventional oils (shale, tar sands, heavy oils) has extended the U.S.' oil dependence. The viability of these kinds of lower-net-energy yielding oils is questionable due to market forces and the tendency of field decline to take place sharply (particularly with natural gas fields). So the "bonanza" for U.S. re-supremacy in world oil is largely hype and unsustainable. It is important to take into account the permanent loss of cheap, high-energy yield oil when considering upgrading and maintaining the vast U.S. infrastructure which is linked to the global infrastructure also built on once-cheap oil. Yet, a "greener" infrastructure using less energy and that facilitates more healthful forms of transport and land-use is a definite possibility that offers major employment.

Categories of Infrastructure Projects

The tragic loss of life and property during Hurricane Katrina in Louisiana in 2005 illustrates the importance of ongoing investment in maintaining the estimated 100,000 miles of levees all over the country. While the original purpose of many of these levees was to protect farmland, new communities are now depending on levees built to a lower farmland standard. Compared with high levees designed and engineered to protect communities, levees built to lower heights and lower standards (e.g., earthen walls rather than concrete) to protect farmlands may lead to flooding in big storm events.

Much of our drinking-water infrastructure is in dire need of replacement. In older cities, some of the water pipes are over 100 years old. According to the American Water Works Association, replacing pipes and other projects for drinking water, wastewater, and stormwater systems will cost more than $1 trillion.[2]

The average age of the nation's over 600,000 bridges is over 40 years old[1] and many need to be replaced. Energy-efficient train services should be expanded. Highway congestion needs to be ameliorated. Investments should be made to America's public transit infrastructure because of its role in connecting millions of people with jobs, medical facilities, schools, shopping, and recreation. Parks and outdoor recreation areas support over 6 million jobs and contribute over $600 billion to the economy.[3] We need more not less safe access to the outdoors.

For commuting by bicycle and getting excise and relaxation on two wheels, the infrastructure is poor in two ways: it is lacking, and its use is threatened by motor vehicles. To expand bike infrastructure tremendously would be a relatively minor expenditure, but it appears to threaten the convenience of maximized car infrastructure. So the U.S. is way behind certain countries with better standards of living and traffic safety. The same applies to pedestrian facilities; much can be improved upon at little cost but with great benefits. With more investment in bicycling and walking infrastructure, less road infrastructure, parking lots, and driveways will be required that have high costs for maintenance.

School construction and maintenance budgets have decreased while the needs have increased. The backlog in projects to modernize and maintain schools is nearly $300 billion.[1] We have an aging energy infrastructure requiring upgrades with better electrical grids, gas pipelines, solar technologies, and other renewable energy innovations. Our nation's dams need proper maintenance to sustain essential benefits such as drinking water, irrigation, hydroelectric power, flood control, and recreation. Our bridges and highways should be maintained for safety, traffic congestion alleviation, and economic growth. Our nation's ports need to be maintained and modernized. With our post-carbon future economy, modernizing the ports means to adapt them for transitioning from tankers powered by bunker fuel to wind powered container cargo vessels, as is being pioneered by the Sail Transport Network.[4]

Trains are not presently running on renewable energy to a significant extent, except for some hydropower capacity for some electric trains. However, trains run on diesel in the U.S., which sounds bad, but are eight times as efficient energy-wise than trucks, and one-eighth as polluting. Nevertheless, renewable energy powered trains are a worthy goal, despite the lower energy yield from renewable technologies compared to oil. Natural gas has a big climate-protection advantage over coal, and somewhat over oil. As gas is a preferred electric power fuel, it can be used for electrified trains. This involves eliminating diesel fuel for train engines across the U.S., a major retooling challenge. Regardless, natural gas supplies are not what industry promoters claim, due to (1) market-price minimums needed for exploitation, and (2) the normal, sudden drop-off of gas-field pressure after peak extraction.

Grand Bargain #28: New Public Infrastructure Investments—$3.6 Trillion from 2016-2025

As the grand bargain for maintaining and expanding our infrastructure and putting people to work, let us devote $3.6 trillion to needed infrastructure projects over the next decade. These will involve systems of communication, transportation, water, and other necessary public works over the next decade, beginning with $50 billion in 2016.

Richard from the garden and many other young and old Americans could find employment with this level of needed infrastructure investment in our future. To make this major investment appealing to budget hawks, I propose to pay the entire bill from the consumption taxes without floating bonds or doing any additional borrowing.

The $50 billion for 2016 will be invested in long deferred infrastructure projects. Considering that 60% of the cost of constructing the infrastructure will go for worker wages, over 600,000 jobs will be created.[a] During the first year of the infrastructure enhancement cam-

---

a $50 billion x 0.6 (60% of company income going to wages) / $47,000 per added worker (projected from Social Security's National Average Wage Index[5]) ≈ 640,000 million new jobs

paign, plans will be drafted by engineers and architects. Spending will subsequently increase as construction workers implement the plans.

Communities may expand upon this public funding for infrastructure. With the elimination of corporate income taxes and other major financial benefits for businesses, companies will net over $800 billion in additional profits in 2016 (Chapters 1 and 21). They can devote some of this to meeting higher demands for products and services, much of which will require infrastructure investments. Companies hording profits in cash reserves rather than investing in more products and services reflects economic uncertainty. Grand Bargains' economic reforms will incentivize businesses to invest and grow. Business-friendly tax and regulatory policies together with Grand Bargains-facilitated elimination of unnecessary bureaucracy and waste will allow for the resources to enable additional infrastructure projects in the private sector and for state and local governments.

For instance, communities may be built in which all services are within walking distances of the residents, without the need for automobiles within the living areas. Older residential areas may be retrofitted to have parks, farmers' markets, sports facilities, schools, entertainment venues, and essential stores all within walking distance. Public transportation could be enhanced to easily connect with more distant attractions. Our cities are now largely car-centric regarding transportation. Much new building or redesign will be needed to enable the transition to the post-carbon economy.

Since ACCs will represent the interests of their members and will train and supply laborers, ACC representatives should partner with government and business leaders to select the projects that will make the largest positive impacts on all stakeholders. Corporate leaders and decision-makers will need the input of ACC leaders and stakeholders to know what projects the community wants to undertake. Businesses will also need to align with ACCs that supply skilled workers to carry out the projects undertaken. Additionally, ACC-affiliated credit unions and savings and loan banks will be a source of financing urban and rural development. With the many influences of ACCs added to the picture, building new communities or revitalizing old ones will be a collaborative process between all community stakeholders rather than predominately investment decisions of developers.

Summary and Conclusion

Our growing backlog of needed infrastructure upgrades threatens safety, economic competitiveness, and 21st Century jobs. With Grand Bargains-based health and economic reform allowing for money to build infrastructure without adding to the national debt, it will be a win, win, win for jobs, the economy, and the country to launch a program to continuously upgrade the U.S. infrastructure. We will strive for making it the best in the world, as was once the case when oil was almost as cheap as water.

Given the realities of conventional oil depletion – the maximum global supply was produced in 2005, and the U.S. peak was 1971 – the present oil-built national infrastructure requires low-cost, low-energy modification and repair. This offers a great potential for jobs for not just building but for restoration of the environment.

Beginning with a public infrastructure investment of $50 billion in 2016, we will aim to spend $3.6 trillion over the next decade. Representatives of ACCs throughout the country will be involved in helping to determine the priorities of projects in their regions of the country.

Chapter 16
Education: ACCs to Foster Experimentation

Since my parents could not afford to pay for my college education, I had to work and borrow. Tuition at San Jose State College in the late 1960s cost me about $100 per year. After living at home and commuting to save money for my freshman year, I moved to a rooming house on campus. I kept careful records of my spending for my entire sophomore year. It totaled about $950.

By 1980, tuition at California State University San Jose—my former "college" elevated to a "university"—cost a little over $200 per year, in keeping with the overall inflation in the economy from the 1960s to 1980. However, tuition at my alma mater in 2011 was $5370 per year, 10 times more than 1980 after adjusting for inflation.[1] This has been the trend throughout higher education in the past three decades.

Education Related to Health and Prosperity

Educational achievement is a major social indicator of health (Chapter 10). People with more education live longer, earn more money, contribute more to their communities, and have a better quality of life. Highly educated people are less likely to receive welfare. Prosperity—not necessarily defined by money—depends on excellence in education.

In part, because of our broken educational system, our competitiveness in the global economy is threatened. Our education system's failure to teach our children good health habits has led to the deterioration of public health (i.e., obesity, type 2 diabetes, chronic diseases of lifestyle, substance abuse, etc.) and further puts the viability of our economy and culture in jeopardy.

Crisis in U.S. Education

"We're losing 1.2 million people from our schools to the streets every year," according to U.S. Education Secretary Arnie Duncan.[2] Mr. Duncan is also concerned that while America once led the world in college graduation rates, it now ranks 12th.

These sobering statistics are reinforced by President Obama's linkage of education to the economy: "It's an economic issue when eight in 10 new jobs will require workforce training or a higher education by the end of this decade. It's an economic issue when we know countries that out-educate us today will out-compete us tomorrow."[2]

Few would dispute that our schools are in serious trouble. Education policymakers and politicians seek an approach to improve education for all Americans. However, no consensus exists about the best way forward for enabling all American students to succeed in education. Maybe different approaches need to be tried to see what works best. It might vary for different students and different communities.

To explore the issues in education, let us first examine the current state of our schools.

As the film documentary *Waiting for Superman* graphically described, our educational system is in crisis:[3]

- The annual cost of prison for an inmate is more than twice that spent on an individual public school student.
- Eight years after the "No Child Left Behind" act, with the goal of 100% proficiency in math and reading, students range between 20% and 30% proficiency.
- 70% of eighth graders cannot read at grade level.

- By 2020, only an estimated 50 million Americans will be qualified to fill 123 million highly skilled, highly paid jobs.
- Among 30 developed countries, the United States ranks 25th in math and 21st in science.

Washington-Centric Prescriptions for Schools

The "No Child Left Behind" program of President George W. Bush emphasized the standardized curricula of math and reading over social, athletic, and artistic development. Teachers, students, and parents complained that it over-stressed testing. It polarized the education community. Students experienced tremendous pressures to pass tests. Teachers felt like scapegoats for dysfunctional families and failed social programs. Test scores and dropout rates did not improve.[4]

As has been shown in many studies, excellence in education requires exceptional teachers.[5] Our challenge is to administer public and private schools in ways that attract, inspire, and reward those teachers. Aye, herein lies the rub. How do we improve the quality of our teachers? President Obama's answer was "Race to the Top."

The Race to the Top plan of the Obama administration sought to transform failing schools into privately run charter schools and rank teachers by their students' test scores. It has met major resistance from teachers' unions, parents, and others. The so-called "value-added method" introduced assesses student performance as a factor in deciding what teachers receive financial bonuses, how much extra money is awarded, and even who gets fired. Supposedly, the value added assessment methodology takes into account differences between children (parents' income, parents' education, English language skills, learning disabilities, etc). It purports to isolate the quality of teaching in the child's educational progress. Value added assessments have been especially controversial.[6]

The limitations of relying on value-added teacher assessments include:

- Teacher scores vary markedly from year to year.
- Students are not randomly assigned to teachers (e.g., principals may deliberately assign slow or fast learners to certain teachers).
- Tests do not measure the social skills that are essential to learning.[7]
- Standardized tests are often poor gauges of student performance.[8]

No Consensus on a "One-Size-Fits-All" Ideal Educational System

Government bureaucracies, however well intended, are not as well-positioned as parents, teachers, and local community leaders to use available resources to optimize the learning of students and to evaluate outcomes of education. Only by harnessing the efforts of the entire community can teachers, parents, and the local neighborhoods best encourage students to learn, become productive, and give back to society.

To improve education outcomes, innovation should be incentivized. For instance, "Freedom Schools" since the summer of 2010, enrolled 9600 children at more than 140 sites around the country. These schools emphasize literacy and include diverse activities. As with the origin of these schools in the civil rights era, Freedom Schools are mostly staffed by young college students.

In the morning, Freedom School teachers present a curriculum that focuses on critical thinking, conflict resolution, social action, healthful eating, creativity in the arts, and physical and mental health. After lunch, students participate in sports, listen to presentations by outside speakers, and go on field trips. Parent participation is an essential part of the program.[9]

We need more flexible funding in education at the local level to foster this kind of innovation and community participation.

Alternatives to Top-Down Approaches to Education

Dissatisfied with public and private education options, some parents home school their children. Some home schooled students do better than their colleagues in public schools and others do worse. It largely depends on the children, the teachers, and the socioeconomic strata of their parents.

Frustrated with top-down administrative bureaucracies in public schools, some teacher-run schools have been launched.[10] It is too soon to compare student performance and graduation rates in these schools with those in public and charter schools.

Some teachers and parents hail programs like "Teach for America" as a way to improve education of at-risk inner city and rural youth. In Teach for America, top college graduates make two-year commitments to teach in the most challenging urban and rural public schools. After a five-week summer in "teaching boot camp," they take full responsibility for classrooms and earn full salaries in difficult-to-fill teaching positions.

My daughter, Molly Thompson, taught middle school science in the south Bronx and high school biology in East Oakland through Teach for America. Biology standardized test pass rates in her East Oakland classes rose to about 12% after they were near 0% before her tenure. While Molly left public school education to enter nursing school, her five years of teaching were of tremendous benefit to her and, I'm sure, her students as well. The experience led her to pursue a career as a teacher of nurses.

Nevertheless, education policy experts disagree on the potential for Teach for America and similar programs to be scaled up to transform U.S. public education for the better.[11]

Educational outcomes are strongly correlated with socioeconomic status of the family and learning opportunities outside of the classroom. Poor, hungry children living in chaotic single-parent households in dangerous communities don't learn well no matter what type of schools they attend. Improving educational outcomes requires innovative ways to enhance learning environments and educational opportunities out-side as well as inside schools.

Higher Education: Rising Tuitions—
Less Value for Money

A book titled "Higher Education? How Colleges Are Wasting Our Money and Failing Our Kids and What We Can Do About It," by An-drew Hacker, PhD and Claudia Dreifus, PhD,[1] details the unsustainable rise in the cost of higher education in the U.S. For example, after adjust-ing for inflation, tuition in elite universities averages about three times more than in 1980:

- Williams College: $41,434 (3.2 times tuition in 1980)
- USC: $41,022 (3.6 times 1980)
- Pomona College: $38,394 (2.9 times 1980)

Rather than the extra tuition and fees going to enhance education, most of this money goes to administration, higher salaries and benefits for senior-faculty, college presidents' compensation, and athletic teams. Examples include the President of Vanderbilt University earning $1.2 million per year and varsity golf at Duke costing the University an estimated $20,405 per player per year. Room and board costs have also skyrocketed (e.g., UCLA room and board costs three times the rate of 1980).

Hiring of junior faculty to reduce the size of introductory classes has lagged. Drs. Hacker and Dreifus argue that a generation of young Americans has been shortchanged by overpaid senior faculty and ad-ministrators in our institutions of higher learning.

Rather than competing to provide high-quality education to more students at lower prices, colleges and universities more often battle each other by constructing more buildings and hiring more faculty.

Most prized are senior celebrity researchers rather than hard-working junior teachers.

Colleges and universities should collaborate more and not hire faculty to cover every subject. Institutions of higher learning should provide our students and their future employers the best education for the money.[12] To a much greater extent than now, competition among colleges and universities should be on value for money.

While government financial support is not keeping pace with the rising cost of college, many colleges and universities are increasing their borrowing and expecting to expand their share in the growing higher education market. Since the Great Recession, college and university education has become less affordable and job prospects for graduates less predictable. So it makes no sense for students and parents to be forced to borrow more heavily for school in support of an education arms race between competing universities.

Unsustainable Student Debt

As of 2014, total student loan debt is over $1.1 trillion.[13] This excessive student debt threatens the ability of young Americans to buy homes, start small businesses, begin families, and save for the future. It hurts the economy. This makes it time to reassess our national policies in education.

According to some economists, the already unsustainable levels of student debt may well lead to a collapse similar to that in the subprime mortgage market. However, unlike homeowners that can default on underwater mortgages and start over, students have much more difficulty legally walking away from their college loan debts.

Parallels exist between the unsustainable costs of health care and education. In both cases, the government funds a large proportion of the services with little regard for promoting cost competition among service providers. Like health care recipients, the major consumers of higher education services—students, parents, government, and private donors—are poorly positioned to drive serious completion among providers of services on cost effectiveness.

Grand Bargain #21: ACCs to Lead Experimentation with the Education System and to Prevent Student Debt

The 21ˢᵗ grand bargain is to give ACCs an education mandate. ACCs will channel U.S. Department of Education funds to communities, supplementing the financial and human resources of public and private schools. Along with the funds comes the authorization for ACCs to find their own supplemental approaches to helping students learn the basics as well as to think critically and innovate. Experimentation will be one of the keys to success. In addition, $50 billion in consumption tax money in 2016 will be channeled through the ACCs with the intention of innovatively supporting college and trade school students so they do not accumulate debt.

With Grand Bargains-based reform, the federal Department of Education will be eliminated. The $66 billion projected to be spent by the Department in 2016 for grants to state and local governments and school districts[14] will instead be allocated by the ACCs. ACC managers—informed by parents, students, teachers, and community leaders—will allocate the government education funds to enhance the educational opportunities of students.

The educational enhancement funds of the ACCs will be risk-adjusted, depending on the number of students enrolled and the socioeconomic strata of the families of ACC members that are in school. For each ACC, the allocation of educational enhancement funds from federal government block grants will be determined collaboratively. Each ACC will design a strategy to enhance the educational opportunities of students, utilizing input of all stakeholders.

Examples of possible areas of ACC spending on primary, secondary, and higher education include:

- tutors,
- teachers' aides,
- salary increases for teachers,
- education enrichment programs (music, art, nature study, etc.),
- internships for college students,
- scholarships, and
- work-study program expansions.

As part of devolving the responsibility and authority for education system policy from the government to the ACCs, federal funds for grants to college students will become administered by ACCs. As mentioned above, current federal funds for students will be supplemented by an additional $50 billion per year to prevent the need for student loans.

ACCs will financially help students to most efficiently use their personal savings, supplemented by part-time jobs (Chapter 12), and funding from charitable organizations. Shifting the partial responsibility for funding higher education from a federal bureaucracy to local ACCs will create beneficial pressure on colleges and universities to trim their bloated budgets and reduce their tuitions.

Since competing ACCs will be major players in funding higher education, they will foster free-market competition among colleges and universities to control costs of higher education while increasing the pressures to enhance quality and relevance of instruction. With ACC pressure, colleges and universities will compete to drive down unnecessary expenditures in administration, athletics, faculty, building construction, and other areas. With this funding clout and flexibility, the ACCs will foster real cost competition among colleges and universities by bargaining for reductions in tuition and other expenses for their students.

For instance, "massive online open classes" (MOOCs) may be an innovative way to improve education outcomes while controlling costs.[15] Free classes from elite universities from the U.S. and abroad promise to revolutionize education. The best students in these classes score better than students from Ivy League universities. The Khan Academy, founded by Sal Khan,[16] promises to enhance learning at all grade levels. It provides online lessons in step-by-step fashion that help each student proceed at his/her own individual pace. Lessons may be paused to ponder difficult concepts or repeated to reinforce learning. Students work at practice problems with computerized help whenever needed.

Since enrollees will have their choice of ACCs, the most effective allocation of ACC education funds will be part of the competition among ACCs. This competition will involve the amount of funds allocated to education, the fairness in distribution, innovation in educational funding priorities, the student debt situation, and the educational outcomes of students.

Good education begins with healthy children. ACCs will compete in finding strategies to encourage parents and others to foster good health habits in children. The ACCs with the best health and education outcomes will persuade more people to become members.

Summary and Conclusion

I call for U.S. Department of Education to be closed and the funds transferred to ACCs. The ACCs will use education funds to work directly with teachers, parents, and students in local K-12 schools, trade schools, colleges, and universities.

The education mandate for ACCs is to improve the quality of the instruction, the relevance of the education provided, and student education outcomes. ACCs will foster competition between education providers to cost effectively achieve these outcomes.

An additional $50 billion per year will be targeted by the ACCs for post high school graduation students to prevent the accumulation of student debt. For students in colleges and universities, the ACCs will become strong bargainers to greatly improve value for money in education. They will force colleges and universities to compete on cost. Over time, this will virtually eliminate student loan debt.

This strategy will shift a significant portion of the responsibility and accountability for education outcomes from the federal and state governments and local school districts to ACCs in local communities. Consequently, we will have many competing experiments to find what works best for different students and diverse communities. This will lead us to reclaim our role as the world's leader in education.

Chapter 17

ACC Enhanced National Security:
International Development Aid

The ultimate weakness of violence is that it is a descending spiral, begetting the very thing it seeks to destroy.... Returning violence for violence multiplies violence, adding deeper darkness to a night already devoid of stars. Darkness cannot drive out darkness; only light can do that. Hate cannot drive out hate; only love can do that.

Dr. Martin Luther King, Jr.

The mission of the Department of Defense has always been "to provide the military forces needed to deter war and to protect the security of our country."[1] However, the characterizations of threats to the security of the U.S. and the nature of military combat have both changed dramatically in the past century, particularly with transnational terrorism in the last decade.

While the U.S. is unequaled in military might, we have performed not so well of late in winning the hearts and minds of people around the world. Consequently, we need to fundamentally reassess how best to protect ourselves from danger coming from outside and inside the borders of the U.S.

Since the Vietnam War, we have been involved in dozens of military conflicts. Many of these interventions clearly turned more people against us than caused people to become U.S. supporters. The perception that we fight wars over resources, particularly oil, has not helped our image in the world, especially since we are by far the planet's biggest consumers of oil and other commodities.

The "War on Terror" Calls for New Strategies

Now we are engaged in the so called, "war on terror," which has no geographic boundaries. The war on terror is an ideological war. Politicians and other partisans with different viewpoints present talking points and propaganda, trying to win hearts and minds of people, particularly young males from 15-30 years old.

Terrorist ideologies are resonating with many disaffected young men and some women in foreign countries as well as some at home. By this measure and others, we are failing at the mission of the Department of Defense—deterring war and terrorism.

Using drones and fighter planes to target suspected terrorists in far off countries with bombs and missiles may kill some dangerous people. However, the collateral damage of dead or injured innocent civilians galvanizes ever more people to fight against us. It also helps spread the terrorists' ideologies.

Accordingly, our approach to defense should shift in large part away from simply focusing on better and better ways to kill more terrorists and towards strategies to combat *terrorist ideologies* and to win friends for the U.S. around the world.

If the U.S. could avoid wars by amassing superior military forces, we would already be in a "Pax Americana." However, wars and terrorism arise from issues about sovereignty, territory, resources, religions, and ideologies.[2] Armaments do not address these issues. To deter war and terrorism, we need to understand the causes of major conflicts at a deep level and proactively work to deal with those causes. By addressing the breeding grounds for extremist ideologies, we can prevent incidents escalating into wars or acts of terrorism. Peace movements need to do more than to expose the futility of war and mount opposition to any war that is not truly defensive for the U.S.' security on its shores. Promoting peace should mean to use our resources, skills, and advocacy to counteract the conditions that make people prone to violent conflicts.

In the modern world, national security amounts to much more than national defense. Our military might assures us that we can militarily defeat any country that attacks us. Even Iran and North Korea, which our leaders consider "rogue nations," would not consider an invasion of U.S. territory. However, no amount of military spending and preparedness will make us safe from terrorist attacks.

Alarmingly, U.S. born and educated terrorists are becoming increasingly common. The principles that we stand for—life, liberty, and the pursuit of happiness—are not ringing true or honest with groups of people at home and around the world. We need to seriously consider why this is, and change our national defense strategy accordingly.

Maybe most people agree with our principles but object to our use of our superior military might to defend our interests around so much of the world. If Third World peoples feel economically exploited by us (e.g., our massive imports of oil and other commodities), their anger may add fuel to existing resentments. Some people may hate us because it suits our economic or other interests to support dictators that repress them. Others may dislike us because we supply military aid to their enemies.

People who feel helpless and hopeless and that they have nothing to lose are particularly susceptible to national liberation movements or even repulsive ideologies. Indeed, our use of the instruments of war attempting to settle disputes in other countries to the U.S.' liking tends to consume scarce resources as well as fuel ideological hatred against us. Our militant actions lead to blowback. Our strategy of devoting huge amounts of resources to military preparedness and wars of choice is making us overall less safe. This leaves fewer resources at home and for creating partnerships abroad—economic, educational, technological, public health, social, cultural, ecological, and developmental—that build friendships and mutual interdependency.

Isolationism is not the answer. We need alternatives to constant war. One part of the Grand Bargains-based alternative to "war as a way to win peace" is federal funding of national security activities to aid development in Third World countries. The federal government already has a relatively small international affairs budget that includes development aid. Let's see what the international affairs budget comprises and then what needs to be added.

International Development Assistance Workers Vital for U.S. Security

International affairs activities, which arguably are as important or more important than military might, include:[3]

1. operating U.S. embassies and consulates throughout the world;
2. providing military assistance to allies (arguably counterproductive);
3. aiding developing nations;
4. dispensing economic assistance to fledgling democracies;
5. promoting U.S. exports abroad;
6. making U.S. payments to international organizations; and
7. contributing to international peacekeeping efforts.

The major agencies involved in international affairs include the Departments of Agriculture, State, and the Treasury; the United States Agency for International Development; and the Millennium Challenge Corporation. Funding for all of these activities, about $46 billion projected for 2016,[4] constitutes less than one tenth of the baseline military budget, not counting war supplements. These funds are supposed to protect our national security by doing everything from contributing to fighting terrorism, to stabilizing weak and fragile states, to driving economic development, to alleviating global poverty, to fighting HIV/AIDS, to expanding educational opportunities and strengthening democratic institutions.[5] Given the challenges facing the U.S. today, and the somewhat established humanitarian role many see for the U.S., the allocation of funds and manpower for international affairs is grossly inadequate. Therefore the challenges are (1) for U.S. aid and peacemaking to be greatly enhanced, (2) to change the nature of the aid to become more attuned with the needs in the world, and (3) to make the aid less self-serving and interfering.

U.S. Government Foreign Aid—Little Value for Money

Development aid from the International Affairs Budget is often in conjunction with U.S. military activities in the same country. This presents huge challenges to the effective delivery of the aid. Afghanistan serves as an example in which our development aid brought little if any benefit because of the conflict and the politics. Ex-President Karzai requested that our aid workers leave Afghanistan.[6a]

International aid groups have also complained about the militarization of U.S. government funded development assistance, noting that it endangers all those associated with humanitarian efforts. Poor people in Third World countries are often understandably suspicious of U.S. government-administered aid. In part, this is due to strings attached that channel funds directly or indirectly to the benefit of U.S. companies. U.S. government allegiances to corrupt, oppressive, dictatorial governments in poor countries also lead to cynicism about U.S. government-administered aid. Unfortunately, our perceived strategic interests often get in the way of our ideals.

---

a   In Afghanistan and other conflict zones involving our armed forces, the association of our military presence with foreign reconstruction aid has tended to negate the potential benefit of the aid. Ex Afghan President Hamid Karzai denounced provincial reconstruction teams as one of a number of Western-created "parallel structures" that undermined the authority of his government. He tried to curtail the operations of private security firms and objected to Western-funded aid projects that bypassed government ministries and funneled money directly to contractors and subcontractors. In an angry speech, after yet another incident of innocent civilians being killed by NATO forces, President Karzai requested that reconstruction and development units supported by the NATO force be phased out.[6]

Zambian economist Dambisa Moyo recently published the book *Dead Aid*, arguing that Africa's dependence on foreign development aid has kept the continent in poverty, distorted economies, and fueled bureaucracy and corruption. Instead of handouts, she advocates encouraging trade, foreign direct investment, microfinancing for enterprises, and seeking funds from capital markets.[7]

Waging Peace as a National Security Strategy: Development Aid to Win the Hearts and Minds of People

We must listen carefully to any people we hope to aid. We should seek to understand their needs, from their perspectives. Deterring war and terrorism means proactively winning the hearts and minds of people.

Success in winning the peace depends on an all out endeavor of millions of Americans working toward a unified purpose. In this 21st Century, waging peace and winning hearts and minds should mean U.S. citizens directly providing unconditional development aid to people in underdeveloped countries. The magnitude of the necessary civilian peace endeavor needs to equal or surpass the U.S. civilian support of the allied forces battling in World War II.

While many people in underdeveloped countries do not trust the U.S. government to provide aid, people-to-people aid has been seen more positively. For example, for the past 10 years or so my friend, Rosalind Russell, has travelled to Nepal to give poor village women pregnant goats. The villagers refer to her as the "goat lady." Women receiving the goats are expected to raise the kids produced and give goats to other poor village women. The standards of living in the villages that have received Rosalind's goats have improved significantly.

Rosalind has also worked with the people of one village to build an elementary school. A second school in an adjacent village is in progress. Parents pay no tuition for girls, and for boys the school charges one-half the rate of government schools. By favoring the education of girls, Rosalind wants to counteract the common practice in Nepal of only sending boys to school. Like many others, she has found that the education of girls leads to village living standards going up and birth rates going down.[8]

New York Times Columnist Nicholas Kristof told the story of a Pakistani woman, Roshaneh Zafar, an American-educated banker who has dedicated her life to empowering some of Pakistan's most impoverished women with microfinance loans. Zafar notes, "Charity is limited, but capitalism isn't." She prefers market-based solutions over handouts. Her bank, Kashf, now has 152 branches in Pakistan and has dispersed more than $200 million to more than 300,000 families. She notes that microfinance and economic opportunity are potent tools to fight terrorism. According to Zafar, "The antonym of 'militant' is often 'job.'"[9]

In most developing countries, job #1 is to provide food security.

Food Security: A Necessity to Prevent Wars

Food security in the U.S. and other countries is a fundamental component of national security.

In the 2011 budget of the United States Department of Agriculture (USDA), about $2.3 billion went for "Farm and Foreign Agricultural Services." This targeted the improvement of food security in developing countries. In part, the USDA rationale was the following:[10]

> . . . In addition to ensuring that the world's children have enough to eat, the United States has a strong interest in promoting strong agricultural systems in the developing world, because failing agricultural systems and food shortages fuel political instability and diminish the economic vitality of developing nations. Working with other Federal partners, the Department is working towards reducing global food insecurity and increasing agriculture-led economic growth in developing coun-

tries. USDA's capacity-building, technical assistance, and food assistance programs are effective tools for improving the capacity of countries to produce what they need and to make that food accessible to those who need it . . . .

Indeed, the U.S. does have an interest in global food security on humanitarian grounds and because of our own self interest. Hunger fuels terrorism and wars.

However, some USDA policies are often counterproductive in promoting food security and peace. The USDA policy of providing crop subsidies to U.S. farmers does not improve our food security but favors high calorie, low nutrient, disease promoting junk-food diets (Chapter 13). Likewise, U.S. government funding for famine relief going exclusively for export of U.S. crops puts farmers in developing countries at a disadvantage in becoming self-sufficient.

In developing countries, we need to greatly increase our funding for agriculture programs because our national security depends on helping people all over the world climb out of poverty to become free from hunger. Third World aid should include local sustainable farming projects of mostly plant-based foods that increase food security.

This will make us friends.

Livestock: A National Security Issue

Since all humans have to eat and most people eat animals, livestock production is a national security issue.

Livestock provides food and income for one billion of the world's poor. Especially in dry areas, livestock may be the only source of livelihoods. The Food and Agriculture Organization (FAO) reported, "Since livestock production is an expression of the poverty of people who have no other options, the huge number of people involved in livestock for lack of alternatives, particularly in Africa and Asia, is a major consideration for policy makers."[11]

Worldwide, the livestock sector is undergoing many technological and geographical changes. In the last 40 years, increases in meat production have greatly exceeded increases in fruits, vegetables, beans, and grains for human consumption. About 80% of growth in the livestock sector comes from industrial production systems, also known as factory farming. The resources required and pollution created makes this trend unsustainable. According to the FAO, worldwide shifts from plant-based to animal-based foods mean that livestock are entering into direct competition for scarce land, water, energy, and other natural resources.

Livestock grazing occupies 26% of the Earth's terrestrial surface, and feed crop production takes about one-third of arable land.[11] Deforestation directly results from the expansion of grazing land for livestock. For instance, about 70% of previously forested land in the Amazon is used as pasture. Feed crops cover a large part of the reminder of recently deforested land. Consequently, much land is degraded from overgrazing, compaction, and erosion. The loss of rainforest decreases the carbon dioxide absorbed by plants. Additionally, livestock production directly increases greenhouse gas emissions (e.g., carbon dioxide and methane). Cow eructation (burping or belching) and flatulence are said to cause more global warming that the world's cars because the cows emit methane, a much more powerful greenhouse gas than carbon dioxide.[12]

According to the FAO, livestock account for 18% of worldwide greenhouse gas emissions while cultivating plants for human consumption generates a much smaller fraction of emissions—plants themselves don't generate the carbon dioxide; they sequester it. Livestock consume increasing amounts of water and energy, especially fossil fuels (Chapters 21 and 22). Pollutants generated by livestock include animal wastes, antibiotics, hormones, chemicals from tanneries, fertilizers and pesticides used for feed crops, and sediments from eroded pastures. The livestock sector also contributes significantly to acid rain and acidification of ecosystems by production of ammonia. Overgrazing of livestock endangers biodiversity by causing habitat loss, threatening the survival of more and more species.

While the status quo environmental consequences of livestock production for food are already dire, the FAO predicts that the production of meat will double from now to 2050.[13] This is a recipe for disaster. As a national and planetary security measure, sustainable-development aid workers in the Third World should help people work towards limiting livestock to land that is unsuitable for growing crops for humans.

Two thirds of the earth is now in the process of turning into desert. Scientists estimate that this process contributes more to climate change than fossil fuels. Most areas that are turning into deserts in the world were previously mostly grasslands. In grasslands, large, hoofed animals graze on the grass—buffalo, zebra, gazelles, wildebeest, etc. The grass and the animals evolved to rely on each other. Consequently, if you take away the grass, the hoofed animals die off. And if you take away the hoofed animals, the grassland turns into a desert. A recent strategy for reversing desertification involves creating or recreating grasslands on deserts by bringing back grazing animals to fertilize the grasslands.[14, 15]

While we need more hoofed animals to prevent the advance of desertification worldwide, we need a game-changer to phase out the industrial livestock industry. Living securely and sustainably with seven billion people now and nine billion people projected for 2050 will require limiting the production of livestock to land that requires hoofed animals to support the ecological health of the land. Otherwise, we need to increase plant-based food for human consumption. This should be a central mission of U.S. funded foreign development aid.

Reassessing Our National Security Priorities

We face an increasing number of threats to worldwide stability and our own security. In our increasingly globalized society and economy, we are at a pivotal moment in our relationships with people around the world. Accordingly, we should re-evaluate the components of our spending for national defense and re-evaluate our overall strategy for national security.

As you might have begun to surmise by now, one of the main Grand Bargains' solutions is to focus more on helping people in foreign countries using our strengths in education, health care, public health, agriculture, infrastructure, technology, and other areas. Deterring war and terrorism should now be mainly about partnering with people around the world to help them develop into middle class lives. However, "middle class" will need to be redefined as omitting the emphasis on cars and much of the non-essential consumer products.

A good example of a middle class emerging without cars or consumer goods is Cuba. As detailed in a presentation by Dr. Richard Feinberg given at the Brookings' Institute, up to 40% of Cuban labor force is already operating, at least part-time in the private sector. Dr. Feinberg gave other reasons to consider Cuba a middle class society despite low consumption of consumer products:[16]

1. Income inequality is very low.
2. A World Bank study classified Latin Americans as middle class if they had 10.4 years of education. The average Cuban has 10.2 years of education.
3. All Cubans have ready access to health care, to family planning and contraception. Cuban women have the lowest fertility rates in the Western Hemisphere.
4. Eighty percent of Cubans own their own homes, although many are dilapidated.
5. Almost all Cubans have coverage by social security.

Cuban-style communism doesn't have to be the only model for development of an economically and ecologically sustainable middle class society. But it does demonstrate that Third World countries can become middle class without overconsumption and excessive pollution.

Fortunately, U.S. citizens are especially able to partner with Third World people to combat poverty, facilitate education, teach sustainable farming methods, build clean drinking water systems, and promote public health. This will foster good will towards us. This will protect us. In this 21st Century world, helping people develop is more powerful than weapons systems and special operations team for national defense. Greatly expanding our capacity to help people is an essential component of a rational national security strategy. However, this does not mean disarmament or dropping our defenses.

Waging peace should not be simply delegated to the expert diplomats of the federal government. While they are well meaning and undoubtedly very intelligent, they have failed repeatedly. If we are to become more secure, we must shift our emphasis on waging wars to the hard work of winning lasting peace. As the Grand Bargains' peace budget recommendations for the next decade will demonstrate, the financial cost of waging peace will be nearly as high as waging wars, but it will not nearly as high as the cost of mutually assured destruction.

Grand Bargain #22: ACC Members to Enhance National Security as Professional Development Workers

The Grand Bargains' strategy for national security is to allocate $50 billion in 2016 to development aid programs run by nonprofit organizations staffed, funded, and monitored through the ACCs. Subsequently, funding will increase over the next decade by $50 billion per year to reach $500 billion in 2025.

Following major conflicts, after humanitarian workers have finished providing the necessary disaster relief, development workers are vital to help communities rebuild. Development aid may be the difference between resurgences of war and sustainable peace. For impoverished people that have not recently been fighting with each other or with their neighbors, development aid can potentially stop wars from occurring.

The budget for the Department of Defense is projected by the Congressional Budget Office to decrease as a percentage of the GDP over the next decade.[17] Hence, the Joint Chiefs of Staff are planning to reduce the number of men and women in military service. While downsizing the U.S. military is laudable, threats that we may face from hungry, uneducated, desperate people in foreign countries mean we need to recruit more Americans to seek careers in the peace promoting aspects of national security. The Grand Bargains' peace offensive will provide much needed jobs for U.S. citizens.

Sustainable-development national-security jobs should be funded by the new consumption taxes and administered through the ACCs. The ACC members taking these jobs will focus on helping Third World people with agriculture, education, public health, health care, infrastructure, business, and more.

This Grand Bargains' national security strategy will involve conservatives, liberals, military personnel, veterans, civilians, recent college graduates, and seniors coming out of retirement. Helping people will give us additional national security that no amount of military armaments or personnel could afford.

ACC Foreign Development Aid to Address Climate Change

The Department of State and U.S. Agency for International Development Budget is projected to devote a mere $500 million in 2016 to fighting climate change. We need a much bigger effort.

Realizing the failures of development aid to foreign countries in the past, the Grand Bargains-based national security strategy will address the major issue expressed by Third World countries at the Copenhagen Climate Change Summit: *Sustainable Development*. Many groups at that conference called for $150 billion per year in sustainable-development aid in compensation for the U.S.' outsized contribution to climate change.[18] To answer this call for social, economic, and environmental justice, ACC development aid projects will focus on the underlying causes of terrorism—poverty, hunger, ignorance, and injustice.

To train people for sustainable-development work, funds will be provided through the ACCs to establish college majors and post-graduation master's degrees in sustainable-development strategies. This will increase overall education funding without increasing student debt. U.S. citizens, some having completed these sustainable-development degrees, will be sent to developing countries to help implement sustainable-development programs. The areas of focus will include health care, agriculture, reforestation, transportation, education, preventive medicine, construction, and business.

Each ACC will distribute sustainable-development funds allocated from federal government consumption taxes to support American ACC development aid workers going to foreign countries. ACCs may partner with the Peace Corps or other existing Third World development organizations. They may also invest in "B" company startups (i.e., benefit companies having social missions, Chapter 24) to expand this work. The funding will pay for the training and salaries of selected ACC members as sustainable-development professionals. The funding will also cover the cost of needed technology, equipment, and supplies to aid in achieving sustainable-development goals in Third World countries. Some sustainable-development professionals may have long careers in providing development aid. Others may work for two or three years as a service to humanity and as a duty to keep our country safe and secure.

Each sustainable-development-aid job, including training, living expenses, and aid funds to administer, will cost about $100,000 on average per year. Compare this with the $1 million cost of deploying a soldier to Afghanistan for a year. In 2016, this $50 billion national security initiative will produce over 500,000 permanent professional jobs.[b] By the end of the first decade, helping poor Third World people climb out of poverty will create an estimated 5 million job for ACC members.

The intent is for conflicts over water, land, and other resources to be reduced and for economic and environmental disasters to be pre-

---

b $50 billion/$100,000 per year per job = 500,000 jobs

vented. The dividends of such a sustainable-development program will help in maintaining a more peaceful world.

Many current and former Department of Defense civilian and military workers may apply to be retrained as sustainable-development workers. Rather than the Joint Chiefs' projected declining employment in the Department of Defense, there will be a massive increase of well-paying jobs over the next decade to facilitate a shift worldwide to sustainable development as part of our national security strategy.

Grand Bargains Four Prong Strategy to Defeat ISIS

After President Obama announced in a speech September 17, 2014 on television that he was ordering air strikes on the Islamic State in Iraq and Syria (ISIS), an NBC News/Wall Street Journal poll found that 62% of Americans supported the decision and 68% thought that it would not work.[19]

Chelsea Manning (formerly Bradley Manning, the Army intelligence officer who is in prison for sending classified documents to Wiki-leaks) proposed a strategy to defeat ISIS that is worth considering. In an article published in the Guardian of London, she wrote:[20]

> Attacking ISIS directly, by air strikes or special operations forces, is a very tempting option available to policymakers, with immediate (but not always good) results. Unfortunately, when the west fights fire with fire, we feed into a cycle of outrage, recruitment, organizing and even more fighting that goes back decades. This is exactly what happened in Iraq during the height of a civil war in 2006 and 2007, and it can only be expected to occur again.

Instead, Manning suggests a strategy of containing ISIS over a period of time while their barbarity and brutality work against them. She concludes by saying,

> ... the world just needs to be disciplined enough to let the ISIS fire die out on its own, intervening carefully and avoiding the cyclic trap of "mission creep". .. ISIS is wielding a sharp, heavy and very deadly double-edged sword. Now just wait for them to fall on it.

In a report on ISIS, the United Nations called for a political rather than military solution to the terror. It called for us to

> "Reach a sustainable solution to the ongoing armed conflict in Syria through an inclusive and Syrian-led political process...recognising that the lack of a political process has allowed extremism to fester, the international community and the Syrian Government cannot further delay this process..."[21]

Notably, the U.N. report did not condone the bombing and droning of ISIS targets by the U.S. or even address American involvement in the war with ISIS. It did not call for U.S. or other countries to commit ground troops to fight ISIS.

Indeed, our involvement in yet another war in the Middle East plays into the hands of the terrorists. It helps greatly in recruiting more jihadists. Paradoxically, our militarism hurts many of the people we claim to want to help. Most military analysts and other Americans believe that our war with ISIS is unwinnable without deploying American boots on the ground. If hundreds of thousands of U.S. boots on the ground in Iraq could not win that war, committing ground troops to another Middle East war will be counterproductive and lead more Third World people to hate us. We need a better plan.

First, we must learn about the history and motivations of our new enemy. As cogently laid out by New York Times columnist Thomas Friedman,[22] the aim of Islamic State or ISIS militants is not to invade the U.S. or foreign countries—at least not now—but to spread and impose its extremist concepts of Islamic society on people in Iraq and Syria. The puritanical and intolerant religious ideology of Wahhabi Islam that they espouse is attracting Muslim youths worldwide through social media.

However, ISIS extremism goes far beyond religious ideology. It originates with the complex, interconnected social and economic problems throughout the Middle East. Those problems include underdevelopment, sectarianism, lack of educational opportunities, oppression of women, and poverty. ISIS has capitalized on all these issues. Although the extremist ideology appeals to very few Muslims, ISIS militants have taken advantage of a power vacuum in parts of the region due to the long-standing wars in Iraq and Syria. Poor, uneducated, angry youths, resentful of enduring ridicule from the rest of Muslim society, have joined with ISIS to fill that power vacuum. Expressing their long-held resentment over their feelings of inferiority, they terrorize local people with whom they have had long-standing grudges.

Will air attacks with bombers and drones address the resentments of these ISIS militants towards their own, mostly Muslim, neighbors? I don't think so. If anything, our attacks will radicalize more disaffected youth.

The Grand Bargains' strategy to defeat ISIS has four components:

1. rather than continuing aerial bombing or launching a counterproductive U.S. military ground war in Iraq and Syria, contain and isolate ISIS until it becomes unpopular even among extremist ideologues,
2. become petroleum independent by taxing fossil fuels and reducing non-renewable energy consumption by 30% (Chapter 22),

3. ramp up the humanitarian relief projects in the areas surround-
    ing ISIS held territories and in Palestine, and
4. hire hundreds of thousands of ACC members as development
    workers to help people around the world.

While containing ISIS and waiting for it to burn out on its own is
required initially, it is not nearly enough to win against ISIS or against
the spread of terrorist ideologies.

More than ever, our national security depends on stopping our dependence on foreign petroleum, especially from the war-torn Middle
East. The U.S.' becoming energy independent is essential to combating
the perception of Americans as overconsuming exploiters of people in
other countries. This energy conservation component of the war on
terror must be fought by all Americans, led by legislators enacting the
Grand Bargains' proposed tax on non-renewable energy (Chapter 22).

Finally, we need to be seen as helping people around the world
rather than engaging in constant wars that primarily hurt civilians.
Initially, we need to mount major increases in humanitarian aid going
to the areas surrounding ISIS-held territory. Refugee camps should be
supported in Iraq, including the Kurdish regions, Saudi Arabia, Turkey, Lebanon, Egypt, and Jordan. As of October 2014, nearly 4 million
people are refugees registered by the United Nations. Donations to
meet the needs of those people are about $2 billion short of the amount
required.[23]

With the long standing crisis in Palestine again escalating in 2014,
the United Nations estimates that there are now about 5 million inter-
nally displaced refugees in Gaza and the West Bank.[24] The UN budget
for humanitarian relief in this area is only about $700 million per year.
An additional $300 million has been requested because of the injuries
and destruction in the 50-day war between Israel and Hamas in the
summer of 2014. Repairing the infrastructure damage in the Palestinian
territories from the war has been estimated to cost about $7 billion.[25]

Humanitarian and development aid in these two areas of the Middle
East might initially cost in the range of $10 billion. As a major part

of the U.S. National Security strategy, we should supply the necessary funds for the humanitarian and development aid required for these refugees. This is critical to our restoring our image in the Middle East and the world, and it is the right thing to do. Aiding people in these two critical areas will be a down payment on the Grand Bargains' proposed development aid for Third World countries that is crucial to combating jihadist terrorist ideologies.

Conclusion

As has become increasingly clear, our budget-busting military spending on optional wars has not brought us the sought after national security. We need a new approach to national security in this age of terrorist threats fueled by widespread anti-American sentiment. We can become safer by helping the poor in underdeveloped countries to sustainably develop their systems of agriculture, education, health care, and infrastructure construction.

By sending millions of sustainable-development teachers, engineers, health workers, and farmers to Third World countries, Americans will not be disliked but rather seen as people who help the poor and disadvantaged. In 2016, a $50 billion investment in development of impoverished countries will employ at least 600,000 Americans in meaningful, well-paying jobs. It will combat the attraction of jihadist ideologies. Helping impoverished people rise toward more comfortable, secure lives—especially educating girls—will tend to reduce unsustainable planetary population growth that also threatens our security. Leadership by the U.S. in development aid to the poor of the world will also foster humanitarian and development aid by people from other countries.

In part, out of our own self-interest in preserving our national security, we can lead the development of people from impoverished nations to the post-carbon, prosperous world that we all want to peacefully share.

Chapter 18
ACC-Based Medical Insurance Reform

I underwent an orthopedic surgical procedure in 2009, requiring an overnight stay in the hospital. In the months that followed, the stack of Anthem Blue Cross explanatory statements and medical bills arriving grew to at least a quarter inch thick. The assistant surgeon, whom I never met, sent a bill to me for a co-payment of $384.41 after Blue Cross paid him $1537.65 for his two hour's work. I reluctantly paid the bill after several invoices and a threat to send the bill to collections. About three months later, Anthem Blue Cross informed me that the assistant surgeon overbilled the insurer, so I was due a refund of $175.35. The surgeon's office had incorrectly used a "billing code modifier" indicating that he was the main surgeon.

I spent no less than three hours on the phone speaking with six unhelpful insurance bureaucrats and office workers over the next two weeks to actually collect the refund. None of them was empowered by their company to resolve the problem. It would have been futile to lodge a complaint against these workers, so I didn't write their employers. Our system of providing medical insurance was the problem, not the workers.

Angela Braly, the CEO of WellPoint, the parent organization of my insurer, earned almost $10 million in 2009.[1] That equates to about $5000 per hour. Obviously, her time is much more valuable than mine.

Something is wrong with this picture.

The Employer Mandate—Bad Medicine

There are many things wrong with employers paying for health care. Employers' bearing the cost of employee health care insurance significantly decreases the international competitiveness of U.S. businesses and increases the trade deficit. Employers' tax deductions for medical insurance of workers unfairly favors insured employees of large corporations and government agencies over employees of small businesses, workers that buy insurance individually, and the medically uninsured. The government loses hundreds of billions of dollars in taxes because health care insurance is a deduction for employers. The tax write-off means that the government subsidizes expensive plans (i.e., Cadillac insurance for the wealthy) more than less expensive plans.

In large part, the high cost of employee health insurance together with tough international competition led to the dramatic fall of automobile companies in the Great Recession. Unsustainable employee health care and other benefit obligations contributed to the bankruptcy of General Motors and Chrysler. Up until the bankruptcy of General Motors in 2009, the health care benefits of retired workers' diverted billions of dollars from developing new models and added $1,400 to the cost of each car compared with those made by Asian and European car makers.[2] For many U.S. companies, health care costs continue cutting into profits, curtailing hiring, and limiting expansion possibilities.

According to health care policy analysts from a spectrum of political viewpoints, employer-based health insurance is unraveling.[3, 4] Many health policy experts and a consensus of business and labor interests want a comprehensive game plan to replace the current, employer-provided health care system.[5, 6] The Obamacare plan did not address getting rid of employer-based health care.

ACC-based health reform will spare employers the approximately $700 billion they are projected to pay for health insurance policies for their employees in 2016.[7] This will spur competitiveness of U.S. industries, provide investors more predictability with asset returns, and increase jobs.

The Insurance Company Dilemma

Americans direct much anger to medical insurance companies about problems with health care cost, treatment denials, mind numbing paperwork, quality of care, and access to providers. The public anger about underwriting practices and determinations of benefit packages by insurance company bureaucrats is understandable, but misplaced. If one insurance company insures too many high-risk patients and approves too many services, the high premiums required combined with the fierce competition from other companies will drive it out of business. The broken health care system itself, rather than the symptom of rapacious insurance industry employees, drives our system's extraordinary administrative burden and deprives millions of appropriate health services.

Of our projected cost of personal medical insurance premiums in 2016, insurance company underwriting, billing, claims adjudication, marketing, taxes, lobbying Congress, executive compensation, profits, and other expenses will consume about 19%[a] ($224 billion).[8] Health care administrative services by the government will add approximately another $47 billion. However, a blizzard of insurance company paperwork flooding health services providers and patients will account for most of the outsized $1 trillion+ we are projected to spend in 2016 for medical administration.[8, 9]

A health care reform proposal by the Physicians for a National Healthcare Program would entirely eliminate the private health care insurance business. It would substitute government-run single-payer health care. According to *Health Care for America Now*, a government-run single-payer system would shift $300 billion to $400 billion from administration to health services providers—theoretically enough to cover the uninsured.[10] However, more money for health services providers would not necessarily improve health outcomes.

---

a   About $224 billion will go for insurance company overhead out of $1156 billion (19.4%) in private insurance premiums projected for 2016

We know from Medicare regional comparison data that low-spending regions have as good or better outcomes as high-spending regions.[11] If we adopted a government-run single-payer system, the loss of jobs for over a million medical insurance industry workers would be devastating for those people and the economy. We need to do the right thing for patients and insurance industry workers. The collection and distribution of trillions of dollars for health care services for patients requires financial professionals like those now working for insurance companies and government agencies.

Current pressures on the insurance industry include integrated health care systems like Kaiser Permanente, self-insured corporations, and competition from alliances of doctors and hospitals.[2] Health plans from insurance companies lost members because of the Great Recession. Insurance companies will also lose customers because Obamacare cuts funding for the Medicare Advantage program that allows almost 11 million people on Medicare to receive additional services through private insurance companies.

For medical insurance companies to become part of fixing our broken health care system, they need to insure all U.S. residents while dramatically cutting the paperwork and cost per person insured. To do that, our way of insuring people for health care needs to change fundamentally.

ACC Administration Utilizing Private Financial Services Companies

With ACC-based health care, private insurance companies will function much differently. Instead of covering about 180 million people as they do now, these companies will cover nearly all 329 million people residing in the U.S. in 2016.[12] However, they will not determine who will be enrolled in an ACC or what will and will not be covered by insurance. They will no longer do underwriting, marketing, sales, and claims adjudication. These functions add way too much to medical insurance overhead.[13]

Instead of performing activities related to approving and denying patients for coverage and determining what medical interventions will be reimbursed, insurance companies will be replaced by ACC-affiliated financial services companies. Customers of the new financial services companies will be the ACC practices rather than employers, individual patients, or government agencies. Accordingly, displaced insurance company employees will be retrained in other functions. The former insurance company employees will take on new roles with duties that encompass:

1. receiving revenue from the government, patient premiums, and employers (private pension contributions, Chapter 23);
2. processing payments for health care, preventive medicine, social services (Chapter 10), legal services (Chapter 11), educational services (Chapter 16), and financial services (Chapter 24) to ACC employees, contractors, and members as directed by ACC management;
3. disbursing Social Security and pension funds to ACC members (Chapter 23);
4. processing disability payouts to ACC members (Chapter 19);
5. paying all other bills incurred by the ACCs;
6. transferring funds to ACC-affiliated credit unions and asset management companies (Chapter 24).

The financial risk management functions of the insurance companies will be transferred to the managers and staffs of each individual ACC. ACC managers will employ the actuaries and accountants to monitor revenues and expenditures in order to advise ACC decision makers about the relationship of the projected costs of services to be delivered to members and the financial resources at hand. From that information, ACC leadership in collaboration all stakeholders will decide what medical, social, and other services to provide in the future and whether to adjust member premiums up or down.

The distribution of federal safety-net and social insurance funds will also be shifted from federal government social services agencies to ACC-affiliated private financial services companies. These financial services companies will not succeed solely by maximizing returns on their financial services. To stay in business, the new ACC-affiliated financial services workers will compete by enacting strategies that optimize benefits to ACC members.

Health care and social services will become seamlessly coordinated as well as financially integrated. The financial administration of these social services by the ACC-affiliated insurance companies will allow more money to go to human services and less to bureaucracy.

Financial Services Companies and Researchers Monitoring Health Interventions, Outcomes, and Costs

As mentioned in Chapter 8, medical effectiveness research must expand far beyond randomized controlled trials involving a relatively small number of patients and few medical research questions. The whole health care system and each component part must be continually analyzed by keeping track of health services provided, costs, and health outcomes. With recent advances in online information technology, we now have the capacity to monitor and analyze health services data in real time.

With ACC-run health care, financial services companies will assume the roles of assuring transparency and accountability in the allocation of funds. Statisticians and other scientists in the public and private sectors will analyze the data gathered on services rendered, health and other outcomes, and costs, assuring that patients will not be individually identified. With this information, specific health care and safety-net interventions and individual ACC practices can be compared. Practicing doctors, researchers, and others performing comparative effectiveness research will promote continuous quality improvement. People wishing to opt out of having their data used for research may do so by paying slightly higher premiums.

The ACC-affiliated financial services companies along with health services researchers will need to do the following:

- Itemize the medical diagnoses, health risk factors, and social risk factors
- Detail the up-to-date basis for a risk-adjusted allocation of federal health and social insurance funds (i.e., accounting for medical diagnoses, age, sex, socio-economic factors, and other insurance payment determinants)
- Receive any charitable donations to the ACC
- Report the types of interventions utilized and funded to address the health issues (sickness care, health promotion, long-term care, social determinants of health etc.)
- Determine the cost of interventions to address medical problems, health risks, and social determinants of health
- Within each ACC, assess the health outcomes of all patients individually, those in various demographic categories (gender, age, location, income, etc.), and disease categories (cancer, diabetes, etc.) and those of each PCP's practice
- Analyze the relationship between the health and social risk factors, the medical and social interventions, the health and social outcomes, and the costs of treatment.

The major new functions of financial services companies regarding cost transparency and data collection (e.g., health interventions and outcomes) will require retraining of potential employees. The former insurance company workers from underwriting, billing, customer service, and marketing will be ideal candidates to move to these new roles. Additionally, displaced insurance industry workers can find employment as actuaries within upper management within ACCs.

Competition Between ACC-Affiliated Financial Services Companies

The price for financial services company services will be determined by competitive bidding. Indices of insurance company performance will be developed (e.g., promptness and accuracy of payments, precision of data collection and analysis, etc.), which could determine financial bonuses or penalties designed by the ACCs to foster competition between financial services companies.

Government Funding for ACCs to be Based on Risk-adjusted Determinations

Based on a patient's age, sex, medical diagnoses, socio-economic factors, and cost of health care in recent years, U.S. Department of Health and Human Services (HHS) experts will determine a fair amount of risk-adjusted insurance money to allocate to the patient's chosen ACC. The Johns Hopkins Adjusted Clinical Groups Case-Mix System will be an excellent tool to use for this purpose, because its ability to predict future health care costs has been validated over tens of millions of patient-years of analysis.[15]

Premiums, risk-adjusted by age, and revenue from federal agencies—risk adjusted by socio-economic factors—will vary widely. For an employed, healthy 25-year-old person, the ACC will receive only about $3910 in 2016 from the person's health insurance premium. However, for a kidney dialysis patient or an Alzheimer's disease patient requiring 24-hour per day care, the ACC may receive up to $100,000 per year from the HSS in addition to any health insurance premium.

Options for ACC practices to keep from exceeding the global budget (i.e., the sum of all health care insurance premiums and federal government risk-adjusted patient funds) include:

- building up financial reserves;
- making wise investments in their communities (e.g., homes, businesses, etc., Chapter 24);
- insuring at least 100,000 people per ACC where possible to spread the risk; and
- involving ACC member representatives on committees to advise what services to cover and which to limit (All members will be able to vote to elect the representatives).

ACC members and staff will be making all financial determinations about their health, welfare, and other services. Until now, these decisions have been made for everyone in one-size-fits-all fashion by legislators, government bureaucrats, and insurance company executives.

Integrating Disability, Unemployment, and Workers' Compensation Benefits into ACCs

Most of the disability claims projected to be paid in 2016 will be through government programs—Social Security disability,[16] workers compensation,[17] and Veterans Administration disability benefits.[18] The bureaucratic processes in these overlapping disability systems leads to frustrating delays and unwarranted denials on the one hand, and unjustified wasteful payment allocations on the other.

As mentioned in Grand Bargain #18 in Chapter 1 and detailed in Chapter 10, we should combine all these overlapping disability programs and assign ACC providers and ACC-affiliated financial services companies to manage them. PCPs will determine which enrollees are disabled and what disabled members can still do. Accordingly, ACC-affiliated financial services companies will administer all disability claims.

ACCs will end the chaos of the current workers' compensation system by ACC providing all the medical care and ACC-affiliated financial services companies providing the indemnity payments.[b19] Government bureaucrats, private and public insurance programs, and the courts will no longer be involved.

Instead of employers' paying for workers' compensation and unemployment benefits, funding will come to the ACCs from the federal government collections of the new consumption taxes (Chapters 21 and 22). Social Security Disability payroll taxes will continue to be collected and deposited with the federal treasury. All of Social Security payroll taxes will be distributed to the ACC-affiliated financial services companies as the ACCs take over the administration of Social Security for their enrollees (Chapter 23). Substantial bureaucracy, duplication, and litigation will be avoided. People wanting supplemental disability insurance—perhaps to protect high incomes—can buy it on the insurance market.

Each ACC will hire appropriate advisors and consultants (e.g., attorneys specializing in health law) to determine appropriate indemnity payments in workers' compensation and other disability cases. ACCs will utilize their affiliated financial services companies to administer the delivery of indemnity payments going to those members with work-related illnesses or injuries.

With ACCs administering disability benefits, workers' compensation, and unemployment benefits, ACC services-providers will have strong incentives to find jobs that disabled people can do (Chapter 12). Savings on these social insurance expenditures will go to additional ACC services and/or reduced ACC health premiums.

Summarizing the above, the financial administration of all government health insurance programs (i.e., Medicare, Medicaid, Veterans Administration Health Care, Military Health Care, Children's Health Insurance Program, Indian Health Service, and Obamacare), welfare (e.g., Food Stamps, Housing and Urban Development), and social in-

---

b   In 2016, U.S. employers will pay about $40 billion for worker's compensation insurance—$14 billion for medical care, $10 billion for indemnity payments (money compensating people for inability to work due to temporary or permanent disabilities), and $16 billion for overhead (underwriting, case management, court costs, attorneys, dividends)

surance programs (disability, workers' compensation, and unemployment) will be shifted to the ACC-affiliated financial services companies. The financial services companies will administer health care and social insurance funds from both public and private insurance sources. This will eliminate many government administrative functions done inefficiently because of the multiplicity of government health agencies and insurance programs.

The Role of Government Regulators

The federal government' health care, welfare, and social insurance administrators' new roles will be limited to the following:

- collecting revenue from income taxes on high earning individuals and new consumption taxes (Chapter 21);
- distributing risk-adjusted block grant funds from the government for health care to private ACC-affiliated financial services companies;
- dispersing welfare revenue to ACC financial services companies—money for food, housing, general assistance, etc.;
- allocating money to ACC financial services companies for social insurance programs—disability, workers' compensation, and unemployment;
- distributing federal revenue to ACC financial services companies for other human services agencies (e.g., Department of Labor, USDA, etc., Chapter 19);
- receiving and analyzing data from ACCs on (1) member risk factors, (2) health and safety-net services provided, (3) costs, and (4) health outcomes.

Electronic medical and financial records will simplify claims processing and eliminate excessive redundancy in public and private insurance programs, saving money.

The new responsibilities of federal health agency scientists and actuaries concerning data on health and human services, costs, and health outcomes will be considerable. The funding for government health care administrative services will remain as projected at about $53 billion for 2016.[14]

Medicare Payroll Taxes and Premiums Replaced by Consumption Taxes

With Grand Bargains-based health care, Medicare patients will become ACC patients in a single expanded health care and human services system. In place of Medicare payroll taxes for workers, premiums for recipients (Medicare Part B and D), and "health fees" in states; targeted consumption taxes (Chapter 21) will cover those costs.[c] ACCs will receive risk-adjusted block grants by the federal government. For people ≥ 65 years old or disabled, ACC premiums will go down in consideration of having paid Medicare payroll taxes. However, ACC premiums costing seniors about $480 per month will offset the following costs:

- costs of the Medicare supplemental premiums (B and D): about $1600 per year (Chapter 25),[21, 22]
- supplemental insurance for co-payments, deductibles, and other charges (i.e., Medigap insurance): about $3000 per year (Chapter 25),[23]

---

c   The 2.9% Medicare tax on wages is projected to cost employees and employers about $250 billion in 2016 (Table 2 from Chapter 1).[20] This is only about 1/3rd the cost of Medicare payouts. The rest of the money comes from the general fund. Likewise, seniors will no longer pay the Part B Medicare premiums of $104.90 per month[21] or Part D premiums for drug coverage averaging about $30 per month (totaling about $70 billion in 2016).[22] At the state level the $150 billion in health fees will be eliminated in 2016 (Tables 1 and 2 from Chapter 1). With ACC-based health care, these taxes and premiums, totaling $470 billion in 2016, will be replaced by consumption taxes (Table 3 from Chapter 1 and Chapter 21).

- adding long-term care coverage (Chapter 6): $2800 per year, and
- dental care coverage (Chapter 6): $400 per year.

ACC Individual Health Insurance Premiums

With the shift to ACC-based medicine, the overall cost of personal health care will remain indefinitely as projected for 2016 at about $3.3 trillion ($1.6 trillion from the government and about $1.7 trillion from private sources).

Out-of-pocket health care costs, paid by patients in addition to health care premiums, will decrease from about $361 billion projected for 2016[7] to roughly $100 billion. This will be done by shifting about $261 billion of out-of-pocket funds into the ACC health insurance premiums paid by ACC members. Out-of-pocket costs will go down because (1) 50 million more people will be insured, (2) people will choose ACCs that cover the services that they want, and (3) ACCs will compete to keep out-of-pocket expenses low. This will assure that people will not need to go into debt to pay the deductibles and copayments and other charges that insurance does not cover.

Most health services will be provided without co-payments or deductibles. However, if directed by the ACC staff, financial services companies will bill patients for co-payments for covered services (e.g., for brand name prescriptions selected instead of generics). Health services not covered by a patient's ACC will still be paid by the patient.

Policies concerning co-payments, deductibles, and other out-of-pocket health care costs for ACC enrollees will depend on the individual ACCs that people choose. As an example, for a family of four, instead of $4400 as projected for 2016 for out-of-pocket co-payments, deductibles, and non evidence-based alternative care,[14] the cost will be roughly $1200 for that average family. Most families and individuals will have no out-of-pocket costs.

ACCs will charge enrollees individual health insurance premiums, which will also cover all the other ACC services. The payment of these premiums will result in the required private funds of $1.7 trillion for financing of health care services ($1.6 trillion for premiums and $100 billion for copayments, uncovered care, etc.). The rest of the ACC revenue will come from the federal government. As is shown in Table 1, the premiums will go up with age; just as health care costs increase as we get older.

These initial premiums include paying for all the administrative inefficiencies and the unnecessary tests and treatments that have crept into our health care system. To drive down premiums while improving quality of care, ACCs will compete to introduce bureaucratic efficiencies and to eliminate unnecessary tests, and treatments.

Table 1. Individual health care premiums to operate ACCs in 2016

Age	Premium per year $	Number in age group (million)	Revenue generated ($ billion)
Child 0-17	2910	78.7	229
18-24	3430	32.4	111
25-29	3870	22.2	86
30-39	4900	42.0	206
40-49	5720	45.1	258
50-59	6870	45.7	314
60-64	7720	18.7	144
65 and up	5730	44.2	253
Out-of-pocket costs	308 (mean)		100
Totals	5170 (mean)	329	1700

For instance, if decision-makers of an ACC decided not to offer any of the medical tests and treatments that I found not to be beneficial (Chapter 8, Table 1) and pass the savings along in lower premiums, the cost for that ACC could be under $1200 per year ($100 per month) for children and under $2400 per year ($200 per month) for young adults. Reducing administrative costs could lower premiums further. Premium costs will also depend on the health care benefits packages chosen by ACC members.

These premium rates will initially generate $1.6 trillion of the status quo $1.7 trillion for personal health care only if there is nearly full employment of a greatly expanded work force. People will need to be able to afford to pay the premiums. As detailed in Chapter 12, the Grand Bargains plan will increase those employed by at least 40 million workers, leaving no more than 2% unemployed of the expanded work force. No more than about $20 billion for premiums will need to be paid from ACC social assistance funds.[d]

For a couple in their 40s with two children receiving employer based insurance, the predicted Grand Bargains-based health care premium compares well with the current cost of the average medical insurance premium (i.e., status quo care: $24,334 projected for 2016[8, 24] versus ACC care: $17,260). The reduction in out-of-pocket costs by 70% will add to the savings. To afford these ACC health premiums, one of the couple might be employed full-time by the ACC in parenting their young children, receiving about $31,000 per year.

The linking of the administration of health care and other human services through ACCs allows for flexibility, innovation, fairness and, if needed, for helping people with the cost of health care insurance premiums.

Philanthropic Spending on Personal Health Care

Philanthropists will donate about $25 billion to personal health care services in 2016.[25] ACCs should compete for these targeted donations. Practices with disproportionately large numbers of people in poverty might attract more of the charity funding. As ACCs develop and pro-

---

d   0.02 (< 2% unemployment goal) x 177.6 million (157.6 million (current civilian labor force) + 20 million (parents and carers added to the official labor force)) ≤ 3.6 million goal for unemployed. 3.6 million x $5500 (average premium of working age adults) = $19.7 billion

vide various benefits to many people, more philanthropic donations may ensue, particularly ACC members donating to their own ACCs.

Summary and Conclusion

In our broken health care system, private health insurance industry workers perform the important tasks of collecting and distributing health care funds for about 180 million people. With ACC-based care, private health insurance companies will become financial services companies. They will individually affiliate with ACCs and collectively add to those covered by health insurance to include almost all U.S. residents. Almost everyone will choose to join an ACC because ACC will employ at least 60 million people (i.e., about one-third of the economy) and will provide many social and other services besides health care. Deciding how to allocate health insurance funds will not reside with ACC-affiliated financial services companies. Instead, the allocation of ACC funds for enrollees will become the responsibility of ACC patient-centered medical homes with input from ACC management, which will take into account the interests of all stakeholders.

Multiple government-financed and -run health insurance programs will also be shifted to ACCs (e.g., Medicare, Medicaid, Veterans Health Care, etc). Likewise, multiple federal and state social services programs (e.g., Food Stamps, Housing and Urban Development, unemployment benefits, women and children services, etc.) will become administered by ACCs. The HHS will assume the new roles of distributing the risk-adjusted health insurance and welfare funds to ACCs as block grants. HHS will also collect and analyze data from ACCs on services rendered and clinical outcomes regarding health and social indices.

The integration of multiple health and social services programs (private and public) within competing ACCs will lead to lower overall administrative costs, expanded services, and lower premiums. And, needless to say, better public health and happiness.

Several million health care administrators will become redundant because of the consolidation of health care and welfare within much more efficient and less bureaucratic ACCs. It will be the responsibility of the ACCs to retain these people for other jobs and find suitable employment for them (Chapter 12).

Chapter 19
Payment Reforms

While teaching and practicing at the Los Angeles County + University of Southern California Medical Center (LA County +USC Medical Center), I directed the "Pain and Palliative Care Service" service for terminally ill cancer and AIDS patients. In doing this work, I found that educating physicians, nurses, and other health care workers about the hospice philosophy and techniques is not enough. While high-tech futile treatments of end-stage patients are lucrative, palliative care is not. We need to change the financial incentives favoring the common practice of favoring excessive high-tech treatments at the expense of neglecting the approach of pain-and-symptom management (Chapter 5).

At my hospital, I began to notice the pattern in the administration's treatment of my own service. The many administrative obstacles I encountered when actually improving palliative care of poor people at LA County + USC Medical Center seemed to be linked to the hospital's financial bottom line. In 1995, I found that Medicaid paid my hospital about $2200 per day for acute care. Medicaid paid about $100 per day for home hospice care. Even that money went to an outside nursing agency rather than to the hospital. My Service treated about 400 cancer and AIDS patients that year. Our treatments and outpatient follow-up care in conjunction with home hospice nurses and social workers reduced patient time in hospital by an estimated 10 days per patient (4000 total days per year). Consequently, our service cost the hospital almost

$9 million in potential Medicaid funds per year.[a] Our Service received no Medicaid reimbursement for any of the 150 outpatients on home hospice programs that we followed at any given time. By instituting state-of-the-art hospice and palliative care services for all terminally ill patients in all six LA County Department of Health Services hospitals would have lost the County hundreds of millions of dollars in potential Medicaid revenue.

Because of a financial crisis, the hospital closed the Pain and Palliative Care Service in 1995. The hospital's financial wellbeing trumped the wellbeing of end-of-life patients. Patients reverted to having longer hospital stays and too frequently endured poor treatment of pain and distressing symptoms. Medicaid reimbursement per acute-care hospital day subsequently rose to $3800, worsening the already huge financial incentive to choose inappropriate heroic treatment for terminally ill patients over hospice and palliative care.

The hospital administration was to blame for the dysfunctional system. Medicaid paid the hospital $3800 per acute-care-day and nothing for out-of-hospital days. Within the dysfunctional payment scheme, economic necessity led hospitals, including LA County + USC Medical Center, to reward physicians in proportion to the beds they filled.

Competition Between Hospitals to Maximize Profits Fosters Overutilization of Hospital Beds—Duh!

The overutilization of acute care beds for futile treatment of terminally ill patients is widespread throughout the country. Dartmouth researchers found an almost 5-fold variation in the amount of physician time utilized in managing patients during their last six-months of life.[1] More in hospital time managing end-of-life patients means more intensive care days, more breathing machines, and more other high-

---

a   400 terminally ill patients x 10 days less in hospital per patient = 4000 acute care days billable to Medicaid. 4000 days x $2200 per day = $8.8 million

tech procedures that may not benefit the dying. Los Angeles, where I practiced, ranked third highest in the country in end-of-life spending.[2]

I came to see a systematic pattern throughout other hospital services, encouraging unnecessary days in hospital for economic reasons. The rampant over-hospitalization at my hospital led me to audit my own inpatient internal medicine service for the month of February 1998. My 104 admitted patients averaged 5.1 days in hospital. Patients from the other 11 internal medicine services averaged 6.9 hospital days. Still, many patients on my service had unnecessary acute care hospital days, and waited days for transfers to specialty wards, tests, consults, and other services. Based on this audit, I recorded that 44% of the days of internal medicine patients at LA County + USC Medical Center were medically unnecessary.[3]

Efficient utilization of acute care hospital beds throughout the entire six hospitals of the LA County Department of Health Services would have bankrupted the Health Department. Indeed, the loss of hundreds of millions of dollars from Medicaid would have bankrupted LA County. Administrators from Medicaid (federal and state) and my hospital were not responsive to my pleas to fix their broken reimbursement system.[4]

My case at LA County + USC Medical Center is not unique. Veterans' Administration employee whistleblowers were ignored for years before the very long waits of veterans for psychiatric and other health services came to the attention of the public in 2014.[5]

Doctors Too Need Health Care Payment Reform

Doctors themselves pay a high price for the culture of medicine that focuses too much on money. Practicing cardiologist Dr. Sandeep Jauhar described the financial pressures on specialists in a telling essay published in the *New York Times*.[6]

It is doubtful that doctors and other medical professionals will voluntarily cut their own income (even if some of it is generated by profligate spending). . . .The rising commercialism (of medicine), driven in part by increasing expenses and decreasing reimbursement, has obvious consequences for the public: ballooning costs, fraying of the traditional doctor-patient relationship. What is not so obvious is the harmful effects on doctors themselves. We were trained to think like caregivers, not businesspeople. The constant intrusion of the marketplace is creating serious and deepening anxiety in the profession.

Dr. Jauhar went on to observe some consequences of the increasing financial pressures on doctors and hospitals: "Supply often dictates demand.... And yet the consequences of this commercial consciousness are troubling. Among my colleagues I sense an emotional emptiness created by the relentless consideration of money."

Dr. Pamela Hartzband and Dr. Jerome Groopman, physicians at Beth Israel Deaconess Medical Center in Boston, expressed a similar sentiment in a commentary for *The New England Journal of Medicine*.[7]

. . . Price tags are being applied to every aspect of a doctor's day, creating an acute awareness of costs and reimbursement. . . . The balance has tipped toward market exchanges at the expense of medicine's communal or social dimension. . . . Physicians are now routinely provided with profit-and-loss reports reflecting their activity, and metrics are calculated to measure the cost-effectiveness of their work.

The reformed health care system should incentivize physicians to focus primarily on patient care rather than on maximizing profit. This means finding ways to pay doctors for good quality of care and health outcomes rather than merely the volume of services rendered. You might ask if doctors that make outsized incomes due to our dysfunctional health care system would fight tooth and nail against reform. In reality, doctors are often beaten down by the system and so unhappy that they desperately want true reform.

ACCs and Affiliated Financial Services Companies— $6 Trillion Enterprises in 2016

Financial services companies contracting with ACCs will receive enrollee health insurance premiums and government funds for health care, social-safety-net services, and social insurance. Fully incorporating health care together with social services and other human services requires integrating the funding of all these services. The financial services companies will distribute the funds to all providers according to the orders of ACC decision-makers. Because of the wide ranging services to be provided by ACCs, the financial services companies will receive several sources of funding. The sources of about $6 trillion in revenue for the ACCs—managed by their financial services partners— in 2016 are presented in Tables 1 and 2 below.

Of these funds, about $4.26 trillion will be revenue for health care and human services for ACC members (Table 1). Table 2 shows the remaining $1.72 trillion that will be allocated to Social Security disbursements to seniors and disabled people, and to ACC-affiliated credit unions and savings and loan banks for loans to ACC members. With Grand Bargains-based reform, about one-third of the economy will be managed by private, competing ACCs through their affiliated financial services companies, credit unions, and savings and loan banks (Chapter 24).[b]

---

b $5980 billion (total revenue of ACCs) / $17,905 (projected GDP in 2016) = 0.335 (≈one-third)

Table 1. Funds to be Administered by ACC through ACC-Affiliated Financial Services Companies

Purpose of funds	Source of funds	$ billions
Health care, preventive medicine, and alternative treatments[8] (Department of Health and Human Services (HHS))	Federal consumption taxes	1606
Health care, preventive medicine, and alternative treatments[8]	Premiums from ACC members	1607
Welfare funds for need-based purposes (food, shelter, etc., HHS Chapter 10) [9]	General federal tax revenue /various federal agencies	500
Unemployment insurance[9] (Department of Labor)	Federal consumption taxes (replacing employer contributions)	140
Workers' compensation[10] (from employers)	Federal consumption taxes (replacing employer contributions)	40
Stimulate employment (Department of Labor)[11, 12]	Federal consumption taxes	64
Support for farmers (Department of Agriculture)[13]	General federal tax revenue	25
Supplemental education programs (Department of Education)[11, 14]	General federal tax revenue	73
Reduce student debt for higher education (new expenditure)	Federal consumption taxes	50
Veterans benefits and social services other than health care[14] (Veteran Affairs Department)	General federal tax revenue	104
Foreign development aid (new expenditure)	Federal consumption taxes	50
Totals		4261

Table 2. Funds to be Administered ACC-Affiliated Credit
Unions/Savings and Loan Banks for ACC Members

Purpose of funds	Source of funds	$ billions
Funds to insure ACCs	Premiums from ACC members	100
Social Security Trust Funds dispersal to ACCs	U.S. Treasury	100
Social Security benefits (old age, Chapter 23)[9]	Social Security insurance taxes	901
Social Security benefits (disability, Chapter 23)[9]	Social Security insurance taxes	173
Federal, state, and local government workers' pension fund deposits (Chapter 24)[15-17]	Federal, state, and local general funds	150
Private employees' employer-sponsored pension funds (Chapter 24)[15-17]	Private employers and employees	300
Totals		1724

Right-Sizing Administrative Costs in Health Care

The total cost of personal health care administration in 2016 is projected to be about $1 trillion.[c] The efficiencies of ACC-based health care will initially bring the costs of health care administration down to as low or lower than in Canada (16.7% of costs[19]), saving up to $500 billion in 2016. Additionally, administering the government safety-net funding through ACCs rather than myriad federal, state, and local agencies will efficiently redirect hundreds of billions more dollars per year of wasted money to increasing beneficial health and social services and to decreasing patient premiums.

Major decreases in administration costs with ACC-based health and social services will help hospitals, medical specialists, other health services providers, and safety-net services providers. Several million

---

c $3.3 trillion (personal health care services in 2016) x 0.31 (31% of health care goes to administration[18]) = $1028 billion

health sector employees will become redundant due to streamlining health care bureaucracy. As mentioned in Chapter 1, health care administration now requires 810 financial managers per $1 billion of revenue verses 50 financial managers for other businesses.[20] By switching from largely fee-for-service medical treatment administered by multiple insurers to ACC-based care in a competitive health care market, health services will require about the same number of financial managers per $1 billion revenue as other businesses. This will mean that many of redundant administrators will be in the realm of health care related financial services.[d]

It will be the responsibility of ACCs to retrain redundant medical administrators in other occupations and to find them jobs (Chapter 12).

Health Care and Welfare Spending Priorities

Federal government health care spending for things other than personal health care (e.g., research and public health) will continue under the U.S. Department of Health and Human Services. As will be detailed in Chapter 20, ACCs will partner with government health agencies in the areas of medical research and public health strategies. Members of the public, through their ACCs, will have a greater role in setting health research and public health priorities. For example, much research will be expected to be about funds allocated by ACCs for health interventions and the health outcomes related to those interventions. Financial services company data will be crucial for that research.

Underfunded health priorities (e.g., nurse training programs, substance abuse prevention and treatment, HIV/AIDS prevention, diet and exercise programs, autism, etc.) will be largely financed through ACCs to best suit the needs of their enrollees. Today's insufficiently financed health care, prevention, and safety-net priorities will be ad-

---

d   810 – 50 finance workers = 760 redundant finance workers per $1 billion in services, 760 redundant workers/$1 billion revenue x $3.3 trillion personal health care costs in 2016 = 2.5 million redundant health care financial administrators.

dressed by ACCs redirecting funds from unnecessary or preventable medical interventions and administrative efficiencies to necessary and beneficial health services.

ACC-Based Payment Reform to Resolve State and Local Government Health and Welfare Funding Crises

Rising health and welfare costs battered state and local government budgets during the Great Recession. To balance state budgets, legislators drastically reduced services to people on Medicaid, the Children's Health Insurance Program (CHIP), and other welfare programs. These cuts threatened the public health in part by increasing use of already overwhelmed emergency rooms.[21] With a continuation of the status quo, draconian cuts in safety-net services (e.g., general relief, job training, child protective services, etc.) during future economic downturns could likewise again put pressure on our fragile social and health safety-net services.

To help alleviate future state and local funding crises during economic downturns, ACC-based care will address all health and welfare needs without money from state and local municipalities. Overall, state and local governments will save over $600 billion that they are projected to pay for in 2016 on personal health care and safety-net services for the indigent—about 24% of state and local budgets (Table 3).[22]

With that money, they can rectify the deficits in public employees' pension obligations (Chapter 24), enhance education spending (Chapter 16), and launch major public infrastructure projects (Chapter 15).

State and local public health departments will remain the responsibility of the states and municipalities. In time, these responsibilities and funds may also shift to ACCs.

Table 3. State and Local Government Budget
Benefits from Grand Bargains' Reforms

Revenue Change with Grand Bargains Reform	Amount changed ($ billions)
Difference in proposed versus status quo revenue in 2016 ($2566 billion – $2711 billion, Tables 1 and 2)	–145
State and local health care costs shifted to federal consumption taxes[23]	+600
Welfare costs shifted to federal consumption taxes and distributed through ACCs (Chapter 10, Table 1)	+109
Unemployment social insurance shifted to federal consumption taxes (Tables 1 and 2)	+ 80
Total change	+644

Fairness in PCP Income and Working Conditions

With any ACC compensation model for PCPs (i.e., fee-for-service, salary, or mixed), PCP income should be no less than current projections for in 2016.[e] The improved working conditions and job satisfaction of becoming direct practice PCPs (Chapter 3) will attract more physicians, nurses, and physician assistants to primary care even without major increases in income.

With ACC-based care, I propose that the overall number of PCPs should increase from about 352,000 in 2016[24-26] to about 475,000 by 2025 or one PCP for every 750 people. This will provide enough doctors for everyone to have a direct practice PCP while significantly improving the working conditions for PCPs.

---

e $250,000 per year for 225,000 primary care physicians[24, 25] and $120,000 for 95,000 primary care nurse practitioners[26] and 32,000 physician assistants[26]

To accomplish the necessary increase in residency training of direct practice primary care physicians and specialist-doctors, residency training positions will need to increase by 30% from 2016 – 2020 (from about 100,000 now to 130,000). The relatively small amount of money to increase medical residency training slots by 30% (about $5 billion/year) can lead to direct practice PCPs leading patient-centered medical homes for everyone. Unfortunately, bills in the U.S. House of Representatives and Senate to add a modest 15,000 residency training slots over the next 5 years are given less than a 1% chance of enactment.[27, 28] The grand bargain of shifting from a fragmented, cost-inefficient health care system to an ACC-based system that saves up to $500 billion in 2016 in administrative costs should resolve this political impasse.

Funding Postgraduate Medical Training via ACCs Rather than Through Hospitals

Currently, postgraduate medical education funding by government agencies (Medicare, Medicaid, Veterans Administration, etc.) and private medical centers is channeled through teaching hospitals that employ physicians-in-training. This biases postgraduate training towards acute hospital treatment and away from out-of-hospital care. It would better serve doctors-in-training and the public if ACCs providing comprehensive health care for patients administered the money.

For decades, Congress has divided government postgraduate training funds as follows:[29]

- direct payments for medical education that cover a share of the stipends paid to residents, salaries of supervising faculty, and other allowable program expenses; and
- indirect medical education adjustment, the goal of which is to cover the added patient-care costs associated with training, including additional tests and treatments ordered by residents

(often unnecessary) and longer hospital stays (again, not to be financially encouraged).

As projected for 2016, teaching hospitals will receive about $26 billion for post graduate training of physicians but will pay only about $4.6 billion for resident salaries, faculty teaching stipends, and educational programs (averaging $46,000 per resident).[f] This has disturbed some in Congress[29, 31] and is probably part of the impasse over additional funding for medical residency positions. Indeed, there is poor if any accounting for the majority of money going to train residents (i.e., indirect medical education funds).

As a grand bargain to break the deadlock in Congress over the funding of the necessary expansions of postgraduate medical education, public funds for the training of postgraduate doctors should be channeled through ACCs. This will also check the overemphasis of hospital-based training over training in outpatient settings. ACCs could then contract with medical and osteopathic schools, hospitals, clinics, home health organizations, and specialty provider groups to provide a proper mixture of inpatient and outpatient clinical experiences for trainees. Residents might be better compensated by ACCs than by teaching-hospitals. Residents would also have less brutalizing work schedules (i.e., 80 hours per week on average now) if employed by ACCs rather than by hospitals.

The Urgent Need for Increased Medical School Enrollment

In 2006, the American Association of Medical Colleges estimated that the U.S. will have a shortage of at least 100,000 physicians by 2020.

---

f   Only 28% goes for direct payments for medical education and fully 72% goes for indirect medical education.[29] In addition to $15 billion of government funding for residency training, private insurers will pay an estimated $11 billion toward postgraduate medical education through the higher payments they negotiated with teaching hospitals on behalf of their patients.[30, 31] However, a negligible amount of that money will go for direct payments for medical education.

The shortage was projected to be about equally divided between primary care physicians and specialists. Because of this projected shortage, medical schools are on track to increase enrollment by 30% by 2018 over the number enrolled in 2006 (about 5,000 new positions all together).[32] However, this is not nearly enough.

About one-quarter of physicians and nurses practicing in the U.S. come from foreign countries, including over 30% of our primary care doctors. Many foreign trained doctors practicing in the U.S. emigrate from poor countries with extreme physician shortages, high infant mortality rates, low life-expectancies, and low immunization rates.[33]

In addition, we need to reduce the horrendous workloads on physicians that lead to burnout, shortened medical careers, and reduced quality of care. Finally, we must account for the increased number of physicians that will be needed to take care of aging baby boomers and the overall increase in the population.

For all these reasons, we should increase medical school graduates each year by an additional 10,000 (from about 20,000 graduates projected for 2016[32] to 30,000 by 2025). This will be necessary over the long term for everyone to have a direct practice PCP.

Public Funding of Medical Education

Medical school training is funded by tuition paid by students, state subsidies, university endowments, government and private grants, and other sources. Books, professional supplies, and living expenses for students are additional. The median debt of a medical student upon graduation in 2012 was $170,000.[34] This high medical school debt has been one of the factors cited as leading students to choose careers in lucrative specialties or other professions than medicine rather than in primary care (Chapter 3). With publicly funded medical school tuition, physicians will be more likely to choose careers in primary care.

Relative to the astronomical cost of medical administration and of unnecessary tests and treatments, the cost of medical education for doctors is small. A federal subsidy amounting to about $8 billion per year,[g] would cover medical school tuition and help entice more doctors to become PCPs.

Medical education in an ACC world may be funded through a small part of the government block grants to ACCs for personal health care for patients. In addition to paying for the medical education of the students, the ACCs could pass part of the federal health care block grant funds along to patients treated by medical students in the form of lower premiums.

Public funding of medical schools will also help medicine compete with law, business, finance, engineering, and education to attract the best and brightest students.

Primary Care for Inner City Areas and Rural America

For decades, rural communities and poor inner-city impoverished areas have been underserved medically. The shortage of primary care providers hits people in these communities especially hard. We need to assist rural and inner-city America in attracting PCPs. Medical students and postgraduate physicians-in-training should be given financial incentives to work in these areas.

Medical students who are primary care providers-in-training who would practice in inner city or rural areas might schedule their clinic time in those areas. They could see new and follow-up patients on a biweekly, monthly, or less frequent basis. The primary care providers-in-training will see patients under the supervision of qualified mentor primary care physicians. On completion of medical school and residency, the new primary care physicians will be ready to move into an established practice with hundreds of patients.

---

g   30,000 medical students in each class x 4 years of study x $70,000 per student/year[35] = $8.4 billion/year

Summary and Conclusion

An ACC-based system with decentralized regulation of health care and human services will provide a revenue-neutral method—i.e., no new taxes—of reforming health and social services. Risk-adjusted payments to self-regulated ACCs by the federal government will more efficiently, flexibly, and fairly allocate resources to suit all health care and welfare stakeholders. By eliminating the multiplicity of private and public health care payers and allocating care through ACCs in a free market, health care administration costs will be reduced by up to $500 billion in 2016. Administration cost will go down further in subsequent years due to competition between ACCs. Further savings will come by eliminating funding for tests and treatments that don't work (Chapter 8).

Despite the elimination of perhaps millions of clerical jobs in insurance companies, health-care provider offices, and hospitals, the overall employment in health care will substantially increase. It will be the responsibility of the ACCs to retrain the displaced administrators for new jobs and assist them in finding employment (Chapter 12).

Reductions in spending on bureaucracy and unnecessary medical tests and treatments will directly benefit all members and staff of ACCs. Consequently, this system will incentivize waste-elimination in human services as a win-win-win-win-win for patients, providers, other businesses, taxpayers, and the economy.

Shifting the delivery of health care to ACCs with direct practice PCPs within patient-centered medical homes will be the cornerstone of addressing the looming physician shortage and the crisis in primary care. Public funding of medical education and postgraduate physician training will help enable the transition. Public funding of health care education will also benefit nurses, physician assistants, and other healers. It will open the healing professions to more low and middle income people without them having to assume oppressive levels of debt. It will do this, in part, by switching the recipient of public funding for medical education from hospitals and medical schools to ACCs. Competing

ACCs with diverse stakeholders will be positioned to assure cost effectiveness and value in health education.

The crisis in recruiting sufficient PCPs will be addressed by making primary care more attractive to physicians, nurses, and physician assistants. ACCs providing direct practice PCPs for all U.S. residents, drastically reducing bureaucracy, and eliminating student loan debt will draw many more health care students to primary care.

Over the next decade, these payment reforms will stabilize the cost of health care and social services at 2016 levels. This will remove the drag on the economy caused by health care and welfare and will facilitate more job growth in other sectors.

Chapter 20
Health Care Cost Control

When I had surgery for an orthopedic problem, I was in the hospital for approximately 28 hours. The hospital charged $26,517.26. Anthem Blue Cross negotiated the fee down 89% to $2933.60. The bills of the surgeon, assistant surgeon, and anesthesiologist were separate. Presumably, an uninsured patient would be responsible for the entire retail cost of the hospitalization. For a procedure or day in the hospital, hospitals and medical specialists generally have a retail price and an insurance company negotiated price. These prices can vary tremendously. Hospitals and providers often hide their negotiated prices with insurance companies.

Price Transparency and Price Competition Now Lacking

The American Medical Association contends that health insurers often pay doctors too little and make it too burdensome to get payments at all, driving doctors outside insurance networks.[1] In many cases, the AMA has a point.

In any market, cost control is impossible if well-informed people are not able to shop for value and cost effectiveness. If price transparency only means having doctors and hospitals post the cost of medical services, it may be effective in ratcheting down the cost of a brief outpatient office visit to a PCP from $75 to $50. However, the result will probably be even shorter PCP visits and more doctors choosing careers in lucrative specialties rather than primary care.

With our current multi-payer system, which is in no way a free market, price transparency will do little for health care's big-ticket items. For instance, most of the decisions to perform invasive coronary artery procedures that now cost over $200 billion per year overall[2-4] are made by people with chest pain in hospital emergency rooms. We are not likely to save much money because of price transparency in emergency rooms if sick patients and their fearful and/or grieving relatives are doing the shopping.

Health policy experts and politicians have recently brought attention to the cost control strategy of having people use their own money to pay more of their medical bills instead of relying entirely on insurance. They argue that the more "skin in the game" that people have, the more they will insist on getting good value for their health care dollar. In a Congressional hearing, Representative Jim McDermott, MD (D-Wash) rejected this idea, "The notion that beneficiaries need to have more 'skin in the game' to encourage smarter health care shopping is ridiculous. It is the physicians who are driving the health care utilization in the system, not the beneficiaries."[5]

In practice, non-medically trained people frequently lack the information, experience, and/or skills required to interpret what constitutes high-quality health care and good value. Even many medical practitioners fail in assessing value in health care.

Dysfunctional Financial Incentives of Hospitals

In an article titled, "Slowing the Growth of Health Care Costs," Dr. Edward Fisher, director of the Center for Health Policy Research, Dartmouth Institute for Health Policy, enumerated the dysfunctional financial incentives regarding hospitals:

Hospitals lose money when they improve care in ways that reduce admissions, and they lose market share when they don't keep pace in the local medical arms race. In this race there are no financial rewards for collaboration, coordination, or conservative practice.

To slow spending growth, we need policies that encourage high-growth (or high-cost) regions to behave more like low-growth, low-cost regions—and that encourage low-cost, slow-growth regions to sustain their current trends. Our ongoing research program (funded in part by the National Institute on Aging) suggests that there are two broad and closely linked strategies for accomplishing these aims: fostering the growth of more organized systems of care and implementing fundamental payment reform.[6]

As Dr. Fisher stated, hospitals employing innovative strategies to improve care and lower costs are penalized by our dysfunctional system. For example, Intermountain Hospital in Utah has an evidence-based medicine research team that continually searches for strategies to improve health outcomes of patients. A particularly successful project involved reducing the premature babies delivered in the birth center by convincing obstetricians not to induce babies before the 39th week of pregnancy. As an unintended consequence of reducing the number of babies requiring intensive care unit treatment with ventilators, Intermountain lost $329,000 in one year.[7]

The Duke University Medical Center cardiology department set up a disease-management system for treating patients with congestive heart failure, coordinating the efforts of cardiologists, primary care doctors, pharmacists, and nurse practitioners. However, it was so successful that it decreased the cost of treatment by 40% in a single year. By reducing hospital readmissions and improving outcomes, the hospital lost tens of millions of dollars relative to the previous uncoordinated system. Insurance companies pocketed most of the savings.[8]

With ACC-based reform of health care, hospitals will not lose money by improving the care of patients. This is because patient choice and provider competition in an ACC self-regulated free market of health services will foster high quality hospital care and cost control.

Irrational Rationing versus Rational Rationing

Many people fear rationing of benefits and/or government-imposed cost controls based on results of randomized trials. This could be called a tyranny by comparative effectiveness researchers. This is a legitimate concern.

Federal legislators and others have proposed having a government appointed expert panel determine an evidence-based standard medical benefits package for use by public and private insurers. This is absurd. No physician or physician panel has the wisdom to prescribe for all patients for all conditions.

Economist Milton Friedman framed the issue of rationing: "There is no such thing as a free lunch. The choice isn't between rationing and not rationing. It's between rationing well and rationing badly."[9] Implicit rationing already occurs widely in U.S. health care. Indeed, our current system rations health care very badly. The high cost of medicine negatively impacts the social determinants of health by decreasing health care access, increasing poverty, and decreasing educational opportunities.

According to a Harvard study, rationing health care by ability to pay has led to 45,000 unnecessary deaths per year.[10] In part, Obamacare was a well meaning reaction to any deaths due to lack of access to health care in the richest country in the world. However, the devil is in the details regarding how health policy options will favorably or adversely influence health outcomes. It's much too soon to claim that the ACA related access to care is saving or will ever save lives.

Guidelines for Cost Control Strategies

Many countries with less than half of our per capita spending on health care have better health outcomes. Clearly, controlling costs can be done while improving quality of care and health outcomes.

Ideally, doctors and patients should work together toward optimum health and maximum cost-effectiveness in the allocation of health care services. To this end, ACC health care professionals and their patients need incentives to avoid tests and treatments that are not beneficial.

The system should be self-adjusting for changes in economic circumstances and new medical research findings. It should be easily and inexpensively administered and transparent. We should be able to track how resource allocation choices of different health and safety-net providers relate to their patients' health outcomes. This will enable us to learn what works well and lead us to foster continuous quality improvement.

Cost containment policies need to result in enhanced value health care and safety-net services. It should also provide appropriate financial incentives for providers. Cost control strategies should be flexible and involve all the stakeholders. Savings from effective cost control efforts should go to patients more than to providers or the government.

Controlling Sickness Care Costs

I designed ACC-based health care reform to foster patients working together with their caregivers toward the mutual goal of cost effectively treating illnesses and injuries. Without sacrificing quality sickness care, methods of improving health outcomes while reducing costs include:

1. supporting healthy nutrition and lifestyles (Chapters 4 and 13)
2. reducing unnecessary hospital days to enhance patient care by
   - offering out-of-hospital births for low risk mothers
   - facilitating end-of-life care at home

- encouraging outpatient surgeries where feasible
- enabling direct practice PCPs within patient-centered medical homes to catch urgent problems before emergency hospitalization is necessary
- mobilizing resources for home hospital care if desired

3. eliminating hospital readmissions due to poor planning
4. cost-effectively referring patients to specialists
5. having patient-centered medical home leaders rather than insurance industry bureaucrats make decisions about services covered by ACCs
6. instituting health promotion retreat centers
7. using price transparency to shop for value among health services
8. monitoring and reporting provider financial relationships with health industries
9. rational rationing of precious health care, social services, and other human services resources

Numbers 2–9 of this list of methods are detailed below.

Hospitalization Dangers: Reasons to Cut Hospital Days

Hospitalization has dangers. Based on a study in Massachusetts, about 23% of hospitalized people report serious adverse events.[11] In 2011, about 1.7 million people in the U.S. developed an infection while in hospital of whom about 99,000 died.[12] The dangers in hospital include errors by providers, bedsores, delirium, medication errors, medication side effects, hospital-acquired infections, falls, anxiety, depression, and adverse reactions from excessive testing and unnecessary treatments.

The safest, most reliable, and least costly way to avoid the risks of hospitalizations is to decrease the number of patients-days in hospital.

Reducing Days in Hospital

Dr. Sandeep Jauhar, a columnist for *The New York Times* and practicing cardiologist, related a conversation with an internist at his hospital about unnecessarily long hospital stays. The internist told him, "I understand why hospitals want to cut down length-of-stay. But if I discharge a patient early, I don't get paid. It's okay if you have enough patients in the hospital, but if you don't, you sometimes have to drag out the stay. I don't like to do it, but sometimes you have to."[13]

According to U.S. government Agency for Healthcare Research and Quality (AHRQ) data, over 4 million Americans were hospitalized *unnecessarily* in 2011 (about 10% of all hospitalizations).[14] Of those people, some required immediate treatment that could have been given on an outpatient basis, and others did not require acute-care level treatment. These figures do not include over 6 million arguably unnecessary hospitalizations for low-risk childbirth that midwives could have assisted outside of hospitals. Nor does it include admissions for other unnecessary medical interventions cited in my previous book, *Money Driven Medicine—Tests and Treatments That Don't Work* (Chapter 8, Table 1).[15]

Hospital-Level Care at Home

Since I had a special interest in hospice medicine/palliative care, I have known many terminally ill people that absolutely dreaded being hospitalized. However, many were admitted repeatedly anyway because of the lack of alternatives. Although most terminally ill people would rather die at home than in a hospital, more than 1.5 million Americans die in hospitals each year—most of whom are elderly and/or chronically ill people.

Particularly for frail elderly people that have acute medical problems, a common sense economical and effective alternative to hospitalization could be to offer acute medical care at home.

In a study of 455 community-dwelling elderly Medicare and Veterans Administration patients that required acute care for pneumonia, cellulitis (a skin infection), or worsening of chronic heart failure, emphysema, or bronchitis; hospital-at-home care was feasible and efficacious in delivering hospital-level treatment. Home-treated patients had fewer clinical complications (particularly delirium), greater satisfaction with care, less treatment time required per acute episode, and lower bills.[16]

Dr. Jack Resnick, an internist in New York, sees many of his frail elderly patients in their homes. When they need acute care, he arranges for hospital-type services to be brought to them at home. For this to work effectively, Dr. Resnick said, "Everyone must have a single doctor in charge of his care. This doctor should know the person intimately, have immediate access to all of their medical information, and must be available around the clock."[17] This model of acute at-home care for the frail elderly and perhaps other appropriate patients will be supported by ACCs.

I see no reason that home acute care could not be used for many patients with cancer, liver failure, heart failure, Alzheimer's disease, and other conditions. Expertly provided home care is less traumatizing to the patient and family, avoids the risk of hospital-acquired infections, and allows for the patient to have more timely and nutritious meals.

Unnecessary Hospital Readmissions

In 2009, a study published in *The New England Journal of Medicine* found that one in three Medicare patients discharged from a hospital was readmitted within three months.[18] The authors found that the causes of these readmissions were things like poor communication, inadequate discharge instructions, incomplete information transfer, and delayed outpatient follow-up. In 2004, the cost to Medicare for these unplanned readmissions was $17.4 billion to hospitals and more to physicians. According to this article, the 30-day Medicare readmission rates have risen nearly 50% over the past three decades.

To reduce the cost of frequent Medicare patient readmissions, Congress and the Obama administration have begun to give bonus payments to hospitals with low readmission rates and penalties to those with high rates. There are at least two problems with this top-down policy approach. Hospitals do not hospitalize patients—doctors do. Reducing readmissions needs to benefit doctors rather than private insurance companies and government agencies. Secondly, Medicare readmissions are highly linked to socioeconomic status. Poor people are readmitted more frequently for a multitude of reasons that are out of the control of hospitals or doctors. Consequently, safety-net hospitals are hurt much more by readmission penalties than hospitals for the affluent.

Coordinated care by direct practice PCPs within patient-centered medical homes in ACCs (Chapter 3) will significantly reduce unnecessary hospital readmissions. ACCs addressing the social indicators of health (poverty, isolation, transportation, health literacy, etc.) will also help keep people from being needlessly hospitalized and rehospitalized.

ACCs will Facilitate Cost Control in Specialists Care

According to the aforementioned cardiologist and *New York Times* columnist Dr. Sandeep Jauhar, "There is plenty of evidence that wasteful expert consultation is adding to health costs and creating redundant care . . . our referral system turns patients into commodities—a way for "cash-strapped doctors to generate business."[19]

Almost half of new patients seen by U.S. doctors are referred by other physicians. We have about twice the rate of referrals to specialists as in the United Kingdom and no better health outcomes.[20] Unnecessary referrals to multiple specialists cause problems for patients. Adverse drug interactions become more likely when several doctors are prescribing for the same patient. Keeping appointments to multiple doctors' offices is a hardship, especially for the frail elderly.

Factors contributing to the high rate of specialist referrals in the U.S. include:

- too many specialists relative to PCPs;
- the lack of time for PCPs to give to complex cases;
- fear of lawsuits over not consulting an expert; and
- possibilities of the referring doctors receiving referrals in return.

As Dr. Jauhar said, "It is hard not to view a referral as an overture from another physician, and it is equally hard not to return the favor."[19]

With ACC-based health care reform, cost control will require competition among ACCs, between hospitals, and between providers who are specialists. Health care provider specialists will compete with each other for referrals from the PCPs based on quality of care and cost. Market forces will determine fair and just compensation for specialist health care providers and facilities. Direct practice PCPs and ACC managers will negotiate payments for services directly with specialists. With ACC-based reform, specialists will be able to significantly reduce their prices for several reasons:

- transparency in pricing—referring PCPs will see charges of selected specialists and those of competing physicians
- universal health care coverage so specialists will be paid for each consultation and treatment—no uncovered care
- medical malpractice system reform (Chapter 11)—no need for costly defensive medicine
- enterprise liability—no need for medical malpractice insurance (Chapter 11)
- reduced administrative burden—less office overhead (Chapter 9)
- public funding of medical training (Chapter 19)—less doctor debt
- price competition with other specialists.

By shifting from uncoordinated fee-for-service medicine to ACC-based care, charges of specialists for evidence-based services will be in line with the value of the services in the local community. PCPs from ACCs will have to authorize payment of each patient's bill for medications, tests, treatments, hospitalizations, and specialist services. The ACC-affiliated financial services companies will pay the bills as directed.

Dr. Fisher from Dartmouth's Institute for Health Policy articulated how financial incentives must encourage physician cost control consciousness:[6]

> First, physicians have an opportunity to lead. Physicians are still almost entirely responsible for determining what treatments their patients receive and where they obtain their care. And, although the increasingly commercial behavior of some physicians may threaten the public perception of the profession, patients still largely trust their own doctors. Leadership is needed at three levels. In their practices, physicians can help patients understand when a more conservative path is likely to be as safe as a more intensive and higher-cost path. In their communities, physicians have the credibility to argue against the need for further growth—whether through hospital expansion, the construction of new imaging centers, or the recruitment of more specialists to oversupplied regions. . . . And physicians can support changes in the health care system that will help their patients and communities get the best possible care at the lowest possible cost.

With ACC-based care, PCPs will be responsible to their patients for maximizing the overall value of health care expenditures. Consequently, each health care professional's incentive to optimize patient benefit and the competition among specialist providers will both reduce referrals to necessary and appropriate levels. Patients will benefit medically and financially from the judicious allocation of health services for everyone. As long as they have adequate time with their PCPs and full support from their patient-centered medical homes, most patients will support the conservative utilization of specialty referrals.

ACCs to Take Charge of Health Services Coverage Decisions

Folotyn, a drug from Allos Therapeutics for advanced cancer of the lymphatic system, costs about $30,000 per month.[21] Since Folotyn is FDA approved, Medicare and Medicaid have to cover it. Once the government insurance programs pay for it, the private insurance companies become pressured to cover it.

With ACC-based care, doctors and not the government or private insurance companies will make funding decisions about Folotyn and other drugs. This will moderate the prices and allow members to choose ACCs that cover the drugs that they want to be covered.

The Patient Protection and Affordable Care Act (ACA) includes funding for acupuncture, chiropractic treatments, dietary supplements, and naturopathic medical providers. Senator Tom Harkin (D-Iowa), chairman of the Senate Health Committee and the leading recipient in Congress of campaign donations from chiropractors and dietary-supplement makers, champions the funding of alternative medicine methods.[22]

While I personally believe that some alternative medical treatments are much better than standard medical interventions, I recognize that my opinions are controversial. Indeed, much in medicine is controversial.

ACC-based care will eliminate the top-down approach of funding decisions being made by U.S. Congress members, FDA bureaucrats, and insurance company executives. ACC health care professionals will be the decision-makers about providing services. U.S. residents will be decision-makers about joining ACCs.

Health Promotion Retreat Centers

To assure adequate reserve revenue for years when unusual amounts of sickness care are required, ACCs should set aside 2% of patient care revenue each year in ACC-affiliated credit unions/savings and loan banks (Chapter 24). After accruing at least $10 million in savings for each 10,000 patients as a buffer for future high-spending years, unspent practice funds should go, in part, to creating, acquiring, or leasing a health promotion-oriented retreat center. Ideally, ACCs should partner with each other in acquiring and utilizing health promotion centers. Located in rural or urban areas, these centers could offer the ACC services of health care including disease prevention and stress reduction, and interventions impacting the social determinants of health. These centers could serve as sites to provide healthy low-tech alternatives for a variety of purposes:

- workshops on healthy-living topics
- pregnancy support
- health promotion activities—healthy diet, aerobic exercise, gardening, exploring nature, etc. (Chapters 4 and 13)
- intensive support for frail elderly, disabled, or chronically ill people (Chapter 25)
- cardiac rehabilitation after cardiovascular events
- recovery from depression, other mental illness, or stress (Chapter 6)
- rehabilitation from orthopedic problems and injuries
- substance abuse rehabilitation
- assisted living/nursing home care
- employment: construction, gardening-farming, food services, health care and social services professions
- rest, relaxation, and socializing
- spiritual practices—prayer, contemplation, meditation, and reflection

- safe and enriched environment for children—music, art, athletics, nature study, etc.
- sustainable retirement living (i.e., minimal autos, local food production, affordable rents, lower overall consumption, higher quality lifestyles)

With ACC-based reform, each PCP will be able to prescribe a stay in a health promotion retreat for patients that need it.

Medical Tourism + Price Transparency = Moderate Costs

PCPs will know the local medical providers of products and services and what they charge. In collaboration with patients and ACC managers, PCPs will make well informed decisions about allocation of resources for personal health services.

Where local prices remain unreasonable, ACCs could economize on exorbitant costs of specialist care and hospitalization by outsourcing to state-of-the-art hospitals in other countries. For example, Bumrungrad Hospital in Bangkok, Thailand treats more foreign patients than any other hospital in the world. More than 500 doctors, most with international training, take care of more than 350,000 international patients a year. Various high-tech surgeries cost about one-eighth as much as in the U.S.

Striving to become the world leader in medical tourism, private hospitals in India charge even less—about 10% of U.S. fees. High-tech procedures include hip and knee replacements with the latest innovations. Treatment includes private-duty nurses for post-op care.[23, 24]

Projecting from a study from the Deloitte Center for Health Solutions,[25] at least 4 million Americans will become medical tourists in 2016. Wouldn't it be better for all to have local care in the U.S. for an affordable price?

The price transparency and other cost control reforms built into ACC-based care will moderate the cost of high-tech medical procedures in the U.S. for the benefit of patients, providers, and the country. ACC-based care will greatly reduce, but probably not entirely eliminate, the need for price-driven medical tourism.

Reporting Financial Relationships with Health Industries

Obamacare includes "sunshine provisions" that are supposed to reveal the financial relationships between the medical industry and doctors. For instance, drug companies have to disclose the payments for speeches and consulting services they make to health care providers, medical researchers, medical institutions, professional medical associations, industry-sponsored foundations, and disease advocacy groups. However, according to health care policy analysts, these provisions are unlikely to work better than past efforts by state legislatures, federal agencies, and academic hospitals.[26]

ACCs will have more clout in requiring that their consultants disclose any financial relationships with providers of medical devices, pharmaceutical companies, or other special interests. ACCs will be in a position to prevent wasting money on services due to special interests paying off providers.

Rational Rationing: Fair Allocation of Medical Services

Optimization of cost effectiveness and fairness in allocating health services will be the responsibility of each person's chosen ACC. ACCs will end rationing of services based on the patient's income or rationing emanating from decisions made by bureaucrats from the government or private insurance companies.

If ACCs deny services because of perceived lack of demonstrated overall benefit to patients, however defined by the ACCs, people could receive those services and pay out-of-pocket. To provide effective checks and balances, ACC personnel will consider patient input and will operate within the oversight of a committee including patient representatives to hear appeals of denied services. Dissatisfied patients may change ACCs. In return for this form of "rational rationing" of health care resources, (1) everyone will be insured, (2) each person will have a direct practice PCP in charge of the allocation of services, (3) health services perceived to be valuable will be greatly expanded, and (4) overall health care costs will be controlled.

Health Care Cost Control over the Long Term with ACC-Based Reform

After the transition to an ACC-centered system, spending on health care will be the same as projected for 2016—$3.5 trillion per year.[27] Federal safety-net services expenditures will also be maintained at the 2016 rate—$500 billion per year.[1] Assuming health care premiums on average remain the same over the next decade, this will save the government and consumers about $14 trillion compared with the status quo projections.[28a] Future welfare spending with our unsustainable status quo is hard to predict.

With ACCs delivering health and human services and the economy growing at only the current 2.5% per year, health care will consume about 15% of the GDP in 2025.[b] Worldwide, the U.S. will still have one of the highest proportions of the economy devoted the health care. However, health care will not become as projected: a drag on the economy and on overall job growth.

---

a $3.5 trillion x 1.062^10 (6.2% per year inflation in health care costs predicted by the Center for Medicare and Medicaid Services) = $6.3 trillion in 2025. Mean cost/year over next decade= ($6.3 trillion + $3.5 trillion) / 2 = $4.9 trillion. Total cost for the decade = $4.9 trillion x 10 = $49 trillion. Total cost for the decade with ACC-based care = $3.5 trillion x 10 = $35 trillion. Health care savings over the decade = $49 trillion – $35 trillion = $14 trillion.

b   With indefinitely continued 2.5%/year GDP growth, projected GDP in 2016 = $17.9 trillion ($16.6 trillion (in 2013[29]) x 1.025^3 = $17.9 trillion). Projected GDP in 2025 $17.9 trillion GDP(projected for 2016) x 1.025^10 (only 2.5% GDP growth per year) = $22.9 trillion. Health care portion of GDP in 2025 with ACC-based care: $3.5 trillion / $22.9 trillion= 15.3%.

Summary and Conclusion

ACC-based reform will put doctors, with input from all stakeholders, in control of deciding what health care interventions are needed and how much they will spend for required health care. Savings from reducing bloated health care administration and unnecessary medical interventions will be redirected toward valuable health and social-safety-net services that will be provided by ACCs. Efficiencies will also lead to reduced health insurance premiums. The projected unsustainable long-term inflation in health care costs will be reversed by these ACC cost control strategies.

The government's contribution to funding personal health care will be permanently frozen at the amount in 2016 ($1.6 trillion[30]). To generate more money for health care and social services, ACCs may raise premiums as tolerated by their patients. The optimal balance in valuing all the components of the complex health-care and human-services systems will be determined by the free market. These strategies will be good for health, health care, patients, providers, and taxpayers. Consequently, we will return health care to being a sustainable and efficient sector of a healthier and more prosperous society.

Chapter 21

Tax Reform: Flat Income Tax and Consumption Taxes

*I*magine *a tax system that promotes businesses, workers, and the environment. Both liberals and conservatives must be happy with* the changes. *To engage conservatives, we embrace* tax reform ideas by Libertarian Republican Congressman and former Vice Presidential candidate Paul Ryan. He introduced a plan called, "*A Roadmap for the Future*," as a bill in the House of Representatives in 2010. The roadmap calls for us to:[1]

- Establish a firm limit on government taxation and spending.
- Eliminate the alternative minimum tax.
- Do not tax savings (no double taxation).
- Replace corporate income taxes with consumption taxes for businesses (8.5% tax on most goods and services).
- *Simplify income tax rates*—10% on adjusted gross income (AGI) up to $100,000 for joint filers and $50,000 for single filers; and 25% on taxable income above these amounts.
- Equate taxable income to gross earnings minus a standard deduction and personal exemption (i.e., no itemized deductions.)

Tax system reform cannot be more pro-business than to begin with eliminating the corporate income tax! For the roughly $2.1 trillion of U.S. corporation dollars now residing in overseas tax havens,[2] the elimination of the corporate income tax will bring the money home to create jobs and stimulate the economy.

The Grand Bargains' second tax reform proposal is to limit the personal income tax to the top 10% of income earners. This consists of individuals earning more than $60,000 and couples earning more than $120,000. While this simplification of income taxes will greatly down-size the IRS, it would still retain the 68% of the current federal and state income tax revenue that comes from high income people.[3] Costs of complying with Internal Revenue Service (IRS) laws and regulations will plummet. As suggested by Congressman Ryan, the tax should be 25% of gross income above the thresholds, with no itemized deductions. This will greatly simplify the system and make it progressive. He boasted that the personal income tax form could be sent to the IRS on a post card.

To compensate for lost income tax revenue and to eliminate unsustainable deficits, consumption taxes will be substituted. Over $1.8 trillion of these taxes will target goods and services for which consuming less will be in the best interests of both the individual and the country. Additionally, employers of undocumented immigrant workers will be required to pay taxes on their wages (Chapter 14).

We need fundamental tax system reform to *make possible the entire interconnected network of Grand Bargains. To accommodate the interests of all stakeholders, several tax reform bipartisan compromises will be required.* The Grand Bargains' deals involving tax reforms are designed to accomplish both liberal and conservative goals. Conservatives will applaud simplifying the tax system and shifting from income taxes to consumption taxes. Liberals will be engaged by the features that address wealth inequality and environmental stewardship. Both sides will appreciate the design of these consumption taxes to promote health and to reduce crony capitalism/corporate welfare. This will appeal to the better natures of partisans of all stripes on tax issues.

Tax reform should (1) simplify the system, (2) reduce the cost of compliance, (3) result in a balanced budget, (4) maintain vital services of the

*government, and (5) generate government revenue equitably. It should
also facilitate the other grand bargains:*

1. *promote wellness*
2. *increase employment*
3. *invest in public infrastructure*
4. *enhance environmental sustainability*
5. *reduce higher education debt*
6. *increase our national security*

Grand Bargains' tax reform will increase the total amount of income taxes generated by high earners by (1) increasing the number of high earners, (2) repatriating tax sheltered personal wealth from offshore tax havens because paying taxes in another country will make no sense, and (3) raising the income and therefore personal income taxes of high earners employed by corporations that will no longer be subject to corporate income tax.

Income Tax Dividends of New Jobs

Chapter 12 detailed how Grand Bargains-based health care and economic reform, including raising the minimum wage to $15 per hour, will create 20 million jobs caring for children and seniors and at least 20 million additional jobs. The second 20 million jobs will be distributed throughout the current mix of occupations throughout the economy. While the care-giving jobs will generally be paid at the $15 per hour (about $31,000 in 2016), the additional net increase of 20+ million jobs will have wages that correspond to those of current U.S. workers (i.e., $47,000 average income projected for 2016[4]). Just as about 10% of the current workers are high earners (> $60,000/year for individuals/>$120,000 for couples) who will be subject to the 25% flat personal income tax,[3] about 2 million of the 20 million new workers in

2016 will be expected to be classified as high earners.[a] Consequently, they will join the approximately 15 million workers that will be required to pay state and federal income tax. This will raise the income tax projected to be collected by about 14%.[b]

Returning Tax Sheltered Offshore Personal Funds

About $400 billion of U.S. citizens' earnings is sheltered by high income individuals to avoid about $60 billion personal income taxes.[5] With simplifying the personal income tax by making it a flat tax, individuals will have no reason to shelter funds abroad. Consequently, the sheltered offshore personal income of high earners will be repatriated, adding $60 billion more to the collection of personal income taxes.

Repatriating Corporate Tax Sheltered Income and Higher Profits Will Generate More Personal Income Taxes

The U.S. has the highest corporate income tax rate in the world, 39.1% (combining federal and state).[6] To avoid high taxes, an estimated $2.1 trillion of U.S. company income in 2014 is sequestered by U.S. companies in countries with lower corporate income tax rates. This exceeds the $1.9 trillion corporate reserves invested domestically.[2] Sheltering these profits allowed the companies to avoid an estimated $140 billion in corporate income taxes.[7]

Grand Bargains-based reforms to make the U.S. more business-friendly will include (1) eliminating the federal and state corporate income tax, (2) relieving businesses of the burden of paying for employee medical insurance (Chapter 18), (3) eliminating most of the social insurance fees (i.e., Medicare, unemployment insurance, and

---

a   20 million x 0.10 = 2 million new taxpayers in the top 10% bracket projected for 2016 (Chapter 12)

b   The 10% top earners of 146 million workers (0.10 x 146 million = 14.6 million). 2 million net new high-income earners/14.6 current high-income earners = 0.137

workers' compensation, Chapter 18), and taking over the management of employee retirement plans (Chapter 23).

Businesses will transfer to ACCs the responsibility of providing health care insurance, unemployment insurance, and workers' compensation. As was explained in Chapter 12, it will be firmly in the best interests of businesses to hire more workers and pay them living wages. It will be in the best interests of ACCs to have members working and healthy.

With these Grand Bargains-based provisions, businesses will net an additional over $800 billion in profits in 2016.[c] Social Security payroll tax will continue to be split between employer and employee.

Because of all these business-friendly changes improving the financial bottom lines of corporations, there will be more local business investments and hiring of workers. This will stimulate economic growth.

Regarding the $140 billion in U.S. corporate income taxes now lost each year due to offshore tax havens, I conservatively project that most of this will be recovered in individual income taxes of high earning corporate investors, contractors, and employees. If only 50% of the additional $800+ billion in corporate profits went to salaries and bonuses for corporate high earners, at least $100 billion would be recouped.[d]

---

c   Projected Savings in 2016 by Businesses with Grand Bargains' Reforms

Expenses changed	Amount of savings ($ billions)
Federal and state corporate income taxes eliminated	557
Employee medical insurance shifted to employees to pay premiums to ACCs	700
Medicare payroll tax (1.45% of wages)	115
Federal and state unemployment insurance shifted to consumption taxes to be allocated to ACCs	140
Higher employee wages due to $15 / hour minimum wage, Chapter 12	– 660
	852

d   Recovery of personal income taxes from additional profits of corporations: $800 billion (low estimate of additional corporate earnings) x 0.50 (estimating that 50% of additional profits go to earnings of high income investors, executives, contractors, and employees) x 0.25 (25% flat income tax on high earning individuals) = $100 billion

Benefits of the Grand Bargains' Tax Reform Plan

By (1) switching to a flat income tax for high income earners only, (2) making business friendly changes in the tax and regulatory code, and (3) adding 40 million jobs (Chapter 12), the personal income tax collections will be nearly as high as without Grand Bargains-based tax reforms ($1408 billion versus the government's optimistic status quo projection of $1648 billion).[e]

Table 1 (below and previously displayed in Chapter 1) shows the status quo projected revenues that will be collected to run the federal, state and local governments in 2016. Table 2 details the Grand Bargains' proposed tax reform revenue projections.

---

e   Grand Bargains-Based Projected Federal Personal Income Taxes in 2016

Components of Grand Bargains-based federal personal income tax[8]	$ billions
$1648 billion status quo federal income tax estimate (Table 1) x 0.683 (68.3%) of total projected federal personal income tax attributed to high earners	1126
Taxes from additional 2 million high earners: $1126 billion x 0.137 = $154 billion (Chapter 12)	154
Taxes from repatriated tax sheltered earnings: $60 billion x 0.80 (80% portion going to federal government = $48 billion	48
Additional income taxes by high earning employees, contractors, and investors of corporations because of over $800 billion additional corporate profits: $100 billion x 0.80 (80% portion going for federal taxes + $80 billion	80
Total projected federal personal income taxes in 2016 with Grand Bargains reforms	1408

Table 1. U.S. Federal, State, and Local Government Status
Quo Revenues Projected for 2016 ($billions)[8]

Sources of U.S. government revenue	2016 projected revenue
Federal funds	4100
Taxes, fees, insurance	3570
Individual income	1648
Corporate income	502
Social insurance	1130
Old age and survivors	690
Disability (SSI)	120
Unemployment	60
Hospital insurance	250
Business and other	60
Ad valorem taxes	220
Excise	60
Transportation	50
Other	110
Borrowing	530
State and local revenue	2711
Individual income	336
Corporate income	55
Social insurance	380
Unemployment	80
Retirement	300
Business and other	370
Utility/liquor	150
Fees and charges	460
Health	150
Ad valorem taxes	1110
Excise	60
Sales	490
Property	420
Transportation	80
Licenses	50
U.S. government taxes + borrowing	6810

Table 2. U.S. Federal, State, and Local Government Revenues Projected
for 2016 ($billions) with ACCs and the Grand Bargains

Sources of U.S. government revenue	2016 revenue
Federal	4684
Taxes, fees, insurance	4684
Individual income	1408
Corporate income	0
Consumption taxes	1862
Trading equities	150
Nonrenewable energy	700
Plastics	150
Tobacco	27
Alcohol	75
Guns	50
Water	300
Systemic risk banks	50
Electronic media	120
Imported goods	240
Immigrant employment	60
Social insurance	1074
Old age	901
Disability (SSI)	173
Unemployment	0
Business & other	60
Ad valorem taxes	220
Excise	60
Transportation	50
Other	110
Borrowing	0
State and local revenue	2568
Individual income	328
Corporate income	0
Social insurance	300
Unemployment	0
Retirement	300
Business and other	370
Fees and charges	460
Health	0
Ad valorem taxes	1110
Excise	60
Sales	490
Property	420
Transportation	80
Licenses	50
Total U.S. Government revenue	7252

This proposed plan will substitute consumption taxes for the corporate income tax, the personal income taxes for all but the top 10% of earners, and employer-paid unemployment taxes and workers' compensation insurance. Other federal, state, and local taxes, fees, and social insurance charges (i.e., Social Security payroll tax) will remain the same as with the status quo.

Based on the calculations of Representative Ryan,[1] substituting consumption taxes for income taxes will save most of the $200 billion per year that it costs Americans to comply with the IRS.

While status quo government projections call for borrowing $530 billion in 2016,[8] the Grand Bargains-based budget (Table 2) includes no borrowing. The consumption taxes and the additional taxes from 40 million more workers will fill the federal deficit.

As an added benefit of Grand Bargains' tax reform, $442 billion in additional projected federal revenue from the above taxes should be invested as shown in Table 3:

Table 3. Allocation of Additional Revenue in 2016 with Grand Bargains Reform

Purpose of funds	Source of funds	$ billions
Replace unemployment insurance taxes	Federal consumption taxes	140
Replace Workers' Compensation employer taxes	Federal consumption taxes	40
New infrastructure projects	Federal consumption taxes	50
College and trade school student grants and part-time jobs	Federal consumption taxes	50
Distribute Social Security Trust Funds to ACCs	Employment taxes from U.S. Treasury	100
Foreign development aid to enhance national security	Federal consumption taxes	50
Allocation at the discretion of Congress	Federal consumption taxes	12
Total		442

As mentioned in Chapter 19, shifting to Grand-Bargains-based health care and human services will allow states and municipalities over $600 billion in revenue for employee pensions (Chapter 24), infrastructure projects (Chapter 15), education (Chapter 16), and other priorities.

Proposed New Consumption Taxes

Basic economics teaches us that any product or service that is taxed will be utilized less than if it is not taxed. Therefore, I propose targeting products and services for taxation that we should be consuming less of for health, environmental, and/or economic reasons. For these commodities and services, reduced consumption will help to prevent chronic illnesses, promote full employment, stimulate economic growth (quantitative and qualitative), and foster environmental sustainability.

To understand how these consumption taxes will work, we need to understand the concept of "price elasticity." Price elasticity means that an increase in overall cost of an item will decrease consumer demand by a certain percentage.[9] Economists express this as the percentage drop in consumption occurring with each 1% increase in the cost of an item or service. For many of the proposed consumption taxes, price elasticity data are available to estimate the effect of the tax on reducing consumption of the product. On average, for each 1% increase in cost, a commodity will be consumed about 0.5% less. However, price elasticity varies considerably. For any commodity, the reduction in consumption intensifies as the price goes up, particularly if it is a long-term increase in price.

The following are the proposed consumption taxes.

Tobacco Tax: $2 per Pack

According to the Center for Disease Control and Prevention,[10] about 44 million people in the U.S. use tobacco. Tobacco causes cancer, heart disease, stroke, and lung diseases. Smoking leads to approximately 443,000 premature deaths annually in the U.S.[11] Tobacco products along with state and federal excise taxes on purchases cost U.S. smokers about $90 billion/year. [12, 13]

The relationship between the cost of tobacco and the number of smokers in a population is very strong. High tobacco taxes work better than anti-tobacco education campaigns in getting smokers to quit and in preventing young people from starting to smoke.[14] Price elasticity studies have shown that, for each 1% increase in the cost of tobacco, there will be a 0.4% decrease in consumption.[14] Given the current average cost of a pack of cigarettes ($5.62),[13] an increase of $2.00 per pack in tobacco taxes will increase the price by 36% and reduce tobacco consumption by about 14%.[f]

This will generate about $27 billion in yearly federal revenue. [12, 13g] The reduction in tobacco use will save consumers about $13 billion on the cost of tobacco.[h] According to data cited in a Surgeon General's Report,[15] this will reduce the costs of health care and tobacco-related low productivity by about $40 billion per year.[i]

For workers who are laid off because of the downsizing of the tobacco industry, ACCs will train them for new jobs and facilitate their reemployment.

Alcohol Tax Hike

The Center for Disease Control links excessive alcohol consumption to liver cirrhosis, premature and underweight babies, various

---

f   An increase of $2.00 per pack in tobacco taxes will increase the price by 36% ($2.00/5.62 = 0.356) and reduce tobacco consumption by about 14% (0.36 x 0.4 (price elasticity) = 0.144.

g $90 billion for retail tobacco x 0.856 (≈14% reduction) x 0.356 (≈36% consumption tax)= $27.4 billion federal revenue generated

h $90 billion for retail tobacco x 0.144 (14% reduction in consumption) = $13.0 billion (reduction in expenditures on tobacco)

i $289 billion per year in tobacco-related medical expenses and reduced productivity (Surgeon General's Report) x 0.14 (14% reduction in tobacco use) = $40.4 billion.

cancers, unintentional injuries, and violence.[16] Alcohol abuse accounts for about 88,000 deaths per year in the U.S.[17] The costs to taxpayers of the complications of alcohol abuse for 2016 are projected to be about $66 billion.[18, 19]

The Community Preventive Services Task Force, formed in Atlanta, GA in conjunction with the Center for Disease Control to evaluate public health strategies to reduce the adverse impacts of alcohol abuse, found strong evidence that raising alcohol taxes reduced the complications of alcohol abuse. For each 1.00% increase in the cost of alcohol, they found a 0.77% decrease in alcohol-related adverse health impacts.[20] Price elasticity studies concerning alcohol consumption show an average price elasticity of alcohol consumption of – 0.50% per 1.00% increase in price.[21] Consequently, raising the overall cost of alcoholic beverages by 50% ($0.85 per average drink) by increasing the excise tax would reduce consumption of alcohol by about 25%.[j] [20]

Based on recent trends in consumption of alcohol by U.S. residents,[22] the cost of alcohol purchases is projected to be about $200 billion in 2016—averaging about $1.70 per drink. Consequently, raising the cost of alcohol by 50% will generate about $75 billion per year in government revenue.[k] This is hardly unreasonable since the Center for Disease Control and Prevention estimates that the cost of excessive alcohol consumption in the United States is about $1.90 per drink, of which about $0.80 per drink is a cost to the taxpayer for health care, law enforcement, and social services.[23]

With this strategy in the U.S., there will be a 25% decrease of alcohol consumption equivalent to about $50 billion before taxes. Even more importantly, the reduction in consumption will save an estimated $75 billion/year on the health and economic costs of alcohol abuse.[24]

---

j   50% increase in cost x – 0.5% change in consumption / 1% increase in cost = – 25% consumption

k $200 billion (alcohol cost projected for 2016) x 0.75 (25% decrease in consumption) = $150 billion consumed. $150 billion consumed x 1.5 (50% increase in cost) = $225 billion for alcohol + consumption tax. Excise tax generated: $225 billion – $150 billion = $75 billion.

Americans will suffer fewer motor-vehicle crashes, less alcohol-related crime, less mortality from liver cirrhosis, and lower all-cause mortality.[25]

A moderate drinker who continues to consume one alcoholic drink per day will pay about $300 more per year. Heavy drinkers will bear the largest burden of the additional tax.

For workers that are laid off because of the downsizing of the beer, wine, and spirits industries, ACCs will train them for new jobs and assist them in finding alternative employment.

Taxing Freshwater from Public Water Systems

U.S. residents enjoy one of the safest public water systems in the world. The Congressional Budget Office (CBO) has estimated that combined water and sewer bills average only 0.5% – 1.0% of household income in this country.[26, 27] When compared to other developed countries, consumers in the United States pay the lowest percentage of income for water and wastewater services in the world. Although the U.S. has about one-quarter of the populations of China or of India, we consume almost as much freshwater as in either of those countries.

My friend Kevin Wattier, Head of the Long Beach Water Department, estimated that Californians, on average, use 10%-20% more water than can be sustainably replenished by rain in the state. The rest of the country also overuses water from aquifers underground. Cheap water constitutes a major subsidy that harms the environment and our security (Chapter 13).

Consequently, a reduction of water consumption of 15% of water use is a reasonable initial goal in order to stabilize groundwater aquifers. Over time, water consumption could safely be reduced much more. This makes for an excellent target for a tax designed to reduce water consumption while raising revenue. A Grand Bargains' tax of $0.004 per gallon of freshwater drawn from public utilities or taken from streams or groundwater wells will generate about $300 billion in 2016.[28]

Given that about 70% of freshwater consumption goes to food production and processing, the major impact of taxing water will be on the

---

price of food. The estimated amount of freshwater tax related to food production will be about $210 billion in 2016.[1] Some foods use many times the average amount of water per pound of food produced (see water footprints of foods, Chapter 13). So these would be consumed less under this tax.

This proposed freshwater tax will have favorable health and environmental benefits. It will encourage consumption of more healthful foods and beverages, along with water conservation in agriculture, landscaping, domestic households, industry, and commerce.

Taxing Plastic

For every pound of human flesh in the U.S., we consume about two pounds of plastic products per year (about 32 million tons in 2011[29]). Almost half of plastics consumed consist of bags and other single-use products. In the United States, the plastics industry employs nearly 900 thousand people and will produce about $400 billion dollars in products in 2016,[30] costing on average about $6 per pound.

My friend Captain Charlie Moore of the Algalita Marine Research Foundation uses his 50 foot Catamaran and volunteer crew to sail the Pacific Ocean to study ocean debris. In a voyage in the 1990s, Charlie and his crew found that the Pacific Ocean contained about six pounds of plastic on average for every pound of zooplankton.[31] His latest research voyage in 2014 showed a much higher level that he hasn't yet quantified. The plastic particles already in the seas will take hundreds of years to break down. This threatens fish, birds, the broader ecosystem, the climate, and people. Because plastics are fossil fuel byproducts, they have a negative effect on climate change. Plastic now comprises about 13% of municipal landfills.[29] Among many health conditions associated with human exposure to plastic pollution are cancer, diabetes, birth defects, and obesity.[32]

---

1 $300 billion total tax on freshwater (Chapter 21) x 0.7 (70% of freshwater goes to food production) = $210 billion

We need strategies to reduce consumption of plastic. Education has shown to help very little. I have a hard time curtailing my use of plastic bags. To different degrees, people realize that plastic pollution harms the environment and are willing to decrease consumption for the sake of good citizenship. However, this is far from enough to avoid the huge environmental damages that will be caused by continuing the overconsumption of plastics and, consequently, ongoing exponential increases in plastic pollution.

To reduce the consumption of plastic while raising revenue, consider a Grand Bargains' tax on plastic products of $3 per pound, raising the cost of plastic products by 50%. This will raise about $150 billion per year in government revenue. It will also save consumers nearly $100 billion by reducing the purchasing of plastic products, particularly the most environmentally damaging single use products.[m]

Equities Trading Tax

Within the past decade, trading on the stock markets of the world has been increasingly taken over by supercomputers that place and then cancel thousands of orders a second. Tech-savvy traders program the computers with statistical algorithms that can predict the upward or downward direction of stocks, allowing them to jump in ahead of big rallies and sell off before big declines. Market fundamentals—value of the companies selling the stocks—have nothing to do with it. Steve Kroft, reporter for 60 Minutes interviewed Joe Saluzzi of Themis Trading LLC, who trades large blocks of stock for institutional investors. Saluzzi called high-frequency traders, "parasites who exploit a technological advantage to suck money out of the market and add no value." When Kroft asked if high frequency trading raises capital for compa-

---

m   Given the price elasticity estimate: – 0.5% per 1% price increase, a 50% increase in price of plastics will reduce consumption by 25% (50% x – 0.5 = –25%). $400 billion (current consumption) x 0.75 (reduce consumption by 25%) = $300 billion. $300 billion x 1.5 (50% increase in cost) = $450 billion cost of plastics + tax – $300 billion cost of plastics = $150 billion in plastics consumption taxes projected for 2016

nies, Saluzzi responded, "Absolutely not. If anything, it's distracting from the capital raising process."[33]

The average stock trades almost five times per year now due to supercomputer churning of the market.[34]

Proponents of high-speed computer trading argue that the technology reduces stock spreads and transaction costs and provides liquidity to the markets. Without short-term traders using high-speed computers, selling stocks would take longer.

However, on the down side of the practice, the speed of transactions has made it difficult for financial regulators to keep track of stock trading. An unintended consequence of high-speed trading was the mini-crash of May 6, 2010, in which the Dow Industrials at one point plunged 600 points for no apparent reason and then recovered within hours. In that case, a mutual fund's supercomputer accidently offered $4.1 billion of securities on the market in a 20-minute period. Other high-frequency traders bought and quickly sold the securities, which triggered a massive selloff by algorithm-programmed computers of yet other traders, spawning fears about the integrity of the entire system.[33]

Using algorithms to determine the upward or downward trajectory of the stocks traded, high-speed computer traders typically earn an extra one or two cents per share traded in addition to the transaction fees. For approximately 600 billion shares exchanged by high-frequency traders in 2010,[35] traders charged investors $6–$12 billion without providing value. The unnecessarily high volume of trades generated by the computer technology lowers transaction fees per trade but adds billions of dollars more in overall transaction fees.

Congressman Peter DeFazio submitted a bill in the House of Representatives to impose a quarter percent (0.25%) equity transfer tax on both the buyer and seller of financial instruments such as stocks, options, and futures.[36] "H.R.1068 - Let Wall Street Pay for Wall Street's Bailout Act of 2009" was a common-sense solution to this predatory trading technology. If the amount of money traded per year dropped from about $80 trillion[35] to $30 trillion (as projected with this tax), this would raise about $150 billion a year.[n] The tax revenue will go to the Federal Treasury.

With the equity transfer tax, if someone has a portfolio turnover of 100% per year, then this tax represents a modest 0.5% per year burden. However, with the current rate of churning stock market investments averaging almost five times per year, the burden would be a more substantial 2.5% per year on the portfolio. Using supercomputers to do multiple trades a day of the same stocks would not be cost effective.[37] Because of a substantial reduction in volume of shares traded, transaction fees per share would go up, but the overall cost of all transactions would go down by billions of dollars per year.

Grand Bargain #29: Preventing Violence by Fixing Mental Health Care and Taxing Guns

As discussed regarding enhancing mental health services in Chapter 6, our epidemic of shooting rampages by mentally ill people and others can't be stopped simply by more laws banning assault weapons or regulations restricting access to guns.

While mental health system improvement is priority #1 in preventing mass shootings and other violence, reduction in the number of guns in circulation (currently about 300 million in the U.S.[38]) is priority #2. Banning guns is not politically achievable or recommended. However, charging a tax on gun purchases and a yearly licensing fee is doable and would definitely reduce the guns in circulation. The case for taxing guns begins with the relationship of poverty and violence.

The Connection between Poverty and Violence

Policy analysts argue that radically reducing gun violence will never happen without eliminating poverty. Poor young men and boys ages

---

n $30 trillion x 0.005 = $150 billion

15-24-years-old living in inner cities are the most likely to be targeted by gun violence as well as to become the perpetrators.[39] Gun violence breeds in a cycle of poverty for youths mired in despair, educational disadvantages, few employment opportunities, depression, poverty, and street violence.[40]

We don't yet know what efforts to strengthen our mental health system will work to prevent gun violence. Competing ACCs will be the perfect laboratories for mental health professionals to experiment with strategies to reduce violence of all kinds.

Racism has a lot to do with the violence, as it does in sending a disproportionate number of people of color to prison and death row. Additionally, rich people are able to avoid prison if having committed violent crimes and convicted. And they rarely go to death row. The wide-ranging services of ACCs in health care, health promotion, human services (social, legal, financial, educational), and employment will be game-changers in overcoming poverty, racism, and the associated violence.

Reducing the number of guns in circulation will help further.

Gun Tax and Yearly Gun Licensing Fee: $300

In conjunction with giving ACCs the human and financial resources to strengthen mental illness prevention and treatment programs (Chapter 6), taxing guns and imposing yearly licensing fees are components of this grand bargain for several reasons. Assessing a high tax on each gun will decrease the number of guns in circulation. A gun tax will likely reduce gun ownership among young, poor people who are most affected by gun violence. Gun taxes and licensing fees also have great potential to raise much needed government revenue for health care, social services, and other services.

I propose a tax of $300 on the purchase of any gun, as well as a yearly licensing fee of $300 for ownership of each gun. If they choose, ACCs will be able to ameliorate or eliminate gun taxes and fees for members. However, it will take a consensus of ACC members to reduce or eliminate them. Refunds of gun taxes and fees to members will come out of the overall revenues of the ACCs that choose to do so. People can choose their ACCs in part on the ACC policies regarding whether to refund gun taxes and fees or not.

Anything short of mental health system reform along with high gun taxes and fees would be unlikely to move the dial on mass murders and other gun violence. With this politically polarizing issue, the involvement of non-governmental organizations (ACCs) in proactively, innovatively, and holistically monitoring the risk of violence and having tools to intervene as appropriate will be a game-changer.

When ACCs differ widely in percentage of gun ownership as might be expected, the levels of gun violence rates in different ACCs can be compared. This may lead to public policy innovations to further reduce gun violence. The idea is to give gun owners some of what they want, give gun opponents some of what they want, raise tax revenue to channel through ACCs, reduce guns in circulation, and to provide a framework for moving further ahead in preventing gun violence.

If about one-third of all guns are sold back to the government as a result of these steep costs of gun ownership, then the taxes and fees on the remaining 200 million guns will return about $60 billion. The net gain in revenue for ACC services after the buyback program will be in the range of $50 billion in 2016.[o]

With the record pace of gun sales since the Newtown, CT massacre,[41, 42] the firearms business (guns, ammunition, ancillary supplies, related goods and services) in 2016 is projected to employ up to 275,000 people, and generate over $40 billion in economic impact. In the absence of data on the price elasticity on guns and the unknown number of gun tax-and-fee rebates that will be granted by the ACCs, consider the price elasticity – 0.25% in volume of gun sales per 1% increase in

---

o   200 million guns in circulation x $300 per year per gun = $60 billion. Gun buyback program cost in 2016 ≈ $10 billion. Net revenue from gun fees: $60 billion – $10 billion = $50 billion.

cost. Consequently, for a 150% increase in cost of firearms, the guns in circulation will decrease by roughly the above mentioned 100 million. [p]

Compared with legislators in Washington, D.C., the state capitals, and the cities, ACC health care and human services providers will be better able to innovate and experiment with gun tax and fee rebates along with holistic violence prevention strategies. Until answers begin to manifest and successful programs replicated, this strategy will be a work in progress.

Gun deaths and injuries occurring in 1977 were estimated to cost U.S. citizens $100 billion.[43] Adjusted for inflation and for the 54% decrease in gun violence now compared with in 1997,[44] gun violence probably still costs us about $100 billion per year. With Grand Bargains' reform removing 100 million guns from circulation particularly among the less affluent that are at greatest risk for violence, the gun taxes and fees should reduce gun violence by one-third and save citizens at least $30 billion per year.[q]

Since stores selling guns and ammunition will be the sites to return guns in buyback programs incentivized by the new taxes and fees on guns, the firearms business will increase in employment and economic impact over several years as an estimated 100 million guns are taken out of circulation.

As a potential violence prevention strategy, ACCs may want to experiment with offering partial gun tax and fee rebates to members that volunteer to be screened by their PCP for suitability for gun ownership. If indicated, PCPs could refer members screened for further evaluation by psychiatrists. ACCs might also give members gun tax and fee rebates for completion of gun safety classes or other violence prevention interventions.

---

p   Adding $60 billion in taxes and fees to the $40 billion firearms industry equates to a 150% increase ($60 billion/$40 billion = 1.50. Assuming – 0.25% price elasticity for each 1% increase in price of guns, 150% increase in gun costs would reduce ownership by a little more than one-third (– 0.25 x 150% = 0.375). 0.375 x 300 million guns = 113 million guns (≈100 million)

q $100 billion (estimated cost of gun violence in 2016) x 0.375 (37.5%) = $37 billion

As in the other domains regarding the comprehensive services provided by ACCs, competition will drive excellence in the prevention and treatment of mental illness and prevention of gun violence.

Too-Big-to-Fail Banks Tax: 0.8% of Holdings per Year

The Editors of Bloomberg News cited studies by leading economists estimating that U.S. taxpayers give the largest Wall Street Banks subsidies totaling about 0.8% of their deposits.[45] The government's financial assistance to the big banks is in the form of implicit guarantees that the government will bail out too-big-to-fail banks ("systemically important financial institutions") that become insolvent. Given over $9 trillion in assets in the largest U.S. banks, this totals over $70 billion per year. This equates to the federal government giving banks about 3 cents of each federal tax dollar collected. Without Congressional action, these government subsidies to financial corporations will cost taxpayers up to $1 trillion over the next decade.

Republicans and Democrats have both drafted legislation that would levy a tax on systemically important financial institutions. However, both sides will probably not resolve the differences between their tax bills in time to make it happen any time soon. Neither plan would impose taxes on big financial institutions that raise anywhere near the cost of those big corporations to taxpayers. The plans differ on relatively trivial issues.[46, 47]

As recommended by Bloomberg News editors, I propose enacting a 0.8% per year tax on assets of systemically important financial institutions that will recover the entire cost of subsidies to those institutions. If those mega-corporations actually pay back the full cost of their government subsidies, many will be pressured to break into smaller, less systemically risky, companies. This would protect the public from the risks of these institutions.

Given that a high tax on too big to fail banks will likely cause some of them to downsize, the proposed tax of 0.8% of assets of the megabanks would raise perhaps $50 billion in 2016. Subsequently, revenue from this tax will depend on decisions by shareholders of these institutions about the breakup of too-big-to-fail institutions.

Electronic Communications Tax

The converging sectors of telecommunication products and services, including broadband media and information technology are increasing in sales at a rate of about 8% per year.[48] In 2016, they are projected to account for nearly $1.5 trillion to the U.S. economy.[49] Of this money, subscriber services for the Internet, smart phones, and television in 2016 are projected to cost about $240 billion. Internet and entertainment services providers offering wireless, cable, or DSL connections compete for market share in this business.

Today's interconnected information, communications, and technology sectors support an estimated 10 million American jobs. Our "information age" with remarkable innovations in electronic media has achieved miracles and has tremendous potential to further benefit individuals and society. However, it also gives rise to public health concerns, particularly for children.

According to the American Academy of Pediatrics, children today spend an average of seven hours a day on entertainment media, including televisions, computers, smart phones and other electronic devices. Much of the content glorifies violence, explicit sex, and unhealthful behaviors (e.g., tobacco, alcohol, junk food, risky sex, etc.). The American Academy of Pediatrics cites studies showing that excessive electronic media use can lead to attention problems, school difficulties, sleep and eating disorders, and obesity. Illicit and risky behaviors of children and teenagers have been related to their exposure to video games, the Internet, and cell phones.[50]

The Academy's policy statement about electronic media expresses concerns about the potential harmful effects of media messages and images.[51] It recommends that parents establish a family home use plan for all media. Additionally, it calls for media influences on children and teenagers to be recognized by schools, policymakers, product advertisers, and entertainment producers.

Many past authoritative policy statements by the American Academy of Pediatrics and others have detailed similar concerns about electronic media content regarding violence, sex, substance use, unwholesome music and music videos. Unfortunately, these policy statements have had little impact on the actions of parents, schools, policymakers, product advertisers, and entertainment producers.

As has been noted in a detailed report by the Future of Children from Princeton's Brookings Institute, government has never done much to protect children from the effect of media marketing. With the First Amendment protections of commercial speech and with rapid changes in electronic media technology and capabilities, the government is unlikely to ever implement what most would consider effective regulations.[52]

Given the influence of diverse, virtually unregulated financial special interests, protecting children from the harmful effects of electronic media requires a couple of game-changers. First, consider a Grand Bargains' electronic media services excise tax based on the duration of use. The electronic media tax will be designed to apply to wireless, cable, and DSL subscription services for computers and mobile devices with wireless and wired connections to the Internet, cell phone towers, and satellite receivers. Telecommunication services covered by the tax will be communications (e.g., smart phones, tablets, IPods, etc.), entertainment (television, movies, etc.), and data transfers.

The Grand Bargains' proposed electronic communications tax will be 50% of the current subscription services fees, raising subscription services from $240 billion in 2016 to $360 billion. Considering all of communication digital technologies, this $120 billion tax with raise the cost of telecommunication products and services by a modest 8%.[r] This will do little to decrease the volume of subscription services.

---

r $120 billion telecommunication services tax / $1.5 trillion total telecommunications products and services in 2016 = 8%

Net-Neutrality or No?—Let ACCs Decide for Members

Yet another polarizing issue will be debated *ad nauseam* in the 114th Congress, beginning in 2015. President Obama and liberal Democrats see net neutrality as sort of an inalienable right. He said, "An open Internet is essential to the American economy and, increasingly, to our very way of life."[53] On the other hand, the telecommunications industry and Republican supporters strongly oppose the tough government regulations meant to assure what they say will stifle innovation and the growth of the Internet. While the Federal Communications Commission is supposedly independent of partisan politics, appointments to the FCC have been made by President Obama and previous Presidents.

Like so many intractable political issues these days, Internet access policy needs a game-changer that is fair to liberals, conservatives, telecommunications professionals, and the public. We need a means for compromise rather than another issue will major winners and losers. Consider a compromise that involves ACCs and open access to unbundled Internet connection services.

Federal legislation requiring Internet service providers to unbundle their products and services and to allow for open usage of cable and fiber optic technologies is stalled in Congress. If enacted, open usage of connections to the Internet will improve competition between providers. Most other countries in the world require open usage of cable and fiber optic Internet access technologies. Subscription prices in those countries are generally lower than ours, their connection speeds faster, and quality of service better than ours.[48]

Naturally, big telecommunication companies (e.g., Verizon, Time Warner, Comcast, etc.) see no benefit to them of sharing their cables or fiber optic wiring and have successfully lobbied against open access regulations. However, these companies may consider unbundling their services in exchange for lack of FCC regulations regarding paying for faster connection speeds. For instance, this way Verizon's FIOS fiber optic cables could be purchased by a customer who uses another Internet service provider for monthly subscription services.

With unbundling Internet services in exchange for dropping regulations against paying for faster connection speeds, ACCs will be in positions to negotiate with Internet services providers and content providers in the best interests of members. Whereas, individuals have little leverage on prices for Internet services because of the near consolidation of the industry with buyouts and mergers, ACCs, representing tens of thousands or hundreds of thousands of members, may be able to broker deals for better prices and services.

The Grand Bargains' subscription Internet connection services proposal is to allow ACCs to represent their members in negotiations with telecommunications companies. ACCs could then negotiate on behalf of their members with competing Internet services providers regarding (1) paying for faster access speeds, (2) content restrictions for children, (3) privacy issues, and (4) prices, and (5) other matters for which individuals have no leverage with telecommunications companies.

With this grand bargain in effect, some ACCs may insist on strict Internet connection speed neutrality and others may not. Content restrictions for children would vary between ACCs. People could have more control over the privacy of their email correspondence and other Internet activities. Prices for Internet connection subscriptions will probably come down due to competition between many more Internet service providers. Innovation and competition will both be accelerated by the decentralization of the regulation of Internet connection services. Given that a quasi-monopoly has evolved in the highly consolidated telecommunications industry,[54, 55] ACCs brokering deals on behalf of members will be a game changer to reinvigorate a genuine free market among Internet services providers.

ACC members, as stakeholders in the availability of Internet services, will offer input into Internet access policies of their ACCs. ACCs will compete in part on how well they represent their members in getting fair and affordable access to the Internet and the related entertainment content and services.

ACCs to Protect Children from Harmful Media

ACC may also assist members in protecting their children and themselves from harmful media influences. Since parents and children will be voluntary members of non-governmental organizations (i.e., ACCs), First Amendment barriers to protect the health and safety of children from dangers of electronic media will not be an issue. Private, competing ACCs will be able to regulate electronic media on behalf of their members (especially children) in ways the government cannot do.

Regarding media content available to children, different ACCs will differ in what programming they want to block and will have different methods of blocking or limiting the exposure of children to offensive content. This multifaceted approach to electronic technology protections will aim to help ACCs and parents limit the harms and maximize the benefits from electronic media. Utilizing local community information technology resources chosen by members, ACCs will have the flexibility, capability, and authority to innovatively work with parents and children.

People will also be at liberty to join ACCs that continued to leave electronic media content available to children solely up to monitoring by the individual parents as is the status quo. As another possible option, ACCs might be able to offer electronic media tax rebates to members for the time that they watch electronic media with content in alignment with a consensus of the membership. For example, children and their parents may not be charged for watching Sesame Street or other wholesome children's programming. In each ACC, all stakeholders could be involved in decision-making about available electronic media content for children. The more united ACC members are about children's media content preferences the more leverage they might exert on media content providers.

The Internet connection services tax will be expected to reduce the time that consumers use their electronic devices. By in large, this will be a good thing. With the assistance of the ACC health, social services, education, and finance professionals of their choice, the Internet connection services taxes will encourage members to be more selective about the content of their viewing and listening.

There is a paucity of information about the price elasticity regarding the use of electronic media. However, the proposed tax, amounting to an additional 8% on the cost of media services, should not substantially reduce the overall use of telecommunication devices. Indeed, volume discounts on electronic media negotiated by ACCs buying media services cooperatively should save some money for their consumers, partially compensating for the tax.

Consumption Taxes on Imports

In 2016, goods imported to the U.S. are projected to cost about $2.7 trillion.[56] Consumption taxes on these imported goods would be appropriate. With Grand Bargains-based economic reform, the cost of products exported will be increased by the consumption taxes on the commodities used to produce the products (e.g., non-renewable energy, plastics, and water). Consequently, costs will go up for foreigners buying products imported from the U.S. because they will indirectly pay U.S. consumption taxes. This will tend to reduce exports to the extent that consumption taxable commodities are used in products. So as not to negatively impact our balance of foreign trade, it is only fair that the new consumption taxes should be levied on imports according to the content of commodities utilized in the production of goods imported.

Almost all of our imported goods carry a heavy carbon footprint due in large part to oil burned for transport. Additionally, there is imbedded energy in the making of industrial machinery and equipment, industrial supplies, computers, computer accessories, telecommunications equipment, and, of course, plastic made from petroleum.

The U.S. is projected to import about $234 billion in petroleum products in 2016.[57] However, with Grand Bargains-based excise taxes on non-renewable energy including petroleum, imported petroleum will be almost eliminated (Chapter 22).

For imported commodities, the estimated average value of the non-renewable energy, freshwater (e.g., in food), and plastics is roughly in the range of 20% of the retail price. Consequently, a 10% consumption tax on imports will be imposed on average, based on consumption taxes appropriate to the composition of the goods.[s] With a price elasticity of – 0.5% for each 1% of tax on average, this will be expected to reduce imported goods other than petroleum products by about 5% or $120 billion. The consumption tax will then raise about $240 billion for the U.S. Treasury in 2016.[t]

The Big Picture on Consumption Taxes

Table 4 below shows the new consumption taxes and the tax on undocumented immigrant labor (Chapter 14). Overall, the taxes will raise over $1.9 trillion while saving consumers about $1 trillion with reduced consumption and other economies. Out of an estimated $200 billion per year in the cost of compliance with income taxes,[1] about $180 billion will be saved in the administration of the IRS. The consumption taxes that replace much of the income taxes will cost no more than half of the administrative costs that we now allocate to the IRS (i.e., about $100 billion in 2016). This will save about $80 billion in 2016.[u] Most of the consumption taxes compliance costs will be with vendors

---

s   For imports that were produced with negligible non-renewable energy, water, and plastics, very little consumption tax would be added. For imports of non-renewable energy, the consumption tax equal to 75% of the value of the energy would be collected—the same as U.S. consumers will pay for domestically extracted fossil fuels and for nuclear energy (Chapter 22). For the average imported commodity with about 20% of the product's value from consumption taxable products, the consumption tax would be in the 10% range (i.e., Increasing price by 1% decreases sales by 0.5%).

t $2.7 trillion (imported goods projected with the status quo) – $238 billion (imported petroleum products largely eliminated by conservation and renewable energy, Chapter 22) = $2.54 trillion. $2.54 trillion x 0.95 (5% reduction in consumption due to the import tax) x 0.10 (10% imports consumption tax on average) ≈ $240 billion consumption tax on imports.

u   Estimated Effect of Grand Bargains Reform of Tax Compliance Costs

Tax compliance costs	$ billions
Current IRS compliance costs	200
Grand Bargains Reform total tax compliance costs	120
Savings with Grand Bargains tax reform	80

of the taxed commodities rather than with the federal government tax collectors.

Table 4. Consumption Taxes to be Levied and Money
to be Saved (Copy from Chapter 1)

Item for the tax	Tax revenue generated ($billions)	Money saved by less consumption ($billions)	Other money saved ($billions)
Tobacco	$27	$14	$40
Alcohol	$75	$50	$60
Nonrenewable energy	$700	$343	$40
Water	$300	$130	-
Plastics	$150	$100	-
Equity trades	$150	$10	-
Guns	$50	-	$30
Systemic risk banks	$50	-	-
Electronic media	$120	-	-
Imported goods	$240	$120	-
Undocumented labor tax ($3/hr)	$60		
Income tax system compliance cost savings			$80
Total	$1922	$767	$250

Immigration reform and the tax on the labor of undocumented immigrants were discussed in Chapter 14. This tax will be fair to undocumented workers, legal immigrants, other workers, and all taxpayers.

Summary and Conclusions

Because of the proposed new consumption taxes, corporate income taxes will be eliminated and personal income taxes will be limited to high earners. These consumption taxes will raise federal government revenue while saving consumers money by reducing the purchase of items with adverse effects on health, the economy, and/or the environment.

Administering these consumption taxes will be much easier than with corporate and personal income taxes. Compliance and fairness will be much better assured. However, disruptions in businesses and employment brought on by these taxes will be major. Tens of millions of workers will become redundant and will need to find new employment. Beginning with the 20 million people employed by ACCs to care for children, the frail elderly, and the disabled, a net increase of 40 million jobs will be expected. For all people able to work, ACCs will guarantee them vocational retraining and will help them find jobs (Chapter 12). A much larger proportion of the population will pay taxes in a taxation system that is more diversified, fair, and equitable.

A non-renewable energy tax, the last consumption tax to be discussed, is a huge topic. It will be the subject of the next chapter.

Chapter 22
Energy Diet for a Sustainable Economy

O ver 20 years ago, I reduced my personal carbon footprint on the earth by adopting a completely plant-based diet and by selling my car. I have since relied on public transportation and my bicycle. Personal transportation and diet are the largest components of the carbon footprint. Compared to the average carbon footprint in the U.S. (about 18 metric tons per year of carbon dioxide), my carbon footprint is less than 3 metric tons/year. These changes in my lifestyle have been good for my health without making me feel impoverished or unduly constrained.

To avoid global average temperature increases of greater than 2° F, the total world carbon footprint will need to drop to the range of 20 billion metric tons of carbon dioxide per year. If the world's population stabilizes at 7 billion, the average carbon footprint per year will need to drop to less than 3 metric tons/year. If the world's population increases to 9 billion people as projected, the average carbon footprint will need to drop to near 2 metric tons/year.

The U.S. holds less than 2% of the world's petroleum reserves and consumes over 22% of the world's oil and 27% of the world's natural gas.[1] The consequences of this long-standing unsustainable situation adversely affect jobs, the economy, the environment, food security, and national security. All the adverse consequences of our overconsumption of oil are on track to get worse. Unrest in the Middle East, unpredictable oil price spikes, pollution of air, water, and soil, and unsustainable trade deficits with other countries are among many reasons to seriously consider enacting strategies designed to reduce fossil fuel consumption.

"Peak Oil" and Skyrocketing Petroleum Prices are Here

In June 2009 for the first time, the U.S. Department of Energy (DOE) reported that global fossil fuel supplies will simply not be able to keep pace with rising world energy demands. Peak oil—the time when the worldwide extraction of oil plateaus before beginning to decrease despite all efforts to extract more—occurred in 2006, according to the International Energy Agency.[2, 3] Price competition for petroleum will become increasingly intense. We cannot continue business as usual in the consumption of energy in the U.S. for many more years.

Using DOE data, the cost of energy in the U.S. for 2016 will be about $1.5 trillion,[4-6] [a] of which $1.3 will be non-renewable energy. As long as we are not independent of energy, other countries will control our future costs of energy and energy supplies. The DOE data indicate that our net fossil fuel imports will be about 20% of our consumption of fossil fuels in 2016.[7, 8] These figures translate to a total projected cost of

---

a   The Projected Consumption of Energy in the U.S. in 2016: Type, Amount, and Cost

Source of Energy	Amount of Energy	Cost ($ Billions)
Petroleum	7.10 billion barrels/298 billion gallons/37.3 quadrillion BTU (British Thermal Units)	976
Ethanol	0.234 billion barrels/9.83 billion gallons/1.23 quadrillion BTU	32.2
Natural gas	26.81 quadrillion BTU	97.3
Coal	1580 billion kilowatt hours /17.17 quadrillion BTU	150.1
Nuclear	808 billion kilowatt hours/8.78 quadrillion BTU	76.8
Renewables	733 billion kilowatt hours/7.96 quadrillion BTU	146.5
Total		1479
Total non-renewables		1332

$297 billion for imported fossil fuels.[b] Energy conservation and renewable energy can eliminate this huge cost.

Non-renewable Energy Subsidies

Estimates of fossil fuel subsidies worldwide range from $400-$600 billion per year by the International Institute for Sustainable Development[9] to $1.9 trillion by the International Monetary Fund.[10] The U.S. accounts for about 25% of fossil fuel subsidies in the world ($100 billion-$500 billion per year).

These subsidies present a huge obstacle to reducing carbon pollution. They keep prices artificially low, distort energy choices, and contribute to carbon emissions. Policymakers justify them based on providing populations with access to low-cost energy sources for basic needs such as heating, cooking, transport, lighting etc. However, these subsidies largely enrich the more affluent and high-consuming segments of the population. The U.S. subsidies for electricity and transport serve as disincentives to energy efficiency, and they work against investment in cleaner sources of energy such as bio-ethanol, wind, and solar.

Subsidies include preferential tax treatment, grants to fossil fuel producers, oil depletion allowances, heating oil payments to low income consumers, road building, and parking facilities. Indirectly, they comprise "negative externalities" such as environmental degradation, public health issues, and traffic congestion.

The push to create clean energy jobs and combat climate change is resisted by members of Congress who represent parts of the country that produce coal and oil or depend on those energy sources for power and manufacturing.[11] Maintaining low energy prices, despite environmental, military, medical, and social costs, has been perceived as an essential component of American economic prosperity for at least a

---

b   Fossil fuel projected net imports projected for 2016:
petroleum: 2.95 billion barrels x $99 per barrel of oil = $292 billion wholesale
natural gas: 1.32 quadrillion BTU x $3.63/1 million BTU=$5 billion
total fossil fuel net imports cost: $292 + $5 billion = $297 billion

century. However, with costly subsidies for fossil fuels to keep prices artificially low, our fossil fuel addiction is a major economic drag that has become ever more clearly unsustainable.

While campaigning for the presidency, Barack Obama promised a new energy policy saying:[12]

> Oil money pays for the bombs going off from Baghdad to Beirut, and the bombast of dictators from Caracas to Tehran. Our nation will not be secure unless we take that leverage away, and our planet will not be safe unless we move decisively toward a clean energy future.

The U.S. needs a plan to achieve energy independence and to control energy costs. Any plan must focus first on conservation and must be good for red states and blue states, people from urban and rural settings, rich and poor. Above all, the plan must create good jobs that people want. They should enable people to not be forced to take jobs they would prefer not to take.

Greenhouse Gas Emissions—The Big Picture

Of the major greenhouse gases emitted by human activity (i.e., carbon dioxide, methane, nitrous oxide, and fluorocarbons), carbon dioxide (CO_2) constitutes about 50% of the total. It is used as a good index of overall greenhouse gas emissions.

Table 1. CO2 Emissions in 2006 by Selected Country[14]

Country	CO2 Emissions per capita (metric tons)	Total CO2 Emissions (billion metric tons)
World	4.2	28.4
China	4.6	6.1
USA	18.7	5.8
European countries	7.8	3.9
Russia	11.0	1.6
India	1.3	1.5
Japan	10.1	1.3
Canada	16.1	0.5
Australia	16.9	0.4
African Continent	1.0	1.0

Three-hundred-fifty (350) parts per million (ppm) of atmospheric CO2 is the maximum that is compatible with a sustainable climate for human habitation on earth, but the earth's atmosphere now has reached 400 ppm of CO2 and will keep rising.[13] Avoiding catastrophic consequences requires that we work to slash greenhouse gas emissions, especially in industrially developed countries like the U.S. where most emissions occur.

With 9 million humans projected on earth in 2050, a stable planet will require an average of about 2 metric tons CO2 emissions per person. Stabilizing the population at 7–8 billion people would allow for slightly higher average CO2 emissions, perhaps 2.5 – 3 metric tons per capita, which would then be sustainable. Obviously, the higher the population size, the more risk of overall emissions being harder to reduce.

Education, economic development, and food security help to bring down high birth rates. Consequently, climate change avoidance and adaptation aid to developing countries should include the education of girls and strategies to improve the status of women. Educated, economically secure women have fewer children. Educating poor girls worldwide is as essential to climate change mitigation as are conservation and renewable energy technology (Chapters 14 and 17).

Needing to curtail energy use and curb deforestation to achieve per capita 2 -metric-ton CO2 is the science community's consensus. However, with positive feedback loops accelerating global warming, additional emissions of carbon dioxide and methane are generated without human effort and are not in the Intergovernmental Panel on Climate Change's models. Thus, it is unknown if the global effort to mitigate climate change will soon require sequestering more carbon dioxide and other greenhouse gases than we emit (e.g., planting trees). Positive feedback loops include the process of sea-ice and glacier loss that results reduces reflectivity, allowing greater absorption of solar heat, thus raising temperatures, thus causing more melting of ice, and so on.

Reducing Non-renewable Energy Consumption

Most Americans believe that climate change and global warming are caused by humans. However, a declining number of people in the U.S. think the earth's climate is being adversely affected by greenhouse gas emissions from burning fossil fuels and other human activities.[15] Never the less, the case for energy conservation does not depend on one's opinion about climate change. Climate change is such a polarizing issue that I think it is best to make the case for fossil fuel consumption reduction based on all major concerns regarding non-renewable energy.

Most people of any and all political and religious persuasions worry about our dependence on foreign countries for oil, about pollution (air, water, and land), and about our unsustainable trade deficit. Forgetting about climate change for a moment, we have overwhelming reasons to reduce fossil fuel consumption.

For instance, the Deep Water Horizon oil spill in the Gulf of Mexico raised concerns about pollution from fossil fuels. Russia is a recent example of energy dependence causing problems. The only effective economic response to Russia's support of separatists in Crimea and eastern Ukraine would be to boycott Russia's petroleum exports. We are calling on European countries to find alternatives to Russian oil. However, we consume more than double the fossil fuel percapita as European countries (Table 3). Even though the U.S. edged out Saudi Arabia and Russia as the producer of the most petroleum of any country in the world,[16] we have none left over to sell to Europe.

We need to align the reduction of non-renewable energy consumption with basic economic policy goals. While there is no consensus, these goals are desired by millions of individuals, a large portion of the business sector, and government agencies. These goals include increasing employment, reducing health care costs, lowering income taxes, fostering more freedom, and promoting economic growth. The good news is that reducing our use of non-renewable energy can mean more jobs, less pollution, energy independence, enhanced national security, and economic prosperity. Everyone can win.

In the Midwestern U.S. where climate change skepticism is the highest, an experiment was sponsored by *The Land Institute*.[17] It endeavored to see if appeals to thrift, patriotism, spiritual conviction, and economic prosperity could persuade residents of six Kansas towns to conserve fossil fuel and use renewable energy. Nancy Jackson, chairwoman of the *Climate and Energy Project*, used a three-pronged strategy.

- Invoke the notion of thrift to persuade towns to compete with one another to become more energy-efficient.
- Work with civic leaders to embrace green jobs as a way of shoring up or rescuing their communities.
- Discuss with local ministers about "creation care," the obligation of Christians to act as stewards of the world that God gave them.

Publicity about the project did not emphasize the threat of climate change.

It worked!

Local farmers volunteered some of their land for windmills for renewable energy to reduce dependency on foreign oil. Savings in electricity bills by households reinforced the project's messages about thrift and land stewardship. Spurred by the competition between towns to conserve, use of energy dropped by about 5% in the region.

Conservation to Create Jobs and Provide Economic and Environmental Sustainability

We need to get real.

Even the U.S. Congress and President cannot repeal the law of supply and demand. Energy imports contribute to our increasing trade deficit with foreign countries, endangering our fragile economy and our security. Not only is reducing our fossil fuel consumption a matter of the utmost urgency for the health of Americans because of the long-term effects of pollution and climate change, but also for immediate economic and national security reasons.

The new world economic reality is that fossil fuel imports cost U.S. jobs, hurt the public health, impair businesses, increase threats to national security, and weaken the government's position in foreign policy negotiations. Enlightened government policies should realign our tax code and government spending priorities in accordance with 21st century realities—economic, political, environmental, public health, and national security.

The bottom line: We need to eliminate fossil fuel imports and change the culture that depends on them!

President Obama should join Republican leaders to call on all Americans to eliminate fossil fuel imports as an urgent matter of national and planetary security. Reducing our non-renewable energy consumption by 30% in 2016 will lower our greenhouse gas emissions to 20% less than 1990 levels,[18] as agreed on in the 1997 world climate summit in Kyoto, Japan. While this reduction will still leave the U.S.

per-capita carbon footprint at over three times the world average,[c] it will position us to make further major reductions in greenhouse gas emissions as advocated by most developed and developing countries. We will then be in a much better position to call on other countries to conserve and do more to shift from non-renewable to renewable forms of energy.

Taxing Non-renewable Energy—$2.40 per Gallon of Gasoline

Relative to the huge fossil fuel subsidies in the U.S., the Obama Administration's $90 billion of stimulus money to promote "clean energy"[19] was hardly significant. To incentivize renewable energy, it is much better to tax non-renewable energy than to pick winners and losers for renewable energy government subsidies.

Mindful of concerns of conservatives about reducing energy consumption causing an economic slowdown, we need strategies to decrease non-renewable energy (fossil fuel and nuclear energy) consumption while increasing renewable energy production, jobs, and economic growth.

A Grand Bargains' non-renewable energy consumption tax will raise revenue, incentivize conservation, and stimulate the renewable energy industry. This tax will increase the overall cost of fossil fuels and nuclear energy by 75%. With an estimated price elasticity factor of – 0.4% decreased consumption for each 1% increase in cost, non-renewable energy consumption should decrease by about 30%.[d] This will begin to level the playing field as to the massive and destructive fossil fuels subsidies, for an energy diet to promote jobs, prosperity, and environmental sustainability.

---

c   18.7 metric tons of carbon dioxide per year per capita (U.S.) x 0.7 (proposed 30% reduction in greenhouse emissions) = 13.1 metric tons of carbon dioxide per year per capita. 13.1 metric tons of carbon dioxide per year / 4.2 (worldwide average carbon footprint) = 3.11 fold more that the carbon dioxide consumed per year per capita.

d   0.75 (75% increase in non-renewable energy cost with consumption tax) x – 0.4 (– 0.4% decreased consumption for each 1% increase in cost) = 0.3 (30% decrease in consumption)

Because of this proposed major change in energy policy, many jobs will be created in agriculture, transportation, green building, and other energy-intensive sectors. The reduction of utilization of fossil fuels and nuclear energy will spur energy-efficient technologies and the need for human labor, thus driving job growth.

As detailed above using U.S. Department of Energy data,[4-6] the cost of non-renewable energy in the U.S. in 2016 will be over $1.3 trillion. Raising the cost of non-renewable energy by 75% will require the following new consumption taxes:

- $2.40 per gallon of gasoline,
- $2.84 / 1 million BTUs of natural gas, and
- $0.071 per kilowatt hour of electricity.

Given a reduction in non-renewable energy consumption of 30%, this will raise about $700 billion in 2016.

A 30% reduction in non-renewable energy consumption, as a consequence of a non-renewable energy tax, will save consumers a projected $400 billion in 2016.[e] This will eliminate our reliance on foreign oil and natural gas and drive down prices considerably on the world energy markets.

Reducing non-renewable energy consumption will both save money and improve health. Burning fossil fuels imposes a cost for the associated human health damage. Based on a report by the National Academy of Science,[20, 21] reducing fossil fuel consumption by 30% would reduce the costs of adverse health effects by an estimated $48 billion in 2016.

The costs of damage other than to health—such as harm to ecosystems, effects of some air pollutants such as mercury, risks to national security, and climate change—have not been monetized. "Externalities" are costs paid not by the corporation or consumer of the corporation's

---

e $1335 billion (total cost of non-renewable energy) x 0.3 (30% reduction in non-renewable energy consumption) ≈ $400 billion (projected savings)

product, but instead paid by society and the ecosystem. It is impossible to put a value on public health and nature.

The above estimates notwithstanding, the DOE fossil fuel cost projections for 2016–2025 are unreliable. The price of oil already spiked to over $140 per barrel in 2008 before declining largely because of reduced demand from the recession. Consequently, the price could easily go to $150–$200 per barrel in 2016 if supplies suddenly decrease due to political instability of oil exporting nations. Battling the Islamic State of Iraq and Syria (ISIS), and Israel's behavioral tendencies and the threats it makes against Iran, might provide that instability in the Middle East. The higher the cost of fossil fuels, the more we have to gain by conservation and incentivizing alternate energy technologies.

Likewise, the health and environmental costs of nuclear energy are too speculative to be quantified. Think about the cost of the Fukushima Daiichi nuclear power plant disaster in 2011. Consequently, the health cost reported by the National Academy of Science was a gross underestimate of the overall externalized costs for non-renewable energy. Nuclear energy is highly subsidized, and the net-energy return from the technology and resource-inputs is among the lowest of all forms of energy.

There is no "technofix" for avoiding deep conservation (curtailment) of energy consumption. This is because alternatives to petroleum do not provide the range of fuels and products so desired by consumers. The U.S. infrastructure, economic growth, and population increase since World War II was achieved with cheap, easy to extract, extremely high net-energy-yielding conventional oil. So, although there are many applications for renewable energy which means employment and reductions in pollution, the decentralized nature of renewable energy will help reshape economic activity to make it much more locally based. This will help ACCs to have a greater role in conservation and with fostering renewables than if cheap oil were still available and had no supply limits.

The confluence of our imported-energy dependence, unsustainable trade deficit, ongoing economic doldrums, and broken health care system creates a perfect opportunity for fundamental change toward a brighter future for the U.S. The non-renewable energy tax can be a game-changer to help lead Americans toward an economic environment that rewards major reductions in fossil fuel burning and wasteful energy consumption overall. With revised expectations and restructuring, we have an opportunity to attain energy independence in a way that fosters all our vital interests—health, health care, social-safety-net services, healthier and more resilient communities, jobs, and environmental sustainability.

A campaign for energy conservation will help us improve national security by stopping our oil dependence on Russia, Venezuela, and Middle Eastern countries while eliminating our balance of trade deficits.

To maximize the effect of the tax on reducing non-renewable energy use, conservation coaches employed by ACCs throughout the nation should help people develop tangible individualized strategies to reduce non-renewable energy consumption. The financial incentive of lower relative cost of renewable energy due to the non-renewable energy tax will unleash American innovation and entrepreneurism in this area.

Benefits of Non-renewable Energy Conservation

Health

A 30% drop in consumption of non-renewable energy will improve health by decreasing motor vehicle use. This will result in less air pollution, fewer accidents, reduced CO_2 emissions, and more active lifestyles. More people will choose to bicycle and walk.

The tax on non-renewable energy will also incentivize home vegetable gardening and the local production of less fossil-fuel intensive plant-based foods. Next to the transportation sector, food production accounts for the largest portion of the U.S. fossil fuel use—18% (Chapter 13).[22] Worldwide, the percentage of fossil fuel use for food is nearer 50%.[23] Consequently, sustainable agriculture is one area that our Third World development aid should be concentrated (Chapter 17).

Economic

In countries with advanced economies like the U.S., subsidies of commodities are usually in the form of taxes that are too low to capture the true costs to society. Economists call these low taxes, "tax subsidies."[10] The low taxes for fossil fuel and nuclear energy fall in this category.

The main externality of nuclear energy is the risk of a catastrophe like in Fukushima, Japan; Chernobyl, Ukraine; or Three Mile Island, Pennsylvania. No private insurance company or coalition of insurance companies has the financial capacity to insure against the small but finite risk of an unprecedented disaster. Consequently, the U.S. government assumes the risk and taxpayers are on the hook if payouts must be made.

In 1957, Congress passed the Price-Anderson act to require nuclear power facilities to carry insurance against catastrophic disaster. However, the entire industry only carries about $10 billion in insurance.[24, 25] Estimates of the costs of the Fukushima-Daiichi nuclear meltdown range from $250-$500 billion.[26]

High demand for energy makes the price of fossil fuels on the world markets rise. Since the U.S. consumes about 25% of the world's energy,[19] reducing non-renewable energy consumption in the U.S. by 30% will decrease overall world demand for energy by an estimated 7.5%.[f] This will drive down prices of fossil fuels on international markets.[g]

The non-renewable energy tax will also reduce the federal deficit and hasten economic recovery by eliminating the need for the government to subsidize alternative fuel research and development. The tax can thus contribute to more green energy jobs in the U.S. and further

---

f   0.25 (U.S. proportion of world's energy consumption) x 0.30 (proposed 30% reduction of U.S. non-renewable energy consumption) = 0.075
g   For each $1 per barrel reduction in the price of petroleum due to our conservation, the U.S. economy will save an additional $5 billion or so per year.[8]

aid the economy with exports of technologies for conservation and alternative energy production.

Another economic damage of energy subsidies is to reinforce wealth inequality. The International Monetary Fund (IMF) found that fossil fuel tax subsidies were much more utilized by upper-income groups compared with middle or low income people.[10] While the rich benefit more than the poor from fossil fuel subsidies, the IMF report warned that fossil fuel subsidy reform should be done in a way that doesn't adversely affect the poor. In this regard, ACC-based fundamental economic system restructuring qualifies since all workers will be assisted by their ACCs to find jobs paying a living wage (Chapter 12). ACCs may also want to invest some social insurance assets (Social Security and pension funds) in energy conservation and renewable energy technologies (Chapter 24).

Using the Department of Energy's estimate that each $1 billion of balance of trade deficit costs 27,000 U.S. jobs, eliminating $297 billion in oil and natural gas imports will create or save about 8 million U.S. jobs.[h]

Environmental

Of the $100 billion-$500 billion of external costs of fossil fuels projected for 2016 in the U.S.,[9, 10] the majority of these adverse effects involve pollution (air, water, and land) and road congestion. Federal and state legislation has provided some environmental protection of air, water, and land pollution. Thankfully, we do not have the air, water, and land pollution problems of China, which has largely neglected the environment in order to drive economic growth.

Our clean air, clean water laws, and environmental regulations are constantly being challenged and new legal loopholes found to get away with pollution. Regulating and lawmaking is a bit like playing "whack a mole." The surest way to protect against environment destruction over the long-term is to shift financial incentives away from investments in

---

h   Net imports of petroleum products and natural gas: $297 billion[4] x 27,000 jobs/$1 billion ≈ 8.0 million jobs

non-renewable energy and towards financial incentives for conservation. Market pressures will then drive investments in renewable energy and in energy conserving technologies.

Incremental approaches to protecting the environment from fossil fuel and nuclear energy damage will not work. We need a fundamental shift in energy policy that has buy in by the vast majority of stakeholders. The non-renewable energy tax in the context of overall Grand Bargains' reform can be just the plan for comprehensive environmental stewardship and energy independence.

ACCs will Foster Lifestyle Changes to Reduce Non-renewable Energy Consumption

Reducing the consumption of non-renewable energy by 30% is a huge but doable task for U.S. residents. Succeeding with this challenge on individual and societal levels requires six ingredients:

1. a financial incentive (i.e., non-renewable energy tax),
2. conservation coaches hired by ACCs to provide practical strategies to lower fossil fuel and electricity consumption,
3. ACC monitoring of energy consumption of enrollees,
4. ACC resources devoted to fossil fuel consumption reduction strategies (e.g., home insulation materials, car pooling networks, public transportation support, bicycle promotion strategies, home energy audits, recycling programs, support for telecommuting for work, support for local vegetable gardening projects, investments in renewable energy projects, etc.), and
5. competition between ACCs to succeed in linking reduced energy consumption with improved lifestyles of enrollees.

According to the Nature Conservancy Carbon Footprint calculator,[11] my fossil fuel energy use is 15.6% of the consumption of the average American (i.e., my carbon footprint = 2.9 metric tons of carbon dioxide per year). My low carbon footprint comes primarily from:

1. not owning a car and renting or borrowing one when necessary,
2. bicycling about 50 miles per week,
3. traveling longer distances by train or bus instead of flying,
4. having an entirely plant-based diet,
5. growing some of my own vegetables,
6. buying organic food,
7. composting all my food scraps in my local community garden,
8. using only about 10 kilowatt hours (Kwh) of electricity per month by employing only a few essential energy efficient appliances, and
9. drying my clothes on a clothes line instead of a natural gas clothes dryer.

Besides saving me thousands of dollars per year, I can attest that these lifestyle choices have greatly improved my health and quality of life.

Table 2 was adapted from National Public Radio's (NPR) Marketplace Sustainability Desk,[20] the Nature Conservancy Carbon Footprint calculator,[i][11] and the U.S. Department of Energy.[6] This table shows the potential steps to take to reduce non-renewable energy consumption with no detriment in quality of life. While the ACC-based economic reform goal is 30% reduction in non-renewable energy use, this table shows that about 42% could be reduced without serious hardship by proper alignment of incentives and dissemination of information on conservation. The Heritage Foundation's Center for Data Analysis forecasts that carbon taxes would have, "severe consequences—including crushing energy costs, millions of jobs lost, and falling household income."[22] If a stiff carbon tax is enacted in isolation, the Heritage Foundation is absolutely right. Their prediction would apply only to

---

i   Per person potential fossil fuel energy consumption reduction based on four people living in a three-bedroom detached house.

the immediate effect on the fossil fuel economy. Adjustments to carbon taxes would occur as a matter of course. The Grand Bargains' strategy is to enact the energy-conserving adjustments in advance and make them into major economy boosters (green jobs, etc). In reality, we do not need the fossil fuel economy, although leaving it ought to be a planned transition instead of clinging to it until it collapses in widespread hunger, unemployment, and civil unrest.

Any new tax in isolation will be detrimental in the context of the current economic environment in the U.S. However, the Grand Bargains-based economic reform includes *dramatically lower business taxes overall and higher corporate profits*. ACCs will also foster the creation of millions of jobs (Chapter 12) that will stimulate economic activity and prosperity in businesses.

Table 2. Lifestyle Changes to Reduce Non-renewable Energy Consumption[8, 27]

Energy Conservation Intervention	Lifestyle Change Level	Non-renewable Energy Reduction %
Increase renewable energy use	Double renewable energy displacing fossil fuels (assuming average consumption increasing to double average)	8.9
Reduce car fuel consumption 88%	10,000 miles/year-20 mpg-driver alone versus 5,000 miles/year-40mpg-driver + 1 passenger	18.4
Reduce air travel	Cut one long trip per year	1.5
Reduce food waste	Eliminate food waste	3.7
Adopt a more plant-based diet	Reduce animal products by half and increase plant food by half	5.9
Switch to organic food	100% organic	0.3
Compost food scraps and yard trimmings	All scraps and trimmings	0.7
Use low energy light bulbs	10 compact fluorescent bulbs replacing incandescent bulbs	0.6

Recycle aluminum, plastic, glass, etc.	Recycle all these items	0.3
Reduce standby power in your home	Unplug unused electrical appliances	0.3
Dry laundry on a clothes line	Clothes line drying less damaging than machine)	0.8
Take steps to heat and cool home efficiently	Cut heating and cooling energy consumption in half of average consumption	0.7
Potential reduction in non-renewable energy with these steps		42.1

With the anticipated elimination of our energy imports, the major loss of jobs due to the proposed non-renewable energy tax will occur primarily in oil and gas industry workers in foreign petroleum exporting nations. This will help the overall creation of jobs within the fundamentally restructured U.S. economy.

Summary and Conclusion

We are reaching a tipping point in our fossil fuel dependence. Heavy use of energy has helped us develop our current economic power, technological sophistication, and public health miracles. However, continuing our rate of non-renewable energy consumption will lead to increasing health, environmental and economic problems due to pollution, climate change, and reduced world-wide competitiveness of our industries.

As part of Grand Bargains-based economic reform, the tax on non-renewable energy will be a win, win, win, win, win strategy for public health, personal health care, economic prosperity, environmental sustainability, and world peace. Even the fossil fuel industry owners will do fine as the margins on sales of their products will be higher as consumption is decreased. Workers displaced from jobs in non-renewable energy will be able to retrain for work with renewable energy or other fields. The proposed non-renewable energy tax will give great incentives for entrepreneurs to develop alternative energy technology.[28]

It is with this appropriate tax on non-renewable energy–to level the playing field by matching the subsidies given non-renewable energy–that solar, wind, biomass, and geothermal energy will become competitive with fossil fuels and nuclear energy.

With the non-renewable energy tax as a game-changer, the amount of renewable energy produced will easily be doubled within a few years. While renewable energy now provides primarily electricity, American entrepreneurs and innovators will find more ways that renewables can replace oil in transportation and other areas.

Because of this major change in energy policy, many jobs will be created in agriculture, public transportation, green building, weatherizing, and other energy-intensive sectors. This will occur both through developing energy-efficient technologies and by employing human labor to make up for the reduction in fossil fuels and nuclear energy. Department of Energy gimmicks like grants, subsidies, and tax rebates will be replaced by market incentives favoring renewable energy.

Fossil fuel and nuclear energy workers laid off by the downsizing of non-renewable energy will be trained for other jobs and helped to find employment by the ACCs. By all accounts, we are an over-consuming society. Lower consumption and more community will be welcome to many. Although the transition will be extremely challenging, the difficulties will be shared and will increase our innovativeness and mutual interdependence. The hurtles we will face as families, communities, and as a nation can bring out our better natures.

Chapter 23
Social Security and Other Retirement Plans

In 1981, the L.A. County Department of Health Services pulled me and its other 22,000 employees out of Social Security. So my employer and I did not pay into Social Security for the last 17 years of my medical career. However, I still receive a small Social Security pension based on my work previous to 1981. I also get some benefits from subsequent moonlighting work for which I paid into Social Security. My Social Security benefits and pension with medical benefits from the L.A. County Department of Health Services allowed me to write this book, two other books, and numerous medical research articles. For this I am grateful. Most retired Americans similarly rely on Social Security and/or their pensions, or they will in the future. For many, it is or will be their only income.

You have choices about whose comprehensive roadmap for the future you want to buy into and support. Your choices are (1) the millionaires in Congress and their wealthy benefactors, (2) the billionaires of Corporate America and the policy think tanks that they fund (e.g., George Soros funding liberal policy options and Charles and David Koch funding conservative causes[1]), (3) marginalized political parties (e.g., Greens, Peace and Freedom, American Independent Party) or (4) a financially tenuous pensioner like me. *Congress members nor politically active plutocrats nor left or right wing ideologues offer any comprehensive plan that could become a consensus on a roadmap for reforming our economic system.* Maybe that leaves you with my Grand Bargains as a frame of reference until something better comes along.

Social Security Funding Projections

About 67 million people receive Social Security benefits, including retired workers, their spouses and children, survivors of deceased workers, and disabled people.[2] A payroll tax of 12.4%, split between employer and employee, finances Social Security. Interest on the money in Social Security trust funds[3] invested in U.S. Treasury Bills generates additional revenue.

With 75 million baby boomers retiring and due to flood Social Security over the next 15 years, the system is in serious trouble.[a] The immunity of Social Security to the federal government's deficits and fiscal instability is illusionary. Social Security depends as much on federal borrowing as the Pentagon or any other discretionary or mandatory federal program.

The decline in Social Security revenue is structural not cyclical. To become financially sustainable, Social Security will need additional income or it will be able to pay less in benefits or a combination of both.[7]

Debate about the Future of Social Security

Social Security is on an unsustainable path. Each year the future obligations increase by hundreds of billions of dollars while the ratio of those paying into Social Security to those receiving benefits falls. Entitlement reform, including Social Security, is essential to eliminating federal government deficit spending and avoiding a U.S. Treasury financial default.

There are two sharply conflicting points of view about what to do concerning the deficits projected in the Social Security system. Liberals advocate strengthening the system by increasing revenue. This could

---

a   In 2016, the cost of benefits and administration of Social Security is projected to total about $952 billion.[4] Social Security payroll tax revenue in 2016 is projected to total $810 billion.[5] The remaining revenue to finance payouts will be made up with interest payments on the Social Security trust funds and from the general fund. Social Security *has projected unfunded obligations over the next 75 years of about $9.6 trillion.*[2, 6]

be accomplished by (1) increasing the payroll tax and/or by removing the cap on income that is subject to the payroll tax—currently a little over $100,000/year, and (2) by reordering spending priorities, such as reducing the Pentagon budget. Conservatives advocate shrinking the system by

- means-testing the payouts so the wealthy receive less money,
- increasing the retirement age, and
- reducing benefits for workers who are retiring more than 10–15 years from now.

The bipartisan budget deficit commission appointed by President Obama and headed by Erskine Bowles and Alan Simpson was split between those that advocated increasing the Social Security payroll tax and those who favored the conservative options.[8]

The Republican initiative to privatize Social Security during the George W. Bush administration was very unpopular with Social Security recipients and others. Consequently, conservatives are now cautious about reintroducing any market-based privatization proposal.

President Obama, drawing political battle lines in one of his weekly national addresses, said, "I'll fight with everything I've got to stop those who would gamble your Social Security on Wall Street, because you shouldn't be worried that a sudden downturn in the stock market will put all you've worked so hard for—all you've earned—at risk."[9]

"Stalemated" best describes the issue of fixing Social Security's projected increasing future deficit.

Grand Bargain #17: ACCs to Administer Social Security for Members

Shifting the administration of Social Security from the federal government to the ACCs will be the entitlement reform game-changer. Social

Security will no longer be a Ponzi scheme. With Grand Bargains-based reform, *Social Security will break the stalemate by being*

- *less costly for businesses and employees than increasing the payroll tax,*
- *more secure than the Social Security privatization proposal of former President Bush, which would channel Social Security retirement funds into Wall Street investments, and*
- *more flexible and person-oriented in providing financial security for the elderly and disabled than the rigidly bureaucratic Social Security Administration.*

With Grand Bargains-based Social Security reform, a worker earning the average wage ($47,000 projected for 2016[10]) will receive about the same monthly stipend as now at age 66 in constant dollars ($1200 per month).[11] This is not very much to live on. Social Security recipients under Grand Bargains will have opportunities to work part or full time in ACC-provided or other jobs. The integration of ACC health care, social services, and other human services will greatly increase the financial security of seniors.

While the economy has been growing at 2% – 2.5% per year over 5-6 years, Social Security Disability benefit payments have been increasing at an unsustainable 5% per year.[4] Out of work people over the age of 40 are increasingly applying for Social Security Disability when unemployment benefits, Workers' Compensation, and personal savings run out.

Compared with the Social Security Administration, ACCs will be better able to control the runaway increases in Social Security Disability benefit payments now going to 11 million recipients.[12] These disabled recipients will be able to earn nearly twice as much money by working at minimum wage jobs than by relying on disability benefits. Likewise, low income Supplemental Security Income (SSI) recipients will have incentives and opportunities to work and earn at least the $15/hour minimum wage.

With Grand Bargains reform, revenue for Social Security from payroll taxes will increase by about 35% more than currently projected Social Security payroll tax revenue.[b] This will result from raising the minimum wage to $15 per hour and having at least 40 million more people working (Chapter 12). Fewer people will require Social Security Disability benefit payments or Supplemental Security Income. In addition, worker payroll deductions will be higher relative to Social Security benefits to be received because of the much higher minimum wage.[c] Consequently, the payroll taxes will not have to be increased, or benefits reduced, or the age to receive benefits put into the future.

Of the 60,000 federal employees working for Social Security, almost all will be laid off or transferred to administering the consumption taxes (Chapter 21). This will leave a few thousand employees remaining to carry out an orderly transition and to channel Social Security payroll taxes to ACCs. Many former Social Security Administration employees will likely move to ACCs to manage Social Security benefits and other pensions.

Social Security Trust Fund Distributions to ACCs

The Social Security Trust Funds currently hold about $2.7 trillion.[3] As part of the ACC administration of Social Security pensions for ACC members, the federal government will be responsible for paying the ACCs the money now in the Social Security Trust Funds. This is in

---

b   ($660 billion (additional income for existing workers with increasing the minimum wage to $15/hour) + $660 billion (minimum wages for 20 million carers for children, frail elderly, and the disabled) + $940 billion Social Security payroll taxes from 20 million additional workers (20 million additional jobs throughout the economy @ $47,000 per year on average = $2280 billion. $2280 billion x $ 0.124 (Social Security payroll tax of 12.4%) = $280 billion.) Projected Social Security revenue for 2016: $1091 billion ($280 billion + $811 billion currently projected revenue) / $811 billion = 1.35 (35% increase in Social Security revenue)

c   The Social Security retirement system is designed to replace a higher percentage of earnings for lower-income workers and their dependents (i.e., a progressive system favoring low-income people).[16] When the minimum wage is more than doubled and payroll Social Security deductions are correspondingly increased, the eventual payouts to recipients will be much less relative to the additional payments into the system.

consideration of the government's future obligations to those who have paid into Social Security.[2]

This money eventually will be paid to Social Security recipients, but needs to be held in secure investments in the mean time. As will be detailed in Chapter 24, I suggest that ACC-affiliated financial services companies (i.e., credit unions and savings and loan companies) receive the money in order to become a major component of stabilizing the U.S. home mortgage market. For 2016, I suggest that ACCs should receive $100 billion for investments in home mortgages or homes for renting to members (i.e., rent-to-buy arrangements). After 2016, the rate of payment of the Social Security Trust Funds to the ACCs may be determined by Congress.

These trust funds may be dispersed to the ACCs over a period of at least 10 years. This will make a significant down payment on eliminating $18 trillion federal debt.[13]

Underfunded Public Servants' Pension Plans

Deposits in pension fund saving accounts for federal, state, and local government employees will reach about $150 billion in 2016.[4, 14] Despite this huge expenditure, many public pension plans are underfunded.[d] Pension fund managers tend to be overly optimistic about returns of pension fund investments.[e]

Government worker pensions have become politicized. Democratic Party liberals believe in the positive uses of government. Their

---

d   As of 2014, public service pensions will be underfunded by $1.4 trillion-$4 trillion over the next 30 years, depending on the assumptions of actuaries about future investment growth.[15] Using more realistic conservative assumptions, the underfunding is in the higher range.

e   For instance, Calpers, California's giant state pension fund, required five times the state's contribution in 2010 as was projected in 1999. Optimistic pension managers had assumed a yearly return on investments of 7.75%. Overall, the unfunded pension liabilities of California's state and local governments exceeded $700 billion in 2010. California state government retirement packages now valued at more than $1.2 million per employee on average are funded by taxpayers who have an average of $60,000 saved for their own retirement.[16]

supporters in public employee unions benefit when Democrats are in power. Politicians that negotiate costly pension benefits with public sector unions are often gone when the burden of those pensions are felt decades later.

Small-government, conservative Republicans oppose unions and their pension demands. It is politically difficult for liberals to oppose excessive union demands or conservatives to agree to needed expansions of government services. Increasingly, cities must cut funds for parks, libraries, street maintenance, and public safety to pay their pension obligations.

Some suggested solutions to deal with underfunded public pensions include:

- moving all new employees to 401(k) retirement plans with fixed employer contributions—despite the valid objections to doing this[17] (discussed later).
- bailouts with tax-free federal government bonds,
- capping pensions,
- raising the retirement age, and
- preventing salary manipulation before retirement to spike pensions.

Republicans in Congress have introduced legislation to bar states from seeking bailouts for underfunded pensions from the federal government.[17] Retrospectively capping public pensions is prohibited by law in many states. Raising the retirement age would decrease job opportunities for younger workers. There are no easy solutions to making public pensions sustainable.

Defined Benefit versus Defined Contribution Pension Plans

Many workers and policy analysts oppose shifting public employee defined-benefit pensions to fixed-contribution 401(k) plans. With defined-benefit plans, you are guaranteed a defined inflation-adjusted monthly income for life. A pensioner with an amount of money saved with a defined-contribution plan must determine how fast to spend that money, not knowing how long he/she will live. When retiring, placing some or all of savings into an annuity[f] will decrease the risk of running out of money before dying. However, compared with 401(k) and other defined-contribution plans, defined pension plans: (1) cost less, (2) attract and retain suitable workers, and (3) help stabilize and benefit the economy.

Bankers and brokers earn tens of billions of dollars off the top with 401(k) plans. Management and investment fees of 401(k) plans are as much as three times higher than with defined-benefit pension plans. Hidden fees can eat up a third or more of one's savings in 401(k) plans. The only way states can save money by switching to 401(k) plans is if they slash retirement benefits. Since public sector employees already earn less than those in the private sector, the public workforce quality may go down without defined-benefit pensions.[19] Defined-benefit pension plans have many advantages. Financial services professionals managing money in pooled pension funds usually get higher returns than workers who manage their own 401(k) accounts. Risk-seeking employees with high turnover rates tend to prefer 401(k) plans, making them less suitable to be ideal public employees.

Compared with traditional pensions and Social Security, 401(k) plans spawn financial bubbles and make recessions worse, fueling an unstable economy. When public sector workers can retire with guaranteed defined-benefit pensions, more jobs will be available for younger workers.[20]

Without defined-benefit pension plans, workers risk (1) poor investment returns, (2) outliving their assets, and (3) inflation that would

---

f   Annuity: an investment product that pays a fixed amount of money to someone each year or other fixed interval. There are two main classes of annuities: annuities certain and contingent annuities. Under an annuity certain, a specified number of payments are made, after which the annuity stops. A "life annuity" is a kind of contingent annuity that continues paying as long as the recipient survives. In a group of people with life annuities, some will not live long enough to receive back all the money they have paid, while others will live long enough to collect more than they have paid.[18]

erode the value of their income in retirement. Compared with defined-benefit pensions, individual savers with 401(k) plans must contribute nearly twice as much to ensure similar monthly retirement incomes, for three reasons: [19]

- First, individuals must save more to protect themselves should they live longer than average. [g]
- Individuals face the risk of retiring during a bear market and losing their assets.
- Portfolio management fees for 401 (k) and other defined contribution retirement plans are higher.

Private Sector Pension Deficits and Risks

Retirement planning in the private sector has changed dramatically over recent decades. Despite the advantages of defined benefit pensions, private businesses more frequently offer 401 (k) and other tax deferred savings plans to employees. However, there are still about 40 million workers or retirees from private businesses with defined benefit pensions. [21]

The Pension Benefits Guarantee Corporation (PBGC) is a federal agency created by the Employee Retirement Income Security Act of 1974 (ERISA). The role of the PBGC is to protect pension benefits in private-sector, traditionally-defined-benefit pension plans. If a participating plan terminates, usually through the sponsor's bankruptcy, without sufficient money to pay all benefits, the PBGC's insurance program will pay the benefits provided by that plan up to the limits set by law. PBGC financing comes from (1) insurance premiums paid by participating companies, (2) the assets taken from defunct pension

---

g   Defined benefit plan payouts are determined by the average life expectancy of people in the group. Defined contribution plan payouts should take into account that you might live to be 100 years old. Consequently, monthly payouts are less.

plans, and (3) recoveries from the companies formerly responsible for the plans.

The PBGC was never supposed to be funded by the American public. However, as of early 2011 PBGC became insolvent with a net deficit of over $30 billion, leaving the American taxpayer holding the bag.[22] Unusually rapid appreciation of stocks on the stock market since 2011 bailed out the PBGC, at least temporarily.

Private sector workers have a difficult time with retirement savings. Workers change employers more frequently than in the past. Multiple pensions are difficult for individuals to manage. Professional management fees are high.

The average duration of survival of a business has been reported as 12.5 years. The average duration of a multinational, big, solid company is only about 40 years.[23] Consequently, defined benefit pensions, while they are superior to defined contribution plans, are quite risky for both private sector employees and employers.

ACC-affiliated financial institutions would be ideal for converting savings in defined contribution plans into secure savings in defined benefit plans.

Grand Bargain #18: ACCs to Manage New Contributions to Public and Private Sector Retirement Plans

Grand Bargains' reform calls for new contributions to public and private sector employer-sponsored retirement plans to be shifted from the employer to the management of ACCs. With this Grand Bargains' strategy, pension fund managers from the public and private sectors will continue to manage the approximately $20 trillion in existing pension funds, annuities, and other retirement plans. Independent retirement accounts (IRAs), life insurance annuities, and other private retirement savings plans will continue to be managed privately. However, new deposits of public sector and private sector employer-related retirement plans will be managed by ACC-affiliated credit unions and savings and loan banks (S&Ls). One justification of this major disruption of the retirement saving industry is the ongoing systemic risk of having so much money managed by too-big-to-fail banks, insurance companies, hedge funds, and other institutions. Another justification is the need for a mechanism to bring about the recovery and stabilization of the housing market.

Most private company retirement plans and some government employee retirement plans are of the defined contribution variety. However, employee retirement plans administered by ACC credit unions/S&Ls will be the defined benefit variety. As is current practice, the amount of pension contributions and the proportions paid by employers versus employees will be negotiated between the employers and employees.

ACC-affiliated credit unions/S&Ls will be in charge of managing approximately $450 billion in new contributions to employee retirement plans.[h] Instead of these funds being managed by Wall Street investment brokers, the money will be invested in a way that will resolve the long-lingering home mortgage crisis in the U.S.: Funds will be invested in mortgages for homes, condos, and farms of ACC members. Chapter 24 will detail the rolls of ACC-affiliated credit unions/S&Ls that will manage the worker pension funds.

Over time, pension managers for private corporations and government agencies will not need to hide their future deficits by assuming that pension funds will earn 6%-8% returns each year. State and local governments will no longer be responsible for funding about $600 billion of health care and welfare. So, they will be in better positions to make good on their previous obligations to their employees for pension plan deposits even based on conservative growth assumptions (Chapter 19). Consequently, governments will not have spending for public

---

h   Status-quo projected employer-based public and private sector retirement plan deposits for 2016: $350 billion[4, 14, 24] (about one-third public sector and two-thirds private sector). Increase of 40 million workers in 2016 will increase retirement plan deposits by at least 27% (186 million workers projected for 2016 / 146 million workers currently = 1.27), all in the private sector.

Total projected employer-sponsored retirement plan deposits in 2016 with Grand Bargains' reform: $350 billion (current projection) x 1.27 (increase by 27%) ≈ $450 billion

services held hostage to continual stock market gains that support the pensions of current and retired employees (Chapter 24).[25]

With ACC-affiliated credit unions/S&Ls managing private sector pensions, businesses will not become insolvent because of their pension obligations.

ACCs should seek to automatically enroll their own employees in pension plans in addition to Social Security. This will include the 20 million people employed by ACCs to care for their own children, frail elderly relatives, or disabled friends or relatives. ACC employees and members will be able to contribute their own additional funds into their ACC-managed defined benefit pension plans according to parameters negotiated with the ACC's management. Ideally, pension plans will be subject to automatic escalation, where the percentage of income saved grows as the worker's salary and years of service increase.[26]

Workers will have their choice of ACCs. A consideration in the selection of an ACC will be the management of employer-sponsored retirement plans of members. Pension benefits provided by ACCs will be integrated with health care, social services, Social Security, and other benefits delivered by the ACCs to maximize enrollee financial security. ACCs will compete, in part, on effectiveness and transparency of managing retirement plans and the integration of retirement savings with overall health and human services. Other ACC-provided retirees services might include locating employment opportunities, enabling bartering, and offering legal, financial, and conservation coaching.

Summary and Conclusion

Social Security will be strengthened by the shift from the federal government management to ACC control. At least 40 million more workers participating in Social Security and most receiving higher wages will make the system more secure and financially sustainable. Informal economy jobs with no Social Security payroll tax or other benefits will become rare.

Delaying retirement, decreasing benefits, or raising the Social Security payroll tax will not be needed. ACCs will be insured against insolvency so that Social Security contributions by workers will be protected in case of the mismanagement and dissolution of an ACC.

The availability of more jobs will reduce the utilization and costs of the Social Security Disability and Supplemental Security Income programs. The additional Social Security payroll taxes and decreased Social Security Disability and Supplemental Security Income disbursements will bring the Social Security system financially in balance without unfunded liabilities.

Public servants' and private company workers' pensions are currently highly vulnerable to underfunding. Without Grand Bargains' reform, downturns in the stock markets will continue to cause waves of pension plan defaults. Shifting public and private sector worker pension programs' administration to the ACCs will give workers financial security while improving the financial stability of public and private sector pensions.

Many current federal government Social Security employees, as well as public and private sector pension managers, will be able to shift their employment to go manage retirement savings of ACC members.

ACCs will compete, in part, on securely providing Social Security beneficiaries with funds integrated with health care, social services (Chapter 10), part-time or full-time jobs (Chapter 12), financial education and counseling (Chapter 24), and other human services.

Investments of Social Security and pension funds by ACC financial services professionals in credit unions/S&Ls will be addressed in the next chapter.

Chapter 24
Personal and National Financial Security

While on a family road trip in 1991, I listened to a book on audio tape called, Your Money or Your Life, by Joe Dominguez. Mr. Dominguez retired from his job as a financial counselor at age 29 and never again accepted money for his work. His mission became to help everyday people become financially independent.

He asserted that with careful planning and saving you can achieve financial independence within a finite period of time. Once financially independent, you will have the time to work on what you feel is most important. You can use your valuable time to help create a better world. In both the audio tape and the best selling print book by the same name that he co-authored with Vicki Robin, they recommend that you employ a nine step plan to accumulate enough money safely invested to have an adequate, stable, secure income for the rest of your life.

I craved this kind of financial independence.

I loved medicine and my jobs of supervising medical residents in clinics and on inpatient wards and directing the Cancer and AIDS Pain Service at LA County + USC Medical Center (Chapter 5). However, I did not feel secure in my position as an attending physician in the Internal Medicine Department. My perception of how to best help patients often did not align with my bosses' notions, hospital policies, or budget priorities.

With some modifications, I utilized the Your Money or Your Life personal financial management program for the past 23 years. Despite being out of work for the past 16 years, it helped me live a full middle class life with an income less than half of that of the average American worker. Without learning to live frugally and minimize my consumption of "stuff," I would have never had the resources and time to research and write this book.

My total direct outlay for financial services (i.e., checking account, credit card, and wiring cash) in 2013 was $150. This was just $75 for wiring money to another country and $75 for using Turbo Tax to file my income tax data with the Internal Revenue Service (IRS). I paid nothing for the services of my credit union and credit card provider. For my approximately $3000 in credit card purchases, the vendors were probably charged about $100. By contrast, the average American spends about $4300 per year directly and indirectly on financial services.[a]

Financial Illiteracy, Wasteful Spending, and Excessive Debt

To improve financial literacy of persons in the United States, Congress established the Financial Literacy and Education Commission (herein the "Commission") under Title V of the Fair and Accurate Credit Transactions Act of 2003.[2] The Secretary of the Treasury Chaired the Commission which was composed of members from 20 federal agencies. This high-sounding Commission had little or no impact on financial illiteracy among U.S. citizens and did not prevent the subprime mortgage disaster and subsequent financial meltdown leading to the Great Recession.

Undaunted after the abject failure of the Commission, the federal government attempted to reinvigorate financial education. On January 22, 2008, an Executive Order by President Bush created the President's Advisory Council on Financial Literacy. This Order established "the policy of the federal government to encourage financial literacy among the American people."[3] The 16-member Council came from diverse organizations, including corporations, nonprofits, faith-based groups,

---

a   Total financial services cost in the U.S. in 2016 = $1.4 trillion.[1] $1.4 trillion / 329 million Americans= $4255 per person

state government agencies, regulatory authorities, and academic institutions.

The initial financial literacy nationwide survey conducted by this partnership showed the following major deficits in the financial knowledge and behavior of consumers:[4]

1. Nearly half of survey respondents reported facing difficulties in covering monthly expenses and paying bills.
2. Most did not have "rainy day" funds set aside for unanticipated financial emergencies.
3. The majority did not plan for predictable life events, such as their children's college education or their own retirement.
4. Over 20% reported engaging in non-bank, alternative borrowing methods such as payday loans, advances on tax refunds or pawn shops.
5. Few appeared to be knowledgeable about the financial products they owned.
6. While many American adults believed they were adept at dealing with day-to-day financial matters, they nevertheless engaged in financial behaviors that generated unnecessary expenses and fees.
7. They exhibited a marked inability to do basic interest calculations and other math-oriented tasks.
8. Few compared the terms of financial products or shopped around before making major financial decisions.

The inability to manage finances was much greater in those with less education, those with household incomes below $25,000 per year, and in blacks and Hispanics. This indicates that poor people with limited education are the most vulnerable to predatory loans and abusive financial products.

Widespread financial illiteracy exploited by financial services providers and other merchants exacerbated the Great Recession. Arguably, the pervasive lack of financial management capacity caused the ongoing financial crisis. Nefarious Wall Street bankers and traders just took advantage of the easy prey. Yet, fraudulent practices by bankers were not always obvious to even educated victims, and were legion until law-enforcement crackdowns.

Much has been said about the financial meltdown in 2008, beginning with the collapse of Lehman Brothers investment bank and quickly spreading to subprime mortgages and beyond. The poorest and most financially illiterate of the middle class that were hurt most by the Great Recession are now even more vulnerable to toxic financial services products. They still receive predatory loans, make risky investments, and are otherwise exploited by financial services providers, although perhaps less blatantly. Due to Congress' enactment of Dodd-Frank regulations on banks, loans are now much harder to obtain by home buyers and business owners.

Now, over six years later, the "too-big-to-fail banks" (systemic risk financial institutions) are even bigger than in 2008. The ingredients present in the run up to the 2008 financial crisis, particularly extensive financial illiteracy, are unabated.

Grand Bargain #16: ACCs to Provide Members Financial Counseling to Promote Member Financial Security

Helping each work-ready member to find a job will be a tremendous help (Chapter 12). However, a well-paying job will not necessarily assure financial security.

As part of ancillary human services, ACCs will hire financial professionals to educate members in money management, to protect them from predatory lenders, and to show them how to save money. Each ACC will have a financial services department charged with educating enrollees about managing money.

Financial services professionals employed by ACCs will also counsel enrollees about major financial decisions such as acquiring credit cards, automobiles, and home mortgages. The financial services counselors will assist clients with planning for retirement, college education for children, and small business creation. Enrollees facing financial stresses will seek ACC financial counselor help in eliminating debt, selling assets, cutting unnecessary expenses on energy and consumer items, and generally living within their means. ACC financial services departments will employ "conservation coaches" to help members reduce their consumption of items subject to the new consumption taxes. For instance, the conservation coaches will work with ACC members to decrease non-renewable energy utilization by auditing home energy use, financing home insulation, promoting alternatives to daily commuting alone in a car (i.e., bicycling, walking, public transit, car pooling, telecommuting, etc.), offering alternatives to plastic products (Chapter 22), and educating people about ways to reduce food waste (Chapter 13).

The ACCs' financial services professionals will be able to coordinate their efforts with other ACC staff. On behalf of ACC members, financial counselors will network with ACC providers of health and social -safety-net services, employment, conservation coaching, educational opportunities, and legal services.

This grassroots approach to financial literacy education and financial counseling will provide substantial protection against old and new predatory financial instruments of the banking and credit services industries.

ACC Strategies to Reduce Personal Debt

With the advent of ACC financial education and counseling services, personal debt in the U.S. will be decreased substantially. The estimated 22,300 payday loan stores nationwide will not be needed. These predatory lenders extract about $30 billion from poor people each year.[5] Credit card interest charges of $38 billion per year[6] and penalty fees of $22.5 billion per year[7] will also be sharply reduced.

Current and former college students owe over $1.1 trillion in outstanding student loans, costing tens of billions of dollars per year in interest payments and financial services fees.[8, 9] In future these costs will be dramatically reduced when ACCs assume a major role in financing the costs of higher education. As large purchasers of higher education services, ACCs will negotiate steep discounts in tuition and fees for students that they help send to colleges and universities. To further help students, ACCs will receive $50 billion in 2016 from the new consumption taxes to support students of higher education. Scholarships and part-time jobs, administered through the ACCs, will assist students in remaining debt-free. As explained in Chapter 16, universities will lower costs in order to compete for students, forcing the cutting of waste in academia, in athletics, and top administrative posts.

ACCs facilitating the reduction of our dependence on fossil fuel and the automobile (Chapter 22) will decrease consumers' cost of living by financing fewer cars. ACCs could also help members switch from owning to sharing cars and could find members local jobs that do not require cars for commuting. Americans will be able to save money while reducing emissions that lead to climate change.

With Grand Bargains-based reform, interest paid by homeowners on mortgages and businesses on loans no longer will be deductible on state and federal personal income taxes (Chapter 21). This will lead to a modest reduction of the $9.4 trillion in home mortgage debt and $13.6 trillion in business loans. Without income tax write-offs, consumers will be more careful about assuming debt.

As will be discussed later, ACCs themselves will own an increasing number of homes for members to rent or buy on favorable terms.

These reforms will lead owners of homes and businesses to have properties with increased equity and less debt. That will help stabilize the entire financial system.

The Financial System's Risk of Another Meltdown

In the U.S., the financial services industry employs about 5.9 million people. It accounts for about 7.7% of the GDP (about $1.4 trillion in earnings projected for 2016).[1, 10] The trends of the financial services sector in employment and proportion consumed of the GDP have been markedly upward over the last 60 years.[b] A similar massive growth in financial sector profits occurred in the U.S. in the decades before the Great Depression of the 1930s.

The financial sector intermediates money and assets flowing across economic sectors. The three basic functions of this intermediation are:

1. to give people places to save,
2. to give them credit to borrow, and
3. to mitigate the risk of a financial collapse of financial institutions and of the entire system.

Are we getting value for our money from the financial sector?

The more that bankers, investors, and venture capitalists spend other people's money on risky high potential growth financial transactions (i.e., selling and buying equities, lending money, etc.) the more money they may earn. The less capital that financial system regulators require for institutions to hold in reserve, the more investors can leverage holdings to earn more profits.

However, as capital in reserve goes down, the risk institutional default goes up. For "too-big-to-fail" banks, institutional default means a risk of financial system-wide meltdown.

The conditions that led to the 2008 worldwide financial meltdown have not gone away. Too-big-to-fail banks are larger than before. Consequently, banking regulations will not protect us against the next shock to the entire financial services system.

---

b   In the early 1950s, only 2.9% of the GDP went to financial services. In 1980, financial services consumed 4.9% of the GDP. Before the 2008 financial meltdown, banks, credit unions, insurance companies, money market funds, pension funds, mutual funds, and leasing companies gobbled up 8.3% of the economy. In 2012, it accounted for about 7.7% of the economy.[1] At the estimated 2.5%/year GDP growth,[10, 11] this projects to $1.4 trillion in financial services profits in 2016.

A Brief History of the Federal Reserve Bank (Fed)

Federal Reserve Act of 1913 created the U.S. central bank, calling it the Federal Reserve Bank (Fed). Congress gave the Fed no mandate for reducing unemployment or controlling inflation and was only charged with providing an "elastic currency" and to act as a lender of last resort for banks.[12] [c]

Because of periodic financial panics, Congress wanted to create an institution that would stabilize the currency. When the system was threatened with periodic regional or national financial crises, they wanted the Fed to provide liquidity to support the failing banks. They called this creating an elastic currency.[14]

In 1977, Congress updated the monetary policy objectives of the Fed, making a tall order:[15]

> The Board of Governors of the Federal Reserve System and the Federal Open Market Committee shall maintain long run growth of the monetary and credit aggregates commensurate with the economy's long run potential to increase production, so as to promote effectively the goals of maximum employment, stable prices, and moderate long-term interest rates.

Given these vague, some say impossible, mandates, how well has the Fed performed since 1977?

Under the Fed's leadership since 1977, the U.S. economy's production has dropped into the recession range on four occasions,[16] unemployment has spiked to over 10% twice,[17] inflation in prices has ranged from – 0.4% to 13.6%,[13] and the Feds' Funds Rate[d] (seeking to influence short-term interest rates) has ranged from 0% to 17%.[19]

---

c   Since winning independence from Great Britain until 1913, there had been virtually no inflation. Inflation began with the Second World War and accelerated after the change from the gold standard to fiat currency in 1971.[13]

d   The Fed controls the short-term interest rates charged by banks by varying the Fed Funds rate. This is a short-term interest rate that banks can fund themselves (i.e.

Role of the Federal Reserve Bank in the Great Recession

Beginning in 2008, the Fed provided credit to financially troubled firms with the Troubled Asset Relief Program (TARP). The Fed still holds many of these toxic assets. The Fed holds most of the mortgage-backed securities issued by Fannie Mae and Freddie Mac that precipitated the financial crisis (i.e., sub-prime home loans issued to unqualified buyers).

After financial markets stabilized, the Fed has continued to purchase mortgage-backed securities and other assets, trying to stimulate GDP growth and job creation. While the Fed's asset purchases have totaled over $4.4 trillion since the financial crisis, including about $1.7 trillion is in mortgage-backed securities,[20] the GDP remains stuck at 2%-2.5% and unemployment and underemployment remain unacceptably high.

The Fed's zero percent short-term-interest loans to banks and their asset purchases from banks sought to stimulate the economy. Fed leaders reasoned that by driving short-term interest rates down and giving banks easy money to lend, it would allow banks to lend more money to home buyers and business owners. However, banks held on to the money rather than lending it. Low short-term interest rates and these other strategies did not return sufficient equity into the housing market to resolve the underwater home mortgage crisis or hike GDP growth.

After these Fed policies failed, the Fed launched "quantitative easing" (QE), in which it made additional purchases of securities and other bank assets. This time the Fed purchased longer-term securities, mostly home mortgages, in an effort to drive long-term interest rates down. Since 2008, three successive rounds of QE (QE1 – QE3) have all failed to resolve the home mortgage crisis or kick start the GDP.

These Fed policies have raised concerns about (1) the stability of the dollar, (2) the likelihood of future hyper-inflation, (3) the prospect of exposing taxpayers to further losses, and (4) even about the financial strength of the Federal Reserve itself.

borrow money from the Fed).[18]

Norbert J. Michel and Stephen Moore of the conservative Heritage Foundation said, "The Fed's monetary policies are looking increasingly futile in terms of creating more jobs or accelerating economic growth."[20] On the liberal side, Larry Summers, President Obama's first choice for Fed Chairman to replace Ben Bernanke, speaking of the Fed, said, "There's no evidence of growth that is restoring equilibrium. One has to be concerned about a policy agenda that is doing less with monetary policy than has been done before, doing less with fiscal policy than has been done before, and is taking steps whose basic purpose is to cause there to be less lending, borrowing and inflated asset prices than there was before."[21]

Both conservatives and liberals would like to see different monetary policies at the Fed.

Too Much Debt Risks Government Insolvency

The other systemic risk to our financial system is U.S. government's $18 trillion debt and ongoing half a trillion dollar per year deficit spending. In great part, government debt is due to subsidies to individuals (e.g., tax breaks and welfare) and special interests (i.e., corporate welfare). However, if government subsidies and deficit spending coaxed the economy into robust sustainable growth, we would not have experienced the Great Recession.[22] The current government economic strategy can be characterized as follows: When subsidies, low interest rates, quantitative easing, and tax breaks causing massive deficit spending all fail to produce job growth and a higher GDP, double down on them and hope for the best.

We need a better way to protect against the systemic risk of the banking system. We need a fundamentally changed financial system that does two things:

1. dramatically reduces the overall debt in the U.S., both governmental and personal[e], and
2. places a substantial proportion of financial assets under the management of more secure financial institutions.

As has been mentioned before, the reduction of personal and governmental debt is built into Grand Bargains' reform. ACCs are designed as reducers of debt and waste throughout the economy.

As will be discussed later, ACC-affiliated financial institutions will greatly decrease systemic financial system risk by their involvement in resolving the housing crisis. However, we need to first make sure that ACCs themselves do not add any financial instability of the economy. The solvency of each ACC needs to be ensured.

Grand Bargain #23: ACCs to Self-Insure Against Bankruptcy

Because of mismanagement or unforeseen financial losses, some ACCs could become insolvent. A mechanism needs to be instituted for the orderly dissolution of bankrupt ACCs so their members can move to successfully managed ACCs. To ensure members against loss of benefits with the closures of their ACCs, each ACC will accumulate reserve funds as self-insurance. In the case of financial stress of an ACC, the reserve funds can be partly or entirely liquidated to cover all promised benefits to members. Financial management practices and member benefits may then be restructured in a sustainable fashion.

As part of Grand Bargains-based reform, ACCs will each set aside about 2.3% of patient care revenue as self-insurance. Collectively, ACCs will set aside about $100 billion of health and human services revenue each year to self-insure against insolvency.[f] As will be discussed later,

---

e   From 1980 to 2014, overall debt in the U.S. (households, businesses, government, and financial institutions) rose from about $4.7 trillion to $59 trillion.[23] Whereas, the debt to GDP ratio in 1980 was about 1.6/1, it is now over 3.3/1.[24]

f $4.3 trillion (health and human services revenue of all ACCs, Chapter 19) x 0.023 (2.3% of ACC revenue for credit unions) ≈ $100 billion this money will earn interest while being utilized to help members find decent, affordable housing.

First, some background on the origins of the housing crisis is in order.

U.S. Home Mortgage Crisis: A Personal Perspective

My mother bought our house in Sunnyvale, California for $11,000 in 1957. Working as an elementary school teacher and using the GI Bill to get a government-subsidized loan, my single mother could afford a new three-bedroom home in what was to become "Silicone Valley." When my mother died in 1985, I sold the house for $175,000.

My then wife and I bought our first home in San Diego, CA for $27,000 in 1977. In 1986, we sold the home for $64,000.

In Long Beach, CA, we bought our second home for $140,000 in 1980 and sold it in 2002 for $380,000. The income tax write-offs for the mortgage interest payments and property taxes on the house (i.e., government subsidies) saved us tens of thousands of tax dollars over those 22 years.

When equity accumulated in our Long Beach home, I refinanced the loan for a lower interest rate and a higher principal. This allowed me to pay for a new car outright without a high-interest, non-tax-deductible car loan. I also used part of the new mortgage loan to max out my contributions to my employer-sponsored, tax-deferred savings plan, with my deposits partially matched by my employer. As my case demonstrates, government housing subsidies can be creatively ma-nipulated by the wealthy.

Two of my daughters have homes in the San Francisco Bay Area. Those homes, purchased with government-subsidized ultra-low inter-est loans in the last few years, have appreciated even faster than the equities in the previous two generations of our family's houses.

So far, my family has been unusually lucky in the purchases and sales of our homes. As the housing crisis over the past few years has shown, tens of millions of other families have not been so lucky. For many, home mortgages led to financial ruin. Maybe we should ask, "Should luck be so important in buying and selling a home? "Should the housing market be run like a casino?

U.S. Home Mortgage Crisis: The Big Picture

Credit unions are not-for-profit member-owned financial institutions that exist to give its members a safe place to save money and receive reasonable rates on loans. **Savings and loan associations** (S&Ls) specialize in accepting savings deposits and making home mortgage and other assorted loans. Depositors and borrowers may be members and have voting rights.[25] S&Ls can be either corporations or mutuals (a type of business where making a deposit is like purchasing stock in the organization). Given that ACCs are cooperatives, the Grand Bargains preference is for mutual S&Ls. **Banks** are community, regional or national for-profit business corporations owned by private investors and governed by a board of directors chosen by the stockholders.[26]

The S&L crisis of the 1980s and 1990s should be studied by anyone endeavoring to design a more secure banking system. The causes of the S&L crisis included:

1. Deregulation of S&Ls in 1980 gave them many of the capabilities of banks, without the same regulations as banks.
2. S&Ls issued long-term loans at fixed interest rates using short-term money.
3. To reduce inflation, the Fed markedly increased short-term interest rates from the late 1970s to the early 1980s.
4. Lax regulatory oversight led to unresolved insolvent S&Ls.
5. Frauds were committed by S&L executives and employees.
6. The Tax Reform Act of 1986 significantly decreased the value of many real estate investments which had been held more for their tax-advantaged status.

7. Much real estate investment prior to 1986 was done by passive investors (i.e., not home owners).
8. Executives from insolvent S&Ls successfully lobbied politicians to delay necessary supervisory actions.
9. The short-term cost of funding mortgages at high interest rates was higher than the return on lower fixed-rate mortgage loans ("asset-liability mismatches"), precipitating S&L failures.

By 1995, the Resolution Trust Corporation had closed 747 failed institutions nationwide, worth over $400 billion. American taxpayers paid an estimated $160 billion.

William Black, PhD served as an S&L bank regulator in the 1980s and early 1990s. He prosecuted many of the executives of the S&Ls that knowingly made fraudulent loans before their institutions went bankrupt. His book, *The Best Way to Rob a Bank Is to Own One: How Corporate Executives and Politicians Looted the S&L Industry*,[27] details the corruption and fraud in the S&L industry that led to the crisis.

His assessment of the sub-prime mortgage crisis leading to the Great Recession suggests that politicians learned nothing from the S&L crisis. Dr. Black noted that, as early as the year 2000, home appraisers were being coerced to fraudulently inflate appraisals or risk losing their jobs. Honest appraisers created a petition stating: "There is an epidemic of lenders who are extorting us to inflate the appraisal, and when we refuse to do so, they blacklist honest appraisers and refuse to use them in the future." This petition was widely circulated and eventually signed by over 11,000 appraisers.[28] However, fraudulent appraisals continued.

In an interview in 2013, Dr. Black indicated that the mortgage industry learned nothing after the Great Recession. His analysis was that mortgage fraud risk is now relatively low only because the economy is so crippled. He predicted that when the economy booms again, the fraudulent loans will re-emerge.

Dr. Black was questioned about the Dodd-Frank Congressional regulations enacted to prevent future mortgage industry melt downs. He said that we remain at high risk because of "too-big-to-fail" banks and a banking culture that fosters epidemics of banking fraud ("criminogenic environment"). He noted that Dodd-Frank did nothing effective in reigning in outsized executive compensation, which he said was the means of looting the banks. The absence of prosecutions of fraudulent bankers by regulators and the U.S. Department of Justice potentially emboldens bankers to continue putting the country at great financial risk. In this environment, when honest bankers refuse to make fraudulent loans, the bankers lose their jobs.

After the predatory lending practices of banks and rising personal indebtedness precipitated the home foreclosure crisis in 2008, the Treasury Department and the Federal Reserve sided more with the profligate financial institutions than the virtually bankrupt and "underwater" homeowners.[29] As a result, the attorneys general of all 50 states, led by Tom Miller of Iowa, mobilized to conduct a joint investigation into the banking practices that had led to the scandal.

The attorneys general wanted more than to bring corrupt bankers to justice and to win a huge settlement on behalf of homeowners: they sought to force the big banks and other loan servicers to institute widespread, systematic mortgage-principal reductions. These principal reductions would have ameliorated the pain of homeowners by sharing the pain with careless and/or corrupt financial services providers and their investors. In the end, the attorneys general failed to bring honesty and fiscal discipline to the system.

Over 9 million home mortgages remained underwater in the second quarter of 2014.[30, 31] The aggregate value of negative equity of the underwater homes is almost $400 billion.[32]

When mortgage interest rates increase to historically normal levels, another wave of falling home valuations and of foreclosures is very likely.[33] Meanwhile, future taxpayers are forced to assume the long-term costs of a relatively few, wealthy home buyers, speculators, and home mortgage refinancers that get 30-year fixed mortgages at historically low interest rates.

Home and Rental Prices Too High

Even before the housing mortgage foreclosure crisis began in 2007-2008, housing costs were unsustainably high and climbing. After adjusting for inflation, mortgage and rental costs now comprise about four times more than in 1940.[34, 35] The portion of home renters facing a severe or moderate financial burden due to housing costs[g] has risen from about 22% in the 1960s to 50% in the 2000s.[36] As the number of very low-income renters has grown, the likelihood of receiving rent assistance has decreased to about 24% of those who request a government subsidy for rent.[h]

The fraudulent banking practices precipitating the S&L bank crisis and the Great Recession also contributed to increasingly unaffordable housing for all but the rich. The additional factors leading to the early 2000s housing bubble and subsequent crash, include:

1. tax policy[38]
    a. exemption of house ownership from capital gains tax
    b. mortgage interest tax write-off
2. historically low interest rates[38]
3. heavily government subsidized mortgage market[i]
4. diminished private sector role in bearing credit risk[42]
5. risk multiplier of overly leveraged financial institutions and overly leveraged buyers[43]
6. speculative fever.

Most of these government subsidies and tax policies benefit the wealthy much more than middle- and low-income people. Taxpayers

g   Moderately financially stressed renter: > 30% of income going to rent. Severely financially stressed renter: > 50% of income going to rent.
h   Examples of Housing and Urban Development (HUD) rent assistance include low-income senior housing subsidies, "Section 8" housing vouchers for low-income families, and subsidies for spouses and parents of people in the armed forces.[37]
i   The government subsidizes mortgages of over 90% of owner-occupied homes and over 65% of rental properties.[39, 40] Government agencies participating in housing subsidies include Fanny Mae, Freddy Mac, Ginnie Mae, the Federal Housing Administration, Veterans Administration, and the U.S. Department of Agriculture (loans on rural properties). The U.S. Department of Housing and Urban Development operates 127 subsidy programs.[41]

pay for all of them. Administrative overhead of government agencies providing subsidies is high, costing about $2 billion per year to operate the Department of Housing and Urban Development.[44]

Solutions being entertained to solve the housing mortgage crisis include privatization of the market and replacing all the government housing mortgage subsidy programs with another government housing mortgage subsidy provider.[39] Neither of these fixes to the mortgage industry would make housing significantly more affordable. We need a better solution to both the mortgage industry and housing affordability.

What the Housing Market Needs

To establish housing market long-term stability, many economists and politicians on the left and right agree that the government's roles in housing subsidies, tax policy, and perhaps regulation need to decrease. A "Housing Commission," drawn up of Republicans and Democrats appointed by the Bipartisan Policy Center has defined objectives for a reformed housing finance system:[42]

1. to protect taxpayers from paying for so many subsidies,
2. to provide for a greater diversity of funding sources by opening mortgage market access to lenders of all types and sizes, including community banks and credit unions,[j]
3. to serve as wide a market as possible, and
4. to assure consumers fair access to sustainable and affordable mortgage credit.

Since the "too-big-to-fail" bank bailouts in 2008-2009, fiscal policies of the federal government (taxing and spending) and monetary policies the Fed (e.g., zero interest rates, printing money, and quantitative easing) have been directed towards trying to aid the recovery in home values. Fiscal and monetary policies also seek to stimulate overall GDP

---

j   The six largest banks in the nation now have 67% of the $14.4 trillion in the U.S. home mortgage financial system.[45] About 7000 banks and credit unions share the remainder of the market.

growth—represented by Wall Street and the stock market—at virtually any cost.

While many economists criticize this approach,[46] they offer no viable alternatives. Generally, Democrats want to keep deficit spending our way to financial health and Republicans prefer draconian austerity to balance the budget. Success with either strategy is hard to imagine.

For a solution to the housing crisis, think outside-the-box. Consider that we may need to pursue policies to benefit all stakeholders—homeowners, renters, taxpayers, the government, and investors. The strategies should not require big increases in housing prices or high GDP growth. Think about a plan that will simultaneously, (1) provide easy access to affordable housing, (2) equitably resolve the underwater home mortgage crisis, (3) reduce overall debt, and (4) eliminate the ever looming risk of overall financial system meltdown.

What about having safer and more secure financial institutions displace too-big-to-fail banks from much of the home mortgage market?

Grand Bargains #24: ACC-Affiliated Credit Unions/S&Ls to Enter the Housing Market and to Manage Pensions

ACCs will affiliate with credit unions that will make mortgage loans for members to purchase homes, condos, or farms. For the same purposes, ACCs will also affiliate with S&Ls.

ACCs will likely partner with existing credit unions/S&Ls but, if needed, could charter new ones. Credit unions/S&Ls are appropriate institutions to manage these funds since they offer mortgages for properties. By design, they are typically managed conservatively for the benefit of members rather than for high profits for speculators. Taking into account the causes and lessons of the S&L insolvency crisis in the 1980s -1990s[47] and the sub-prime mortgage lending precipitating the Great Recession, ACC-affiliated S&Ls will be tightly watched by government regulators and, even more importantly, closely overseen by ACC stakeholders.

For funding of ACC-affiliated credit union/S&Ls, the Grand Bargains' approach will be to use ACC self-insurance funds, Social Security

Trust Fund dispersements, and pension fund deposits. ACC member saving account deposits will also be welcome. Funding mortgages primarily with retirement savings managed by competing, nonprofit, cooperative institutions, accountable to members, will facilitate stability, security, and efficiency.

To take advantage of ACC-administered housing subsidies (i.e., Housing and Urban Development funds transferred to ACCs, Chapter 19) people will need to obtain mortgages from their own ACC-affiliated credit unions/S&Ls. This way, there won't be a race to the bottom in interest rates and other loan parameters. This race to the bottom usually favors loan brokers shopping among the government subsidized too-big-to-fail banks to the detriment of unsubsidized credit union/S&Ls.

Home mortgage interest rates of ACC-affiliated credit unions/S&Ls and ACC policies on housing subsidies should be considered by people when choosing an ACC. Likewise, people saving for retirement should notice interest rates paid on pensions and Social Security deposits when choosing an ACC. ACC financial services experts will have to balance the desires of home buyers for low interest rates with the needs of pensioners and Social Security recipients for reasonable interest rates on their retirement savings.

New deposits in 2016 to the ACC-affiliated credit unions/S&Ls totaling at least $650 billion will come from the following combination of sources (Chapter 23):

1. ACC reserve revenue set aside as insurance against insolvency ($100 billion in 2016),
2. Social Security Reserve Fund dispersements from the U.S. Treasury ($100 billion in 2016),
3. Pension deposits of government workers ($150 billion in 2016),
4. Pensions of private company employees ($300 billion in 2016), and
5. Deposits of ACC members.

With these funds, ACC-affiliated credit unions/S&Ls will participate in the housing market. They will provide affordable mortgages for members to purchase properties. Additionally, ACCs-affiliated credit unions/S&Ls will themselves purchase homes and apartments to rent to members.

Options for ACC members to rent will include:

1. Younger people may enter into rent-to-buy arrangements for ACC-owned homes and apartments while they save for down payments to buy the properties from their ACCs.
2. Older people that own their own homes may sell them to the ACC-affiliated credit unions/S&Ls for retirement income and continue in the same dwellings as renters.
3. ACC-affiliated credit unions/S&Ls may purchase underwater properties at foreclosure auctions or short sales and allow the former property owners to remain as renters.

As of 2014, U.S. residents owed about $11 trillion in mortgages on their homes, multi-family residences, and farms.[23] Of that mortgage debt, at least $2 trillion worth of those loans had negative equity (underwater mortgages). ACC-affiliated credit unions/S&Ls will seek to buy those properties as soon as possible to stabilize the housing market while helping to make housing affordable to buy and rent for their members. ACC involvement with mortgages will tend to lower average home prices throughout the country. The depressant effect on the GDP of home prices stabilizing at more affordable levels will be offset by increased employment and higher wages (Chapter 12). With ACCs in charge of administering housing subsidies and ACC-affiliated credit unions/S&Ls involved in the housing market, hyperinflation in home values and rents will not recur.

Historically on average, about $500 billion-$600 billion worth of mortgage loans, new purchases or refinances, on homes, multifamily residences, and farms are acquired each year.[23] ACC-affiliated credit unions/S&Ls will have the funding necessary to enter this market, serving low- and middle-income buyers. Private banks are efficiently serving high income home buyers now and can continue to provide mortgages for these people.

In comparison with home mortgage interest rates in 2014 of 3.5%-4.5%, ACC-affiliated credit union/S&L mortgage loans at 5%-6% annual interest will significantly lower home market values. This adjustment is necessary for the long-term stability and affordability of homes and rentals. ACC members saving for retirement or contributing to college funds for their children will receive reasonable and secure returns on those savings (i.e. 4-5%).

Whereas, most government subsidies for homes now go to the relatively wealthy, ACCs will be tasked with targeting housing subsidies to low- and middle-income people to buy or rent homes, condos, or farms. ACCs will have maximum flexibility in administering those subsidies. In addition, ACC-affiliated credit unions/S&Ls will be able to compete with too-big-to-fail banks to provide virtually all mortgages of lower than average cost homes, condos, and farms. When indicated, ACC-affiliated credit unions/S&Ls will be able to collaborate with ACC social services and financial services departments to innovatively integrate subsidies into home mortgage loan packages.

Even more social justice will be brought to the home mortgage market playing field by the consumption tax on too-big-to-fail banks of 0.8% of overall equities (Chapter 21). This will tend to raise mortgage interest rates and consequently lower the value of higher end homes, counteracting future housing bubbles.

ACC-Affiliated Credit Unions/S&Ls Lending to Businesses Including Social Benefit Corporations

After accommodating the home mortgage needs of ACC members and buying the accumulated mortgage-backed securities from the Fed, ACC-affiliated credit unions/S&Ls will likely have funds available for other borrowers. Since loans for small businesses have been very difficult to obtain throughout the financial crisis, businesses should be first in line for ACC-affiliated credit union/S&L loans. As cooperatives chartered to benefit all members, ACCs and their affiliated credit unions/S&Ls will likely favor lending to startup and established businesses with social purposes. Social benefit companies or "B" companies are a relatively new type of company that uses the power of business to address social and environmental problems.[48] In addition they are intended to make money for owners, investors, and employees. B corporations are chartered in 26 states in the U.S.

An example of a B corporation might be conservation coaching. Conservation coaches may help clients find ways to reduce their consumption of non-renewable energy, water, plastics, and other commodities subject to the new consumption taxes. B corps might also be chartered to help clients adopt healthful diets and lifestyles, to advise ACC members on legal issues, to serve as financial planning educators, or to clean up pollution in their local environments.

Competition Between ACCs on Quality of Financial Services

ACCs will compete with each other, in part, on their financial services. These will include financial counseling, financial education, ACC-affiliated credit union/S&L mortgages and loans, scholarships, part-time jobs for college students, and management of retirement savings (Social Security and pensions). The quality of ACC financial services could be measured by whatever financial yardsticks that appeal to the ACC stakeholders. Financial services measurement tools could include:

1. debt free higher education opportunities for students,
2. financial security of retirees,
3. the affordability and accessibility of ACC-affiliated credit union/S&L mortgages,
4. the return on investments of retirement funds (Social Security and pensions),
5. the fairness of ACC utilization of risk-adjusted government block grants for housing and other ACC services,
6. quality of jobs created, and
7. the low frequencies of bankruptcies and home foreclosures of ACC members.

In an environment of ACCs' competing on financial successes of enrollees, the ACC financial services professionals, including those staffing ACC-affiliated credit unions/S&Ls will be responsible for enrollees' fully utilizing their high-value financial services. The most talented of financial services professionals would do well to choose rewarding careers with ACCs helping people achieve financial security. ACCs may well provide start-up loans or grants to affiliated financial services companies that commit to providing financial counseling services.

Monetary Policies: Directed by ACCs Instead of the Fed

Given the widespread dissatisfaction with the Federal Reserve Bank, consider retaining the Fed for its original purpose—to provide elastic currency and serve as the lender of last resort to banks. Then, think about having national monetary policy determined by a federation of ACC-affiliated monetary policy experts. An elected committee of the ACC monetary policy experts would replace the Federal Open Market Committee and the Federal Reserve Chairperson (currently Janet Yellen) in making monetary policy decisions by the Fed.

Compared with the Federal Open Market Committee, the advantages of ACC directed monetary policies would include:

1. decentralization of monetary policies
   a. Each ACC will decide what short-term and long-term interest rates for ACC-affiliated credit unions/S&Ls to charge.
   b. Each ACC will determine what strategies work best for it to maximize employment.
2. greater capacity of a network of competing ACCs to maximize employment that a group of high-powered financial wonks,
3. greater ability of a network of ACCs to stabilize prices:
   a. ACC-affiliated credit unions/S&Ls will participate in credit markets.
   b. ACCs will influence members in terms of supply and demand for goods and services.
   c. As employers of over 60 million health and human services providers and the determiners of what health and human

services will be offered, ACCs collectively will be able to guard against excessive inflation or deflation in the economy.
4. more direct influences over long-term interest rates
    a. Each ACC-affiliated credit union/S&L will set long-term interest rates of mortgages on homes, condos, and farms.
    b. Growth of ACC member pensions and Social Security funds will be determined by long-term interest rates.

It makes a lot of sense to have decentralized ACCs manage the U.S.' monetary policy instead of a few high-level bankers. The Fed's elite monetary policy experts will be able to move to individual ACC-affiliated credit unions/S&Ls where their performances may be compared with other bankers. The best performing bankers may then be elected to a committee of ACC-affiliated bankers that will be charged with determining (1) the Fed's short-term interest rate for bank loans, (2) the amount of currency in circulation, and (3) other decisions made by the Fed.

ACC Monetary Policy: Stop the Fed's Printing Money and Low Interest Rates and Reverse Quantitative Easing

Decades of well-meaning but misguided government housing subsidies strongly contributed to inflated home prices that made buying or renting houses difficult for poor people. It was these inflated home values that helped to fuel the housing bubble in another way: Consumers with some equity could borrow more and spend more until the bubble burst. ACCs' administration of federal, state, and local housing subsidies will more effectively target the low end of the housing market without creating housing bubbles.

Grand Bargains' economic reform calls for (1) stopping the Federal Reserve Bank's policies of zero percent interest rates for short-term loans to banks, (2) decreasing the money in circulation (base money), and (3) reversing quantitative easing (over time selling off the Fed's $1.7 trillion in mortgage-backed securities accumulated to spur growth). With ACC-affiliated credit unions/S&Ls in place in the housing market, these three reforms will safely drive down inflated home prices and lead to long-term housing market stability.

Once ACC-affiliated credit unions/S&Ls buy up the vast majority of homes with underwater mortgages, the Grand Bargains-strategy is for the credit unions/S&Ls to buy back from the Fed the $1.7 trillion in mortgage-backed securities. Purchasing those mortgage-backed securities from the Fed at real market rates will financially strengthen the ACCs. This will also make the Fed and federal government much more financially secure.

By reversing these ineffective monetary policies of the Fed, long-term interest rates will rise to more normal levels (5%-6% per year). This will allow the retirement savings of ACC members to grow securely at adequate rates of interest. This will also inspire confidence in the Fed and the solvency of the U.S. Government.

Downsizing the Financial Services Sector

A government-sponsored enterprise (GSE) is a financial services corporation created by the United States Congress. Loans made by GSEs comprise almost $8 trillion of financial sector debt out of the approximately $59 trillion credit market.[23] This provides a huge government subsidy to the financial services sector. Most prominent among the GSEs are the government backed home mortgage companies (Fanny Mae, Freddy Mac, Federal Housing Administration (FHA), etc). With Grand Bargains' reform, the relatively few GSEs will be eliminated and their roles assumed by the many, decentralized ACCs. ACC-affiliated financial services companies will take over the government's roles of assisting individuals and groups that for decades have received financial subsidies (e.g., farmers, students, and low-income home buyers). Eliminating GSEs will reduce the debt of the government, of companies, and of individuals. Additional government financing of ACC-affiliated credit unions/S&Ls to assume the rolls of GSEs will not be needed. The $650 billion/year from pensions and the Social Security Trust Funds to the ACCs will be much more than the GSEs have been getting from the government.

Regarding government debt, Grand Bargains-based reform will mean not borrowing the projected $530 billion to balance the federal budget in 2016 (Chapter 21, Tables 1 and 2) and subsequently. It will also mean that the Social Security Administration will transfer close to $3 trillion of Social Security Trust Funds to ACCs over the next decade and thereby reduce the federal debt by that amount (Chapter 23). This adds a national debt-reduction role for ACCs along with their other advantages for social progress and healing.

With the elimination of the corporate income tax and simplification of the personal income tax code (Chapter 21), the cost of financial services related to federal and state income tax compliance will be reduced by about 90%.[k] The consumption taxes detailed in Chapter 21 and 22 are designed to reduce consumption of the items taxed. If enacted, reduced consumption of these items will save consumers almost $800 billion in 2016 (Chapter 21, Table 3). Reducing purchases of these commodities will mean less need for financing purchases and less debt.

Individual investors and banks naturally seek the highest returns on their investments. Currently, emerging markets in third world countries may return higher yields on funds than do U.S. investments. Consequently, job creation in the U.S. suffers. However, with local-community-based ACCs controlling investments of privatized Social Security revenues and pension funds (Chapter 23), the tendency of investment dollars to go overseas will be reduced.

As mentioned before, ACCs will provide members with financial professionals charged with helping members:

1. reduce their borrowing,
2. moderate spending on luxuries,
3. conserve on items subject to consumption taxes, and
4. save for the usual contingencies (retirement, kids' college education, home down payments, etc.).

---

k   IRS compliance costs reduced from about $200 billion to about $20 billion. For the new consumption taxes, the compliance costs will be no more than half of the current IRS compliance costs (i.e., $100 billion per year).

Consequently, the overall cost of financial services will be further reduced.

All of the above strategies to decrease public and private debt will lead to a significant downsizing of the financial services sector over the next few years. Personal savings will increase substantially, perhaps from about 5% of personal income in the 2000s to the 10% range maintained in the 1950s to early 1980s[49] before our unsustainable accumulation of debt. ACC financial services specialists who help members manage financial assets will tend to shift money to high-value economic activities that create jobs, strengthen communities, and help the environment.

A downsized financial services industry will continue to thrive but will consume a much lower portion of the income of families. Fewer financial workers will be needed and their average incomes will probably go down to levels closer to the pay of other professionals. Reducing the net cost of financial services by hundreds of billions of dollars per year will strengthen the rest of the economy and make almost everyone better off.

Instead of the overall credit market debt in the U.S. increasing by about $3 trillion in 2016 as projected,[23] it will not increase at all and may decrease modestly. With all of the above reforms, public and private sector debt will decline much more over time while savings increase.

Financial services now consume about 7.7% of the GDP.[1, 10] With Grand Bargains' reform, we will conservatively aim for the financial services sector net profits to comprise about 5% of the GDP in 2025 (about the same as in 1980).

Grand Bargains-Related GDP Growth: Unpredictable

The U.S. Congressional Budget Office (CBO) in April 2014 projected that the 2016 U.S. GDP will be $19.0 trillion.[50] The CBO based this estimate on the optimistic assumption that the GDP will grow by 4.5% per year from 2014 to 2016. If we more realistically assume that the current slower rate of GDP growth (2.5% per year[10]) will continue, as forecast by the International Monetary Fund,[11] the status-quo projected 2016 GDP will be about $17.9 trillion. However, it could be somewhat higher or lower.

Predicting the effect of Grand Bargains' reforms on the U.S. GDP in 2016 will be difficult. Factors that will tend to increase GDP growth through 2016 via Grand Bargains' reforms include:

- 40 million net increase in jobs throughout the economy: at least $2.3 trillion projected additional income (Chapter 12)[1]
- repatriating offshore corporate profits: $2.1 trillion (Chapter 21)
- repatriating individual earnings: $400 billion (Chapter 21)
- immigration reform attracting highly educated and skilled workers from other countries (Chapter 14)
- new infrastructure spending: $100 billion (Chapter 15)
- new education spending on part-time work and grants to college and trade school students to eliminate new student-debt: $50 billion (Chapter 16)
- new national security spending: $50 billion (Chapter 17)
- shifting $100 billion of the Social Security Trust Funds from the U.S. Treasury to ACC-affiliated credit unions/S&Ls to lend to ACC members

Factors that will tend to decrease GDP growth via the Grand Bargains are more difficult to quantify:

- Consumption taxes reducing sales of commodities that are taxed: $767 billion (Chapter 21)
- IRS income tax compliance costs decreased: $80 billion (Chapter 21)
- Fewer legal services due to enterprise malpractice liability and other Grand Bargains' legal system reforms: unknown

---

1   The $660 billion in wages paid to 20 million parents and caregivers for the elderly and disabled doesn't add to GDP because the work was previously unpaid. For the 20 million additional workers with incomes that average the same as other workers ($47,000 per year[51]), the wages will be $940 billion ($47,000 x 20 million workers = $940 billion). The final added value of their products and services is assumed to derive from wages (60%) and other factors (40%). Therefore, the GDP growth estimate from these new jobs is $940 billion wages / 0.6 (fraction of added value going to wages) = $1567 billion

- Fewer financial services costs due to less debt: unknown
- Housing valuation reduced due to a reversal of Federal Reserve Bank's economy stimulating policies (i.e., printing money, low interest rates, quantitative easing, etc.): unknown
- Stock market valuation also reduced because of higher interest rates: unknown

The net change in projected 2016 GDP with the major disruptions of Grand Bargains' reforms is impossible to predict due to so many moving parts of the economy. The GDP could go up or down a few percentage points initially. Whatever the GDP, people will be much better off because of the 40 million net increase in jobs, higher minimum wages, more progressive tax system.

The combination of these reforms will result in a major redistribution of income from the 1% to the 99%. With Grand Bargains' tax reform, the 1% highest earners will pay over 50% of all personal income taxes[m] while the lowest 90% of earners pay no income taxes (Chapter 21). The consumption taxes will strongly impact both the poor and the rich. Compared with rich people, the poor will be under more financial pressure to quit smoking, to limit alcohol consumption, to eat a more healthful diet (i.e., less processed food and more plant-based whole foods), to conserve energy, and limit use of electronic media. ACC human services providers (health, social, financial, legal, etc.) can help people of all income levels to embrace lifestyle changes that will help individuals and the society as a whole.

The Grand Bargains' reform-related decreases in spending on human services (health, welfare, legal and financial), and less spending on housing and items subject to the new consumption taxes, may reduce the GDP initially. However, these reforms will help move us toward widespread prosperity over the long term.

---

m   Currently, the top 1% of earners pay 35.1% of all personal income taxes.[52] With Grand Bargains' reform, the top 10% of earners will pay 68.3% of the projected total of the status quo personal income taxes in 2016. So the top 1% will pay 51% of the total personal income taxes (0.351 (35.1% of all personal income taxes currently paid by top 1%) / 0.683 (68.3% of projected status quo taxes to be paid by the top 10% of earners with Grand Bargains' reform) = 0.513 (51% of the projected total of personal income taxes in 2016 paid by the top 1% of earners).

With ACC-directed U.S. monetary policies, GDP growth will be less cyclical because of the moderating influence of ACC-affiliated credit unions/S&Ls. Over the intermediate and long terms, the GDP will rise at least modestly as ACCs maintain high employment, stabilize the housing market, foster affordable higher education (Chapter 16), and reduce the over-incarceration of U.S. residents (Chapter 11). Whatever the GDP will be at the end of 2016 and subsequently, the economy will become more stable, less subject to commodities bubbles, and much more protected from the kind of financial meltdown we experienced in the Great Recession.

Much study and advocacy have gone into adopting a better measure of economic well-being than the GDP. The Gross National Happiness Index and the Genuine Progress Indicator are the main contenders to the GDP for an agreed-upon, more sensible measurement that does not translate pollution and other wasteful activity as good things because they represent "growth."[53]

The success of Grand Bargains' reforms will not depend on maintaining high GDP growth. If GDP growth continues at 2.5% as it has been for several years, this might be a seamless transition. Indeed, if GDP growth decreases to 0%, it would not create a disastrous meltdown or massive job layoffs. Consequently, the economic growth projections used in this book (GDP = 2.5% increase/year and pensions = 4%-5% earnings/year) are conservative. If GDP growth becomes higher (e.g., > 4%), venture capitalists, entrepreneurs, technology innovators, investors, and owners of wide ranging businesses will do especially well. Extra financial benefits may trickle down to workers and pensioners. However, even with modest or no GDP growth, individual citizens and the country will remain financially secure.

Summary and Conclusion

Widespread financial illiteracy, excessive debt, waste, greed, and inefficiency throughout the sectors of the economy have squandered our wealth and brought the U.S. Government to the verge of insolvency.

Adding 40 million jobs that will pay at least $1.5 trillion in workers' income in 2016 (Chapter 12) will mean economic recovery for more than just the rich. However, continued waste and inefficiency throughout the economic sectors could squander the benefits of more jobs and higher pay. One way of improving society's economic security is fostering individual financial security. This requires teaching financial literacy skills and fiscal discipline throughout the country. ACC financial educators and counselors will help members reduce debt, decrease unnecessary spending, live within their means, and save for the future.

ACC financial literacy education will begin with informing members to use their stakeholder statuses to influence ACC health and human services spending policies. ACCs will establish their own benefits packages regarding health care, social services, and other human services. Based on what services are offered and how efficiently services are delivered, ACCs will decide what premiums to charge members. All stakeholders will be impacted by and therefore involved in these decisions.

Using funds transferred for management from the Social Security Trust Funds and from deposits into public and private sector pensions, ACC-affiliated credit unions/S&Ls will provide loans to members for mortgages (homes, multi-family residences, condominiums, and farms) and businesses. These ACC-affiliated financial services companies will also buy up many of the over 9 million homes with underwater mortgages and purchase much of the inventory of the Fed's $1.7 trillion in quantitative-easing-related mortgage-backed securities.

ACC-affiliated credit unions/S&Ls will also provide loans for startup and established businesses for members. Preferences will likely be given to "B" corporations with social purposes (e.g., health enhancement, environmental protection, etc.) in addition to making money for business owners and investors. ACCs, as employers of more than 60 million people (i.e., one-third of the economy), will need to facilitate the creation and growth of many B corporations that provide health and human services for ACC members.

ACC-affiliated credit unions/S&Ls entering the credit market will help

1. ACC members get mortgages and other loans
2. provide members with secure retirement income,

3. strengthen the Fed, and

4. reduce the risk of insolvency of the U.S. Government.

No one will be financially secure if the entire financial system melts down again because of risky financial services practices. Too-big-to-fail banks now control more financial assets than in 2007. ACC-affiliated credit unions/S&Ls entering the home mortgage market will help eliminate this very real systemic financial risk. The Grand Bargains' strategy for eliminating overall financial system risk is to decentralize U.S. monetary policy. Each ACC will develop its own monetary policies. Each ACC affiliated credit union/S&L will determine its own interest rates charged on mortgages. Correspondingly, growth rates of pensions and Social Security deposits will be set.

An elected committee of ACC monetary policy experts from throughout the country will then assume the roles of the Federal Open Market Committee and the Fed Chairperson. However, the Committee's function will be limited to setting the interest rate that the Fed charges banks for short-term loans and determining the money in circulation (base money).

By using competition between ACCs to combat excessive debt, waste, bureaucracy, and inefficiency; we will empower individuals and communities to grow in financial security and stability. Grand Bargains' reforms will result in a much downsized financial services sector that no longer poses a major systemic risk to our economy. We will no longer have a casino economy with borrowing-fueled commodity bubbles followed by deep recessions.

Less public and private debt, and more personal and systemic financial security, will contribute to improvements in health indices, environmental indicators, infrastructure development, social justice, and jobs.

Chapter 25
Better Care for Seniors and People with Disabilities

The California budget deficit during the Great Recession[a] forced severe cuts in health and welfare services. I attended a forum to discuss the impact of the cuts on seniors hosted by my California State Assemblywoman, Bonnie Lowenthal from Long Beach. Lowenthal chaired the Assembly Committee on Aging and Long-Term Care. The lively meeting featured five panelists that were each directors of service agencies or high-ranking administrators. Each of them excepting the director of volunteer services for seniors recited how many thousands of dollars each agency was cut and how the cuts had impacted their services.

At one point in the conversation, Assemblywoman Lowenthal asked the panel where seniors should call in Long Beach for efficient access to all services available. The panelists looked at each other. Someone finally said to call any of them. There was no one agency charged with coordinating approximately 70 government, nonprofit, and for-profit agencies in Long Beach serving seniors and people with disabilities. This lack of coordination shocked me because many of the agencies provided similar services.

The California Health and Human Services Department agencies that provide services to seniors are divided between the Department of Social Services, Department of Aging, and the Department of Health Services. Coordination seemed to be lacking at the state level.

---

a $60 billion deficit over two-years

After the panelist presentations, representatives of many of the 70+ senior service agencies lined up to comment on the adverse impact of the cuts on their clients and staff. Many complained that they weren't properly funded even before the cuts, so their reductions were especially severe. They all promised to do the best they could under the difficult circumstances. No one had anything good to say about how Governor Swartzenegger handled his difficult role of balancing the California budget.

In the long line of agency representatives, no physician spoke. In fact, I heard no reference to the doctors of the seniors who were receiving the health and social services. I found it odd that physicians did not seem to have a visible role in the network of providers of services for the elderly.

In the tabling area for service providers, I found the representative for the nonprofit providing Alzheimer's disease education and support. I asked him if physicians frequently referred patients to them. He told me that physician referrals were rare and that family members usually called his agency seeking help with forgetful relatives. He said that the Alzheimer's disease nonprofit generally referred clients to neurologists and other physician specialists rather than the other way around. PCPs were not involved at all.

After the forum, I conferred with gerontologist Pamela Mokler, MS, who had invited me to the event partly to show me the lack of co-ordination of services for the aged. She served as executive director of the Orange County Office on Aging and tried to better coordinate the fragmented and often duplicative services. She received considerable resistance from the bureaucracy, especially upper-level administrators over her attempts to streamline care and cut redundant services. A battle ensued over the County's intention to restructure services to the aged in a manner that Ms. Mokler believed was both illegal and threatening to state and federal funding. In 2003, she was unlawfully terminated and won a whistleblower retaliation suit against Orange County. [1]

Ms. Mokler's comment at the forum about the urgent need to integrate all funding streams for the aged was applauded loudly by the audience but received no substantive comment from Assemblywoman Lowenthal or the panelists. It amazed me that, in those bleak fiscal times, policymakers were not especially concerned about eliminating duplicative administrative functions and programs to make the system more efficient in order to better serve seniors and the disabled.

Like Long Beach, CA, numerous municipalities in the country have many well-intentioned individuals, government agencies, and private foundations working to provide social services. However, with the increased need and decreased resources brought on by the economic downturn, agencies with uncoordinated and therefore inefficient social service agencies are overwhelmed. One impasse is that social services providers naturally defend the value of their programs and question the wisdom and intent of any reformers.

Against the powerful inertia of the status quo, ACC care will be the game-changer. ACCs will encourage a culture of innovation throughout organizations and communities by efficiently providing integrated social services. Charitable organizations, volunteers, ACC staff, and private social services agency professionals will work together to best serve those in need. If they don't do so, they will not compete for members well with other ACCs.

Health Care Costs per Medicare Patient: $45,000 in 2016

Seniors and disabled people face incredible health care costs. In 2016, government funding for Medicare patients will average about $18,000 per Medicare recipient.[b2-4] Remarkably, these government funding sources comprise less than half of the actual medical, long-term care, and out-of-pocket cost of seniors and people with disabilities. Additional costs include health insurance premiums, co-payments, deductibles, uncovered services, and long-term care. Long-term care

b   Costs of U.S. Government Medical Care for Seniors/Disabled People 2016

Funding Source	Overall $ (billions)	Per person $
Medicare	715	12,770
Medicaid	248	4430
Veterans' Administration	44	790
Total	1007	17,990

includes nursing home costs paid by the Medicare enrollee, costs of home care not reimbursed by insurance, and the value of unpaid family and friend caregivers.

The total health care cost per capita for Medicare recipients (insurance covered, out-of-pocket, and value of unpaid friends and family members providing home care) will be over $45,000 in 2016.[c]

Social-Safety-Net Services Costs: $4800 per Medicare Recipient

As explained in Chapter 10, social determinants of health (income, education, race, location, diet, lifestyle, etc.) are major factors in determining health outcomes. Social-safety-net services or welfare (food, housing, child care, transportation, financial aid, etc.) for the poor attempt to prevent bad health outcomes due to poverty. In Long Beach, CA and elsewhere, many different public and private agencies provide those welfare services.

Most safety-net spending goes for children, people with disabilities, and seniors. For a conservative estimate, let's assume that Medicare recipients (17% of the total population) receive government welfare at three times the rate as the rest of the population. In 2016, welfare

c   Health care costs for 56 million seniors and disabled people in 2016

Types of treatments	Overall $ billion	Per person $
Out-of-pocket costs[5, 6] • co-payments • deductibles • Medicare Parts B and D • "Medigap" supplemental insurance • employee health benefits • non-covered health services	448	8000
Long-term care costs • nursing home care payment made by the recipient • value of home care by unpaid family and friends @$15/hour	1087 64 1023	19,400
Government programs	1007	18,000
Total	2542	45,400

spending will average about $4800 per Medicare recipient on top of health care costs.[d 7, 8]

Totaling health and welfare costs for seniors and the disabled gives an estimate of about $50,000 on average projected for 2016. With the status quo health and social services systems, the health and safety-net spending for seniors and people with disabilities will be managed largely by hundreds of federal, state, and local agencies, each with substantial overhead. In most cases, no one will be in charge of coordinating health care and social services. The extremely expensive and wasteful status quo health and welfare systems have big problems with quality and outcomes. Lack of coordination of care and lack of accountability for the overall delivery of health and social services are the central problems with quality, outcomes, and costs.

On the other hand, with ACC-based expanded care, each disabled person and senior will have a direct practice PCP within a patient-centered medical home to manage all his/her health and social-safety-net services.

ACCs Offer Seniors More Health Care Services, Less Cost

For seniors and disabled people, comparing the current status quo with ACC-based health care and social services costs is quite complicated. The analysis must take into account changes in medical premiums and taxes. These will differ depending on income and spending of the person. Average savings will be almost $3000 per Medicare recipient.[e]

d   Safety-Net Services for 56 million Seniors and Disabled People for 2016

Types of Safety-Net Services	Overall welfare $ billion	To seniors / disabled $billion	Per person $
Government welfare	500	255	
Charitable giving	26	13	
Totals	526	268	4786

e   Changes in health care spending of seniors and disabled people with ACC based care:

Savings

Each adult over 65 years-old and disabled person will no longer pay the Part B and D premiums: saving $1600 in 2016.[17, 18]

For those earning less than $60,000 per year or $120,000 per couple, personal income taxes will be eliminated (Chapter 16).

No supplemental insurance for co-payments, deductibles, and other charges will be required (i.e., Medigap insurance): saving $2800 in 2016.[9]

For individuals earning less than $60,000 per year and couples earning less than $120,000, eliminating income taxes will save additional money.

Over half of out-of-pocket costs in both cases will be in the value of unpaid family and friends as caregivers for long-term care. Unlike with the status quo, ACCs will have funds to cover a considerable amount of the long-term care at home provided by family members and friends (Chapter 6).

For current Medicare recipients, the net cost of ACC care will vary depending on income bracket, consumption taxes paid, employment by ACC (e.g., child care), etc. For seniors and disabled people who are willing and able to work full-time or part-time, ACCs will provide job opportunities.

Additionally, at the discretion of the selected ACC, further assistance may be provided in the form food, housing, transportation, etc.

Summary and Conclusion

The net financial benefit of ACC-based health care and social services for seniors and disabled people will average almost $3000 per person in 2016. Low- and moderate-income people will benefit more

---

Long-term care from currently unpaid caregivers will be partly covered, saving about $7000 in 2016: $331 billion (long-term care at home: 10 million full-time equivalent care giving jobs x $33,100 per year = $331 billion) + $64 billion (nursing home uncovered fees) = $395 billion. $395 billion / 56 million Medicare recipients ≈ long-term care saving on average $7000 in 2016.

Dental, vision, and hearing services covered by ACC care: saving $3000 in 2016.

Approximate average total savings: $1600 + $2800 + $7000 + $3000 = $14,400

Additional costs

Health premiums to ACCs for seniors (Chapter 18): $5730 in 2016.

Health premiums for younger people with disabilities: up to $7720 in 2016. Consumption taxes (with an average of 30% reduction in spending on items subject to the new taxes: $5842 per year ($1922 billion consumption taxes / 329 million U.S. residents (Chapters 1 and 21).

Approximate average total additional costs per senior or disabled person with ACC based care: $5730 + $5842 = $11,572

Approximate net average health care cost savings: $14,400 (savings) – $11,572 (additional costs) = $2828 in 2016. This does not include paying no personal income taxes for 90% of Medicare recipients.

financially because they will no longer pay personal income taxes and will probably pay less in consumption taxes (Chapter 21).

For frail seniors and disabled people, PCPs from ACCs will be authorized to pay $15 per hour for in-home care by family members and/ or friends. Consequently, those served will be more likely to remain at home rather than to be institutionalized. Caregivers will be less likely to burn out. ACCs could choose to increase funds for caregivers for the frail elderly and disabled in the future.

Given the competing demands on limited money, we should integrate and consolidate all health care and social services funding for seniors and people with disabilities to create one streamlined system. ACCs will do that. They will efficiently provide health and social services to seniors and disabled people because of coordination of care by patient-centered medical homes led by direct practice PCPs. This will be good for seniors and people with disabilities and the many well-trained, dedicated, and hardworking health-care and social-services providers. Consequently, more services may be provided at a lower cost.

Since the elderly and people with disabilities are the highest per-capita consumers of health and welfare services, ACC-based reform will benefit Medicare patients the most in decreasing net out-of-pocket costs while greatly increasing health and safety-net services received.

Chapter 26
Grand Bargains: The Urgency of Now

We have become increasingly divided as decades of worsening inequality, record waste, blatant corruption and citizen disempowerment rage on. Government regulation and corporate power strongly influence if not control health care, social services, education, agriculture, food distribution, financial services, the legal system, and other sectors. Government stalemate, gridlock, and corruption by corporate special interests are rampant. The resulting public policy quagmire has prevented actions to decentralize much power and authority now held by the government and corporations. In the mean time, government agencies and large corporations have exerted increasingly oppressive economic power over people. We need bold, decisive action to unify people around the country toward a practical, non-violent way of taking back decision-making power and authority regarding issues that directly affect them.

Congressional legislation to enact the Grand Bargains' plan to implement communitarian ACCs will be a game-changer. A Grand Bargains' bill in Congress will be perfect to focus attention on this tangible alternative to the status quo of polarized, corporate-money-funded politics. The bill doesn't have to be written by the staff of any member of Congress. Independent political policy analysts could do a great job of adapting this book to the format of Congressional legislation. The overview of the ACC portion of the legislation will be summarized in this chapter.

From now until the year 2016, U.S. society is at a crossroads: multiplying crises worse than stagnation, or an historical opportunity for a fundamental reorganization of health care and a shift to a sustainable economy. The interrelated grand bargains outlined in this book are designed to change the political and policy conversations. They will simultaneously address all of our most pressing interconnected health, social, and economic problems. These problems can only be addressed with a comprehensive network of reforms.

Led by our dysfunctional and bankrupt health-care system, the economy approaches an abyss. We need to embrace a fundamentally new economic paradigm. Moreover, a culture change toward stronger community and cooperation must commence for general healing and solving our crisis of ecological sustainability.

The Much Needed Way Forward

The network of grand bargains here described will deliver universal high value health care, dramatically increase employment, and eliminate deficit spending while also *increasing* human services. The proposed reforms in health care, welfare, and other sectors can improve public health, strengthen communities, and remove major environmental threats. With communitarianism within ACCs controlling one-third of the economy, the interconnected grand bargains will undo much institutionalized waste and inefficiencies in the public and private sectors. Simultaneously, reinvigorated free-market capitalism elsewhere in the economy will support sound economics for the general welfare.

Table 1 shows the spending projections for 2016 with status-quo assumptions contrasted with Grand Bargains-based reform. The table also presents spending projections for components of the GDP in 2025 with the Grand Bargains' plan in place. A conservative estimate for GDP growth (2.5% per year) is used. If GDP growth is higher, the benefits of Grand Bargains' reform are understated. If the GDP stalls at less than 2.5% growth, the benefits will remain strongly in force. By at least 2017, GDP is likely to be higher as 40 million new well-paying jobs are created.

Table 1. U.S. Selected GDP Projections for 2016 and 2025
Spending with Status Quo Versus Grand Bargains' Reform.

Economic Sectors	Status Quo 2016 $ (% GDP)	Grand Bargains 2016 $ (% GDP)	Grand Bargains 2025 $ (% GDP)
GDP projections	17,905 (100)	17,905 (100)	22,921 (100)
Health care[1]	3458 (19.3)	3458 (19.3)	3458 (15.1)
Social-safety-net[2] and social insurance	957 (5.3)	957 (5.3)	957 (4.2)
ACC added services			
Child care	0 (0)	333 (1.9)	425 (1.9)
Caregivers for elderly and disabled	0 (0)	333 (1.9)	425 (1.9)
Education	0 (0)	50 (0.3)	50 (0.3)
Third world country development	0 (0)	50 (0.3)	500 (2.2)
Infrastructure	0 (0)	50 (0.3)	400 (1.7)
Social Security[3]	952 (5.3)	952 (5.3)	1591 (6.9)
Housing[4,5]	2916 (16.3)	2916 (16.3)	2916 (12.7)
Financial services[6]	1400 (7.8)	1300 (7.3)	1146 (5.0)
Legal system[7]	340 (1.9)	323 (1.8)	229 (1.0)
Transportation[8]	1707 (9.5)	1807 (10.1)	1800 (7.6)
Wireless Internet (with Connection Fees)[9]	240 (1.3)	360 (2.0)	460 (2.0)
Education[10-13]	1413 (7.9)	1413 (7.9)	1811 (7.9)
Agriculture and food services[14]	1670 (9.3)	2210 (12.3)	2820 (12.3)
Military operations[15]	584 (3.3)	584 (3.3)	550 (2.4)
Other economic activity	2268 (12.7)	2109 (11.8)	4583 (20.0)

Let your imagination guess where the GDP will go in 2025 with no real reform and the status-quo policies in place.

The funding for health care, social-safety-net services, and social insurance are projected above to be frozen at 2016 levels through 2025. Medical guidelines-decentralization and major reduction in bureaucracy and ineffective medical interventions will be able to cut medical premiums while adding and/or expanding medical and social services. Waste reduction will begin with direct practice PCPs taking charge of improving health outcomes and quality of care while controlling costs. ACCs will be empowered to lead citizens in cooperatively addressing their portions of the $3.3 trillion health-related expenditures. ACCs will compete to eliminate the non-beneficial tests and treatments along with the useless bureaucracy. Money saved will thus be put to good use in providing other health and human services and lowering ACC-member premiums.

With increasing efficiencies over the next decade, ACCs will be able to increase funds for parents and caregivers at the rate of projected GDP growth (2.5%/year), allocating $425 billion for each by 2025.

The shift from government management of welfare to ACC control of social-safety-net funds will allow for tremendous waste reduction as well as increased services to those in need (Chapter 10). Rather than government welfare fostering dependence and paradoxically *increasing* unemployment, ACCs will have the resources and the mandate to administer social-safety-net spending to promote independence and the growth of well-paying jobs.

To maximize cost-effectiveness and quality of education, and minimize student debt, ACCs will experiment and innovate. ACCs will also administer an additional $50 billion per year for college and trade school students, derived from reducing health care waste and inefficiency. Additionally, national security funding administered by ACCs will include funding for post-graduate training for students planning foreign development assistance careers (Chapter 17). Education funding will keep up with the increase in GDP and will be boosted by the extra ACC-administered $50 billion per year to eliminate student debt.

The government has projected that future military expenditures will decrease as a portion of GDP over the next several years.[15] The Grand Bargains' plan would not increase or decrease those government projections. However, national security will be greatly enhanced by foreign development assistance funded through the ACCs, increasing by $50 billion per year—from $50 billion in 2016 to $500 billion in

2025 (Chapter 17). Consumption taxes will fund this vitally important program to protect our security.

Modernizing the U.S. infrastructure will employ millions of workers and make us stronger and safer. Long-term economic prosperity will depend in great part on modernizing the infrastructure and shifting it to be ready for the post carbon future.

In keeping with the retirement of baby boomers, Social Security payouts will rise about 67% over the decade without devastating consequences. No increase in payroll deductions will be needed because:

1. Forty million more workers will pay into Social Security.
2. Worker payroll deductions will be higher relative to Social Security benefits to be received because of the much higher minimum wage (Chapter 23).
3. Fewer people will receive Social Security Disability and Social Security Supplemental Income.

The average projected cost per household for housing is $23,000 annually for 2016.[4] This constitutes 45% of the income of a median income household.[a] With Grand Bargains' reform, government subsidies (mortgage interest tax write-offs, Fanny Mae and Freddie Mac loans, etc.) will no longer go to above-median-income households. This will moderate the value of high-end housing. Returning mortgage interest rates to historical norms, consistent with reasonable retirement savings rates (i.e., 4-6%), will lower all home values. Over several years, ACC-affiliated credit unions/S&Ls will buy up homes with underwater mortgages from banks (about $2 trillion) and the mortgage-backed securities that the Fed bought in quantitative easing programs (about $1.7 trillion, Chapter 24). ACCs acquiring these mortgages and writing the new mortgage loans for the low-end housing will lower the cost of low-end housing.

---

a   Housing costs: $2.9 trillion.[4] Number of households projected for the U.S. in 2016: 128 million. Median household income: $51,400.[16] The proportion of income going to housing for a median income household living in an average cost home in 2016: 45% (average cost of housing per household: $2.9 trillion / 128 million households = $23,200 per year. $23,200 /$51,400 = 0.45)

When ACC-affiliated credit unions/S&Ls are granting the new mortgages, home appraisers will no longer be pressured to fraudulently inflate appraisals. To be fair to all members, ACC-affiliated credit unions/S&Ls will have every incentive to be conservative in the valuing of properties. So, housing costs will likely remain frozen over the decade. The proportion of the GDP going to housing costs will drop from about 16.3% in 2016 to an estimated 12.7% in 2025. If citizens' median incomes increase by 2.5% per year from 2016-2025, the housing cost for the median income household living in an average cost house will drop from 45% of income now to about 35% of their income.[b]

In keeping with the projected major decrease in overall debt; personal, corporate, and governmental, financial services costs should decrease by about $250 billion/year over the next decade. With Grand Bargains' financial system reforms, the intent is for financial services to comprise no more than 5% of GDP in 2025, as it was in 1980 (Chapter 24). These reforms will serve to reduce personal, corporate, and governmental debt and to narrow the income-inequality gap.

ACCs will facilitate full employment and provide basic legal services. Enterprise liability will largely supplant medico-legal court room activities. Consequently, the overall cost of legal services is intended to decrease to 1%, as in other developed countries (Chapter 11).

The 75% tax on nonrenewable energy should reduce consumption of fossil fuels by 30% (Chapter 22). Accordingly, the transportation industry will downsize substantially with major shifts to mass transportation, bicycles, walking, and telecommuting. With innovations and financial incentives, ACCs will help members reduce their commute distances. Congestion will be greatly relieved and quality of life will improve for millions of us. The increased cost of transportation fuel (about $200 billion in 2016) will be largely offset by the decrease in automobile use and cost of traffic congestion, leaving perhaps only about a $100 billion increase in overall transportation costs (6%) in 2016.

---

b   Projected median household income in 2025 (2.5%/year increases in income): $57,900. Projected number of households in the U.S. in 2025: 144 million[17] The proportion of income going to housing for a median income household in 2025: 35% (average cost of housing per household: $2.9 trillion / 144 million households = $20,100 per year. $20,100 /$57,900 (median household income)= 0.35)

Ongoing financial incentives to decrease non-renewable energy use along with political and public pressure will further reduce fossil fuel and nuclear energy. The amount could decrease by about 5% per year from 2017-2025. Correspondingly, renewable energy production will be projected to increase by 15% per year. This concerted weaning off of fossil fuels together with innovations in energy conservation will be estimated to freeze the cost of transportation over the next decade at 2016 levels.

Agriculture and food-services costs will increase about 30% in 2016 because of the taxes on the utilization of water and non-renewable energy in producing food (Chapter 13). The increased labor costs due to the higher minimum wage and more workers needed to improve farm work conditions will also add to the cost of food. Food production and services costs are projected to increase at the rate of inflation over the next decade as ongoing ACC promotion of less food processing, more organic, labor-intensive, diversified farms and a more plant-based diet take hold. ACCs will have the responsibility of administering food subsidies, farm subsidies, and of improving the diets of members. They will be well positioned to reduce the costs of bringing fresh, healthful, affordable foods from farms and community gardens to people. The goal will be to radically reduce the $2.5 trillion per year cost to ACCs for treatment of diet and lifestyle related diseases.

Synergistic Benefits of Interconnected Grand Bargains' Reforms

The Grand Bargains' reforms are free-market oriented, but less subject to corruption by greed, crony capitalism, or special interests. The key component to this economic *and* culture change is to provide everyone with the opportunity to join an ACC (Chapter 2). Shifting about $6 trillion of our $17.9 trillion projected GDP (i.e., one-third) to competing ACCs within the private sector will empower like-minded citizens at the local level to work together. For each ACC, members and staff will get things done for the benefit of all members in ways that hyperpartisan politicians cannot do for the benefit of a sharply divided, disenfranchised, marginalized citizenry. This will allow us to move the nation ahead by reaching widespread consensus within individual ACCs on many polarizing issues in our extremely diverse country.

ACC roles in agriculture, education, financial services, legal services, and conservation will unleash American entrepreneurial innovation. ACC-affiliated B corporations (public benefit) can be created to address needs for any and all health and human services (Chapter 24). Credit union/S&Ls can provide necessary funding. ACC employment departments can find the workers.

As more and more health- and welfare-promoting ACC resources get into place, the stakeholders of each ACC will work toward optimizing available services to achieve mutually determined goals. This will create a just, fair, and sustainable course to healthful and prosperous ACC member outcomes. In this way, intractable problems can be addressed, including obesity, type 2 diabetes, drug abuse, poverty, unemployment, crime, excessive litigation, financial illiteracy, over-consumption, immigration, retirement security, deficit spending, over population, violence, and counterproductive military adventures.

Our current severe problems in health care and the overall economy will not yield to more government deficit spending or purely market solutions. Instead, our problems can be overcome by self-regulated, innovative ACCs, creating jobs and helping members improve unhealthful lifestyles. On a broader level, Grand Bargains-based reforms will allow much government spending to be shifted to ACCs while deficits are eliminated.

By creating fiscal discipline in the U.S. government, this proposed network of grand bargains can also serve as an alternative to dead-end draconian austerity measures. Each of these grand bargains provides benefits for diverse groups of stakeholders. Each seeks to find common ground that can be embraced by people of all political persuasions.

Through alignments with like-minded people in diverse ACCs, people will work compatibly toward goals that they select and that will benefit them. This will help us all and enhance environmental stewardship. The great potential for the U.S. is too precious to lose. We need Grand Bargains-based reform now.

References

Introduction

1. Cundiff DK. **Euthanasia Is Not The Answer -- A Hospice Physician's View.** 1992 Humana Press. Available at: http://www. amazon.com/Euthanasia-Not-Answer-Hospice-Physicians/ dp/089603237X#reader_089603237X

2. Cundiff DK, McCarthy ME. **The Right Medicine --How To Make Health Care Reform Work Today.** 1994 Humana Press Inc. Available at: http://www.amazon. com/Right-Medicine-Health-Reform-Today/dp/0896032841/ref=sr_1_1?s=b ooks&ie=UTF8&qid=1402703374&sr=1-1&keywords=9780896032842#read er_0896032841

3. Cundiff DK. **The Story Behind a Whistleblower Doctor License Reinstatement Hearing** KevinMD.com medical weblog; January 6, 2010. http://www. kevinmd.com/blog/2010/01/story-whistleblower-doctor-license-reinstatement-hearing.html

4. Cundiff DK. **Whistleblower Doctor--The Politics and Economics of Pain and Dying** Lighening Source Books; 2010. http://www.amazon.com/ Whistleblower-Doctor-The-Politics-Economics-Dying/dp/0976157136

5. Cundiff DK. **Money Driven Medicine--Tests and Treatments That Don't Work.** Long Beach, CA; 2006. http://thehealtheconomy.com/MDM/ExecSum-MDM.pdf

6. Diao D, Wright JM, Cundiff DK, Gueyffier F. **Pharmacotherapy for Mild Hypertension.** *Cochrane Database of Systematic Reviews.* 2012; (Issue 8):CD006742. Available at: http://onlinelibrary.wiley.com/ doi/10.1002/14651858.CD006742.pub2/abstract

7. Cundiff DK. **Anticoagulants for Non Valvular Atrial Fibrillation (NVAF) - Drug Review.** *Medscape General Medicine.* 2003; 5(1):4. Available at: http:// www.medscape.com/viewarticle/448817

8. Cundiff DK, Manyemba J, Pezzullo JC. **Anticoagulants Versus Non-steroidal Anti-inflammatories or Placebo for Treatment of Venous Thromboembolism.** *The Cochrane Database of Systematic Reviews.* 2006; **Issue 1. Art. No.: CD003746.** http://www.mrw.interscience.wiley.com/cochrane/clsysrev/articles/CD003746/frame.html

Chapter 1

1. **Culture: definition.** Wikiquote; 11 August 2013. http://en.wikiquote.org/wiki/Culture

2. **Chronic Disease Prevention and Health Promotion.** Center for Disease Control and Prevention Services HaH, 2014 Washington, D.C. . http://www.cdc.gov/chronicdisease/ Accessed January 15, 2014

3. Krupa C. **IOM Presents Blueprint to Combat Chronic Disease.** Feb. 13, 2012

4. **Soft power.** Wikipedia. November 4, 2014. Available at: http://en.wikipedia.org/wiki/Soft_power. Accessed November 11, 2014

5. Nuvark J. **Thomas Jefferson Quotes.** Free Republic Blog; November 30, 2005. http://www.freerepublic.com/focus/news/1531520/posts

6. **Promise of Value-Based Purchasing in Health Care Remains to Be Demonstrated.** RAND Corporation. March 4, 2014. Available at: http://www.rand.org/news/press/2014/03/04.html. Accessed May 8, 2014

7. **Statement on the Co-operative Identity.** International Co-operative Alliance. Available at: http://www.ica.coop/coop/principles.html. Accessed November 13, 2010

8. Vespa J, Lewis JM, Kreider RM: **Population Characteristics: America's Families and Living Arrangements.** Census Bureau U.S. Department of Commerce, 2013. http://www.census.gov/prod/2013pubs/p20-570.pdf Accessed July 11, 2014

9. **Legacies, Clouds, Uncertainties--Chapter 2: Country and Regional Perspectives.** World Economic Outlook (WEO): International Monetary Fund; October 2014. Available at: http://www.imf.org/external/pubs/ft/weo/2014/02/ Access date October 15, 2014

10. **The Future of Patient-Centered Medical Homes: Foundation for a Better Health Care System.** National Center for Quality Assurance. February 2014. Available at: http://www.ncqa.org/Portals/0/Public%20Policy/2014%20Comment%20Letters/The_Future_of_PCMH.pdf. Accessed March 11, 2014

11. Pelzman FN. **Patient-Centered Medical Homes: Is the Devil in the Details?** MedPage Today; Mar 13, 2014. http://www.medpagetoday.com/ PatientCenteredMedicalHome/PatientCenteredMedicalHome/44754

12. Pittman D. **MedPAC Iffy on Patient-Centered Medical Homes.** MedPage Today; Mar 8, 2014. http://www.medpagetoday.com/Washington-Watch/ Reform/44680

13. **CPI Inflation Calculator.** Bureau of Labor Statistics. 2014. Available at: http:// www.bls.gov/data/inflation_calculator.htm. Accessed October 12, 2014

14. **National Health Expenditures Aggregate, Per Capita Amounts, Percent Distribution, and Average Annual Percent Growth, by Source of Funds: Selected Calendar Years 1960-2008.** 2009 Center for Medicare and Medicaid Services. Department of Health and Human Services. Available at: http://www. cms.hhs.gov/NationalHealthExpendData/downloads/tables.pdf. Accessed February 6, 2010

15. Jacobson R, Feinstein A. **Oxygen as a cause of blindness in premature infants: "autopsy" of a decade of errors in clinical epidemiologic research.** *J Clin Epidemiol. .* 1992; **45**(11):1265-1287. Available at: http://www.ncbi.nlm.nih. gov/pubmed/1432008

16. Cundiff D. **Pay Health Care Aides to Jump-Start the Economy.** Health Beat; February 6, 2009. http://www.healthbeatblog.com/2009/02/pay-health-care- aides-to-jumpstart-the-economy.html.

17. Daitz B. **Filling a Need (and a Tooth) in America's Poorest Pockets.** *NY Times.* April 12, 2005. Available at: http://www.nytimes.com/2005/04/12/ health/12teet.html?pagewanted=all&position=

18. Berenson A. **Boom Times for Dentists, but Not for Teeth.** *NY Times.* October 11, 2007. Available at: http://www.nytimes.com/2007/10/11/business/11decay.ht ml?ei=5087&em=&en=39838c7fa5c22b6f&ex=1192248000&pagewanted=all

19. **World Health Organization: Social Determinants of Health.** 2009. Available at: http://www.who.int/social_determinants/en/. Accessed April 19, 2011

20. Cuckler GA, Sisko AM, Keehan SP, et al. **National Health Expenditure Projections, 2012–22: Slow Growth Until Coverage Expands And Economy Improves.** *Health Affairs.* 2013; **32**(10):1820-1831. Available at: http://content. healthaffairs.org/content/early/2013/09/13/hlthaff.2013.0721.abstract

21. Chantrill C. **Time Series Chart of U.S. Government Spending.** USGovern- mentSpending.com. 2014. Available at: http://www.usgovernmentspending. com/charts.html. Accessed April 17, 2014

22. **The Healthcare Imperative: Lowering Costs and Improving Outcomes: Workshop Series Summary.** *Excess Administrative Costs* National Academy of Sciences. 2010 http://www.ncbi.nlm.nih.gov/books/NBK53942/

23. **Employment Projections: 2012-2022 Summary.** Bureau of Labor Statistics Deparment of Labor, 2013 Washington, D.C. http://www.bls.gov/news.release/ecopro.nr0.htm Accessed June 16, 2015

24. **Liability: Patient-Centered and Safety-Focused, Nonjudicial Compensation.** In: J. M. Corrigan, A. Greiner, and S. M. Erickson,, ed. *Fostering Rapid Advances in Health Care: Learning from System Demonstrations.* Washington, D.C.: National Academy Press; 2003:81– 90. http://books.nap.edu/books/0309087074/html/81.html#pagetop.

25. **U.S. Tort Costs: 2011 Update Trends and Findings on the Cost of the U.S. Tort System.** Towers Perrin Tillinghaus. 2012. Available at: http://www.towerswatson.com/en/Insights/IC-Types/Survey-Research-Results/2012/01/2011-Update-on-US-Tort-Cost-Trends. Accessed May 13, 2014

26. **Common Good: The Problem--Drowning in Law.** 2011. Available at: http://www.commongood.org/pages/the-problem. Accessed May 13, 2014

27. Roosevelt FD. **FDR Inaugural Address, March 4, 1933.** In: Rosenman S, ed. *The Public Papers of Franklin D. Roosevelt: Volume Two: The Year of Crisis, 1933.* New York: Random House; 1938:11–16. http://historymatters.gmu.edu/d/5057/

28. **Employment Situation Summary Table A. Household data, seasonally adjusted.** Bureau of Labor Statistics Department of Labor, October 2014 Washington, D.C. http://www.bls.gov/news.release/empsit.nr0.htm Accessed November 11, 2014

29. **Historical Tables Budget of the U.S. Government.** Office of Management and Budget White House, 2014 U.S. Government Printing Office Washington, D.C. http://www.whitehouse.gov/sites/default/files/omb/budget/fy2015/assets/hist.pdf Accessed October 12, 2014

30. Choi C, Fahey J. **Workers' Protests Highlight Fast-Food Economics.** Associated Press; September 1, 2013. http://finance.yahoo.com/news/workers-protests-highlight-fast-food-130129184.html

31. Allegretto S, Doussard M, Graham-Squire D, Jacobs K, Thompson D, Thompson J. **Fast Food, Poverty Wages: The Public Cost of Low-Wage Jobs in the Fast-Food Industry.** Berkeley, CA UC Berkeley Labor Center; Center for Labor Research and Education, October 15, 2013. Available at: http://laborcenter.

berkeley.edu/publiccosts/fastfoodpovertywages.shtml Access date November 2, 2014

32. Glasmeier AK. **Living Wage Calculator**. 2014 Massachusetts Institute of Technology. Available at: http://livingwage.mit.edu/. Accessed August 6, 2014

33. de Graaf J, Wann D, Naylor TH. **Affluenza: The All-Consuming Epidemic**: Berrett-Koehler Publishers, Inc.; 2005 http://www.barnesandnoble.com/w/affluenza-john-de-graaf/1110852069?ean=9781576753576

34. **The Widening Gap Update: Issue Brief**. June 2012. Available at: http://www.pewstates.org/uploadedFiles/PCS_Assets/2012/Pew_Pensions_Update.pdf. Accessed May 10, 2014

35. Fritz M. **Pension Reform or Else**. *LA Times*. January 18, 2011. Available at: http://www.latimes.com/news/opinion/la-oe-fritz-pension-reform-20110118,0,6116807.story?track=rss

36. **The Pension Benefits Guarantee Corporation**. Unfunded Liabilities and the Coming Class War. September 21, 2009. Available at: http://unfundedliabilities-andclasswar.blogspot.com/2009/09/pension-benefits-guarantee-corporation.html. Accessed October 14, 2010

37. Chantrill C. **Time Series Chart of U.S. Government Revenue**. U.S. Government Revenue. 2014. Available at: http://www.usgovernmentrevenue.com/custom_chart. Accessed April 17, 2014

Chapter 2

1. Pittman D. **MedPAC Iffy on Patient-Centered Medical Homes**. MedPage Today; Mar 8, 2014. http://www.medpagetoday.com/Washington-Watch/Reform/44680

2. **Employment Projections: 2012-2022 Summary**. Bureau of Labor Statistics Deparment of Labor, 2013 Washington, D.C. http://www.bls.gov/news.release/ecopro.nr0.htm Accessed June 16, 2015

3. Kliff S. **When Squirrels Attack! There's a Medical Code for That**. *Washington Post*. February 14, 2014. Available at: http://www.washingtonpost.com/blogs/wonkblog/wp/2014/02/14/when-squirrels-attack-theres-a-medical-code-for-that/

4. **Statement on the Co-operative Identity**. International Co-operative Alliance. Available at: http://www.ica.coop/coop/principles.html. Accessed November 13, 2010

5. Smith M. **Is There an Rx for High Drug Prices?** MedPage Today; Jun 16, 2014. http://www.medpagetoday.com/InfectiousDisease/Hepatitis/46346

6. Pittman D. **Focus on Medicare Cost Drivers, Congress Told.** MedPage Today; May 21, 2013. http://www.medpagetoday.com/PublicHealthPolicy/Medicare/39315

7. Hamburger T, Geiger K. **Healthcare Provision Seeks to Embrace Prayer Treatments.** *LA Times.* November 3, 2009. Available at: http://www.latimes.com/features/health/la-na-health-religion3-2009nov03,0,6879249,full.story

Chapter 3

1. Sommer E. **Doctor Shortage Looms as Primary Care Loses its Pull.** *USA TODAY.* 8/18/2009. Available at: http://www.usatoday.com/news/health/2009-08-17-doctor-gp-shortage_N.htm

2. Hauer KE, Durning SJ, Kernan WN, et al. **Factors Associated With Medical Students' Career Choices Regarding Internal Medicine.** *JAMA.* 300(10):1154-1164. Available at: http://jama.ama-assn.org/cgi/content/abstract/300/10/1154

3. Kelleher K. **"Who" Not "How": The Real First Step in Health Care Reform - Primary Care Docs are Becoming an Endangered Species. Here's How to Save Them.** Manhattan Institute. July 31, 2008. Available at: http://www.medicalprogresstoday.com/spotlight/spotlight_indarchive.php?id=1760. Accessed August 25, 2009

4. Starfield B, Shi L, Grover A, Macinko J. **The Effects Of Specialist Supply On Populations' Health: Assessing The Evidence.** *Health Aff (Millwood).*http://content.healthaffairs.org/cgi/content/abstract/hlthaff.w5.97v91

5. Physicians' Foundation. **National Survey Finds Numerous Problems Facing Primary Care Doctors, Predicts Escalating Shortage Ahead.** November 18, 2008. Available at: http://www.physiciansfoundation.org/uploads/default/PF_Medical_Practice_Report_2008.pdf. Accessed June 18, 2014

6. **Primary Care Poll Results.** WebMD. August 2009. Available at: http://www.medscape.com/px/instantpollservlet/result?PollID=3192&BackURL=/px/instantpollservlet/result?PollID=3192. Accessed August 24, 2009

7. Zuger A. **Being a Patient - For a Retainer, Lavish Care by 'Boutique Doctors'.** *NY Times.* October 30, 2005. Available at: http://www.nytimes.com/2005/10/30/health/30patient.html?ei=5094&en=4dda454678e09295&hp=&ex=1130644800&partner=homepage&pagewanted=all

8. Alexander GC, Kurlander J, Wynia MK. **Physicians in Retainer ("Concierge") Practice - A National Survey of Physician, Patient, and Practice Characteristics.** *Journal of General Internal Medicine.* 2005; **20**(12):1079-1083. Available at: http://www.ncbi.nlm.nih.gov/pubmed/16423094

9. **The Patient-Centered Medical Home: A Purchaser Guide.** National Business Coalition on Health. 2008. Available at: http://www.nbch.org/documents/pcpcc_guide_070908.pdf. Accessed September 2, 2009

10. Pelzman FN. **Patient-Centered Medical Homes: Is the Devil in the Details?** MedPage Today; Mar 13, 2014. http://www.medpagetoday.com/PatientCenteredMedicalHome/PatientCenteredMedicalHome/44754

11. O'Kane ME, Barrett P. **Sneak Preview: 2014 Patient-Centered Medical Home Recognition.** National Commission on Quality Assurance. March 10, 2014. Available at: https://www.ncqa.org/Portals/0/Newsroom/2014/PCMH%20 2014%20Press%20Preview%20FINAL%20Slides.pdf. Accessed March 11, 2014

12. Zimlich R. **The Costs of Becoming Patient-Centered.** Medical Economics. MAY 25, 2013. Available at: http://medicaleconomics.modernmedicine.com/medical-economics/news/costs-becoming-patient-centered?page=full. Accessed March 11, 2014

13. **Study Finds Higher Morale, Job Satisfaction Associated With PCMH Model: Increased Chance of Physician Burnout Also a Result.** American Academy of Family Physicians. March 14, 2012. Available at: http://www.aafp.org/news/practice-professional-issues/20120314pcmhmorale.html. Accessed March 13, 2014

14. Pittman D. **MedPAC Iffy on Patient-Centered Medical Homes.** MedPage Today; Mar 8, 2014. http://www.medpagetoday.com/Washington-Watch/Reform/44680

15. Chen PW. **Medical Student Distress and the Risk of Doctor Suicide.** *NY Times. http://www.nytimes.com/2010/10/07/health/views/07chen. html?hpw=&pagewanted=all.* October 7, 2010

16. Dyrbye LN, Massie FS, Jr, Eacker A, et al. **Relationship Between Burnout and Professional Conduct and Attitudes Among U.S. Medical Students.** *JAMA.* 2010; **304**(11):1173-1180. Available at: http://jama.ama-assn.org/cgi/content/abstract/304/11/1173

17. Schwenk TL, Davis L, Wimsatt LA. **Depression, Stigma, and Suicidal Ideation in Medical Students.** *JAMA.* 2010; **304**(11):1181-1190. Available at: http://jama.ama-assn.org/cgi/content/abstract/304/11/1181

18. **Reviews & Ratings for "Doctors' Wives" (1971).** IMDb picks; 2014. http://www.imdb.com/title/tt0067004/reviews

19. Dean Ornish MD. **Dr. Dean Ornish's Program for Reversing Heart Disease.** New York, NY: Ballantine Books; 1990.

20. Ornish D, Scherwitz LW, Billings JH, et al. **Intensive Lifestyle Changes for Reversal of Coronary Heart Disease.** *JAMA.* 1998; **280**(23):2001-2007. Available at: http://jama.jamanetwork.com/article.aspx?articleid=188274

21. Ornish D, Brown SE, Scherwitz LW, et al. **Can Lifestyle Changes Reverse Coronary Heart D? The Lifestyle Heart Trial.** *Lancet.* 1990; **336**(8708):129-133

Chapter 4

1. Ornish D, Scherwitz LW, Billings JH, et al. **Intensive Lifestyle Changes for Reversal of Coronary Heart Disease.** *JAMA.* 1998; **280**(23):2001-2007. Available at: http://jama.jamanetwork.com/article.aspx?articleid=188274

2. Dean Ornish MD. **Dr. Dean Ornish's Program for Reversing Heart Disease.** New York, NY: Ballantine Books; 1990.

3. Williams KA. **CardioBuzz: Vegan Diet, Healthy Heart?** MedPage Today; July 21, 2014. http://www.medpagetoday.com/Cardiology/Prevention/46860

4. Ornish D. **CardioBuzz: 'Lifestyle Medicine'.** MedPage Today; July 31, 2014. http://www.medpagetoday.com/Cardiology/Prevention/47018

5. **Survey: Is There Enough Evidence to Recommend that Patients Eat a Vegan Diet to Prevent and Reverse Heart Disease?** MedPage Today; July 25, 2014. http://www.medpagetoday.com/survey.cfm?tbid=46940

6. Hellmich N. **Government Requires More Fruits, Veggies for School Lunches.** *USA TODAY.* January 25, 2012. Available at: http://yourlife.usatoday.com/fitness-food/diet-nutrition/story/2012-01-24/Government-requires-more-fruits-veggies-for-school-lunches/52779404/1

7. ElBoghdady D. **Schools to Serve More-Nutritious Meals Under New Guidelines.** Washington Post. January 25, 2012. Available at: http://www.washingtonpost.com/business/economy/schools-to-serve-more-nutritious-meals-under-new-guidelines/2012/01/25/gIQAFYGzQQ_story.html

8. Wickline S. **Docs to Congress: First Lady Has It Right.** MedPage Today; June 19, 2014 http://www.medpagetoday.com/PrimaryCare/DietNutrition/46402

9. Watanabe T. **Solutions Sought to Reduce Food Waste at Schools.** *Los Angeles Times.* April 1, 2014. Available at: www.latimes.com/local/la-me-lausd-waste-20140402%2C0%2C373444.story

10. Taber DR, Chriqui JF, Powell L, Chaloupka FJ. **Association Between State Laws Governing School Meal Nutrition Content and Student Weight Status: Implications for New USDA School Meal Standards**. *JAMA Pediatrics*. 2013; **167**(6):513-519. Available at: http://dx.doi.org/10.1001/jamapediatrics.2013.399

11. Wickline S. **Mrs. Obama's Lunch Plan: Not So Fast**. MedPage Today; June 23, 2014. http://www.medpagetoday.com/Pediatrics/Obesity/46459

12. Alderman L. **For Many, Health Law Offers a Chance for Preventive Care**. *NY Times*. April 9, 2010. Available at: http://www.nytimes.com/2010/04/10/health/10patient.html?_r=0

13. Russell LB. **Prevention Will Reduce Medical Costs: A Persistent Myth**. The Hastings Center. June 17, 2009. Available at: http://www.thehastingscenter. org/HealthCareCostMonitor/Default.aspx?id=3578&blogid=87870. Accessed September 3, 2009

14. Cohen JT, Neumann PJ, Weinstein MC. **Does Preventive Care Save Money? Health Economics and the Presidential Candidates**. *N Engl J Med*. 2008; **358**(7):661-663. Available at: http://www.nejm.org/doi/full/10.1056/ NEJMp0708558

15. **Medicare Reimbursement for Intensive Cardiac Rehabilitation Programs**. Preventive Medicine Research Institute. Available at: http://www.pmri.org/certified_programs.html. Accessed December 13, 2010

16. Pear R. **New Health Initiatives Put Spotlight on Prevention**. *NY Times*. April 4, 2010. Available at: http://www.nytimes.com/2010/04/05/health/policy/05health.html

17. Hook J. **Insurance Discounts for Healthy Habits Spur Debate in Washington**. *LA Times*. November 4, 2009. Available at: http://www.latimes.com/news/ nationworld/nation/la-na-wellness4-2009nov04,0,5260362.story

18. Andrews M. **Does the Law Encourage Preventive Care?** *NY Times*. May 7, 2010. Available at: http://prescriptions.blogs.nytimes.com/2010/05/07/ does-the-law-encourage-preventive-care/?hpw

19. Pear R. **Health Plans Must Provide Some Tests at No Cost**. *NY Times*. July 14, 2010. Available at: http://www.nytimes.com/2010/07/15/health/policy/15health. html?hpw

Chapter 5

1. Temel JS, Greer JA, Muzikansky A, et al. **Early Palliative Care for Patients with Metastatic Non–Small-Cell Lung Cancer**. *New England Journal of*

Medicine. 2010; **363**(8):733-742. Available at: http://www.nejm.org/doi/full/10.1056/NEJMoa1000678

2. McNeil DG. Jr. **Palliative Care Extends Life, Study Finds**. *NY Times.* August 18, 2010. Available at: http://www.nytimes.com/2010/08/19/health/19care.html?_r=1

3. **National Health Expenditures Aggregate, Per Capita Amounts, Percent Distribution, and Average Annual Percent Growth, by Source of Funds: Selected Calendar Years 1960-2008.** 2009 Center for Medicare and Medicaid Services. Department of Health and Human Services. Available at: http://www.cms.hhs.gov/NationalHealthExpendData/downloads/tables.pdf. Accessed February 6, 2010

4. **National Health Expenditure Projections 2012-2022 Forecast Summary.** Center for Medicare and Medicaid Services U.S. Department of Health and Human Services, Washington, D.C. http://www.cms.gov/Research-Statistics-Data-and-Systems/Statistics-Trends-and-Reports/NationalHealthExpendData/downloads/proj2012.pdf Accessed June 19, 2014

5. From Sally Lee (Chief Medi-Cal Operations Division) to Jonathan B. Weisbuch M **Memo Regarding a Proposed Hospice Ward at the LA County + USC Medical Center.** December 11, 1992. http://thehealtheconomy.com/WD/app27.pdf

6. Fenig EC. **'Death Panels' in Oregon?** The American Thinker. August 11, 2009. Available at: http://www.americanthinker.com/blog/2009/08/death_panels_in_oregon.html

7. Pear R. **Obama Returns to End-of-Life Plan That Caused Stir**. *NY Times.* December 25, 2010. Available at: http://www.nytimes.com/2010/12/26/us/politics/26death.html?_r=1&hp=&pagewanted=all

8. Hoffman J. **Being a Patient - Doctors' Delicate Balance in Keeping Hope Alive** *NY Times.* Dec 24, 2005. Available at: http://www.nytimes.com/2005/12/24/health/24patient.html?pagewanted=all&_r=0

9. Sack K. **In Hospice Care, Longer Lives Mean Money Lost**. November 27, 2007. Available at: http://www.nytimes.com/2007/11/27/us/27hospice.html?pagewanted=all&_r=0

10. Parker-Pope T. **Treating Dementia, but Overlooking Its Physical Toll**. *NY Times.* October 19, 2009. Available at: http://www.nytimes.com/2009/10/20/health/20well.html?ref=health

11. Cundiff DK. **Euthanasia Is Not The Answer -- A Hospice Physi-cian's View**. 1992 Humana Press. Available at: http://www. amazon.com/Euthanasia-Not-Answer-Hospice-Physicians/ dp/089603237X#reader_089603237X

12. Fisher ES, Wennberg DE, Stukel TA, Gottlieb DJ, Lucas FL, Pinder EL. **The Implications of Regional Variations in Medicare Spending. Part 1: The Content, Quality, and Accessibility of Care**. *Ann Intern Med.* 2003; 138(4):273-287. Available at: http://www.annals.org/cgi/content/abstract/138/4/273

13. Welch WP, Miller ME, Welch HG. **Geographic variation in expenditures for physicians' services in the United States**. *N Engl J Med.* 1993; 328:621– 627. Available at: http://www.nejm.org/doi/full/10.1056/ NEJM199303043280906

14. Pritchard RS, Fisher ES, Teno JM. **Influence of patient preferences and local health system characteristics on the place of death. SUPPORT Investigators. Study to Understand Prognoses and Preferences for Risks and Outcomes of Treatment**. *J Am Geriatr Soc.* 1998; 46:1242–1250. Available at: http:// europepmc.org/abstract/MED/9777906

15. Wennberg JE, Freeman JL, Shelton RM,. **Hospital use and mortality among Medicare beneficiaries in Boston and New Haven**. *N Engl J Med.* 1989; 321:1168 –1173. Available at: http://www.ncbi.nlm.nih.gov/ pubmed/2677726

16. Fisher ES, Wennberg JE, Stukel TA. **Hospital readmission rates for cohorts of Medicare beneficiaries in Boston and New Haven**. *N Engl J Med.* 1994; 331:989 –995. Available at: http://www.nejm.org/doi/full/10.1056/ NEJM199410133311506

17. Gatsonis CA, Epstein AM, Newhouse JP. **Variations in the utilization of coronary angiography for elderly patients with an acute myocardial infarction. An analysis using hierarchical logistic regression**. *Med Care.* 1995; 33:625– 642. Available at: http://www.ncbi.nlm.nih.gov/pubmed/7760578

18. Sirovich BE, Gottlieb DJ, Welch HG. **Variation in the tendency of primary care physicians to intervene**. *Arch Intern Med.* 2005; 165:2252–2256. Available at: http://archinte.jamanetwork.com/article.aspx?articleid=486758

19. Sirovich BE, Gallagher P, Wennberg DE. **Does local health care spending reflect the decisions made by individual physicians?** *J General Intern Med.* 2005; 20(Suppl 1):77

20. Barnato AE, Herndon MB, Anthony DL, et al. **Are regional variations in end-of-life care intensity explained by patient preferences?: A Study of the US Medicare Population.** *Med Care.* 2007; 45:386-393. Available at: http://www.ncbi.nlm.nih.gov/pmc/articles/PMC2147061/

21. Gawande A. **The Cost Conundrum: What a Texas town can teach us about health care.** *The New Yorker.* Available at: http://www.newyorker.com/reporting/2009/06/01/090601fa_fact_gawande?currentPage=all

22. Wennberg JE, Cooper M. **The Dartmouth Atlas of Health Care.** Center for the Evaluative Clinical Sciences, Dartmouth Medical School. 2007. Available at: www.dartmouthatlas.org. Accessed October 3, 2009

23. Nichols LM, Weinberg M, Barnes J. **Grand Junction Colorado: A Health Community That Works.** New America Foundation. August 2009. Available at: http://www.newamerica.net/files/GrandJunctionCOHealthCommunityWorks.pdf. Accessed October 3, 2009

24. **Dartmouth Atlas of Health Care.** Dartmouth Institute of Health Policy and Clinical Practice. Available at: http://www.dartmouthatlas.org. Accessed October 4, 2009

Chapter 6

1. Miller B. **Motivational Interviewing.** Available at: http://www.motivationalinterview.org/Documents/1%20A%20MI%20Definition%20Principles%20&%20Approach%20V4%20012911.pdf. Accessed July 19, 2014

2. Pittman D. **Pay and Practice: Mental Health Reform Gets Lost.** MedPage Today; Dec 18, 2013. http://murphy.house.gov/uploads/Families%20in%20Mental%20Health%20Crisis%20Act.pdf

3. , House of Representatives 113 Congress 1st session: **Helping Families in Mental Health Crisis Act of 2013,** Introduced by: Tim Murphy, December 19, 2013, Accessed July 19, 2014 http://murphy.house.gov/uploads/Families%20in%20Mental%20Health%20Crisis%20Act.pdf

4. Kupelian D. **How Evil Works.** New York, NY: Threshold Editions: a Division of Simon and Schuster; 2010. http://superstore.wnd.com/books/HOW-EVIL-WORKS-Autographed-Hardcover

5. Kupelian D. **Newtown Massacre: The Giant, Gaping Hole in Sandy Hook Reporting.** WND Commentary. January 6, 2013. Available at: http://www.wnd.com/2013/01/the-giant-gaping-hole-in-sandy-hook-reporting/

6. Kohls GG. **The Sandy Hook Massacre: The Official Cover-up Continues. Who and/or What Messed up Adam Lanza's Brain?** Global Research; December 04, 2013. http://www.globalresearch.ca/the-sandy-hook-massacre-the-official-cover-up-continues-who-andor-what-messed-up-adam-lanzas-brain/5360186

7. MindFreedom. **MindFreedom Support Coalition International. Available at: http://mindfreedom.org/about.shtml. Accessed April 28, 2006.;**

8. Krishnamurti J. **"It is no measure of health to be well adjusted to a profoundly sick society.".** Good Reads. http://www.goodreads.com/quotes/13620-it-is-no-measure-of-health-to-be-well-adjusted

9. **2013 National Drug Control Strategy.** Office of National Drug Control Policy. National Institute of Mental Health, 2014 Washington, D.C. http://www.white-house.gov/ondcp/national-drug-control-strategy Accessed June 25, 2014

10. Roan S. **At Addiction Centers, Longer Treatment Programs are Proving Key to Ending the Relapse-Rehab Cycle.** *LA Times.* November 10, 2008. Available at: http://www.latimes.com/features/health/la-he-addiction10-2008nov10,0,1225784.story

11. **Crossing the Quality Chasm: A New Health System for the 21st Century:** The Institute of Medicine of the National Academy of Sciences; 2001. Available at: http://www.iom.edu/report.asp?id=5432 Access date

12. Morgan S. **Can Electronic Medical Records Save You Money?** *WSJ.* August 24, 2009. Available at: http://www.smartmoney.com/personal-finance/health-care/can-electronic-medical-records-save-you-money/

13. Goozner M. **Why Computerize Your Medical Records?** *AARP Bulletin,* **46**(8):24. September 2005. Available at: http://www.angelfire.com/tx6/emedical-records/aarp.html

14. Pho K. **Electronic Medical Records Obstruct Patient Interaction.** MedPage Today; February 15, 2014. http://www.kevinmd.com/blog/2014/02/electronic-medical-records-obstruct-patient-interaction.html

15. Cundiff DK. **Alternative Health Care--Tests and Treatments That Don't Work.** pages 23-42, 146-148, 217-224. Long Beach, CA; 2006. http://theheal-theconomy.com/MDM/ChaptersMDM.pdf

16. Johnson KC, Daviss B-A. **Outcomes of Planned Home Births with Certified Professional Midwives: Large Prospective Study in North America.** *BMJ.* 2005; **330**(7505):1416. Available at: http://bmj.bmjjournals.com/cgi/content/full/330/7505/1416

17. Reeves KD, Hassanein K. **Randomized Prospective Double-Blind Placebo-Controlled Study of Dextrose Prolotherapy for Knee Osteoarthritis with or without ACL Laxity.** *Altern Ther Health Med.* 2000; 6(2):68-74. Available at: http://online.liebertpub.com/doi/abs/10.1089/10755530050120673

18. Uthman I, Raynauld J-P, Haraoui B. **Intra-articular Therapy in Osteoarthritis.** *Postgrad Med J.* 2003; 79(934):449-453. Available at: http://pmj.bmjjournals.com/cgi/content/abstract/79/934/449

19. Ornish D. **CardioBuzz: 'Lifestyle Medicine'.** MedPage Today; July 31, 2014. http://www.medpagetoday.com/Cardiology/Prevention/47018

20. Buescher AS, Cidav Z, Knapp M, Mandell DS. **Costs of Autism Spectrum Disorders in the United Kingdom and the United States.** *JAMA Pediatrics.* 2014; 168(8):721-728. Available at: http://dx.doi.org/10.1001/jamapediatrics.2014.210

21. Smith M. **Autism Costs U.S. Billions a Year.** MedPage Today; June 10, 2014. http://www.medpagetoday.com/Neurology/Autism/46243

22. Alderman L. **Acupuncture Is Popular, but You'll Need to Pay.** *NY Times.* May 1, 2010. Available at: http://www.nytimes.com/2010/05/08/health/08patient.html?hpw

23. Harris G. **Where Cancer Progress Is Rare, One Man Says No.** *NY Times.* September 15, 2009. Available at: http://www.nytimes.com/2009/09/16/health/policy/16cancer.html?_r=1&hp

24. Roan S. **Exploring Fibromyalgia's Mysteries, Researchers Look to the Central Nervous System, Gaining Deeper Insight nto Why we Suffer.** *LA Times.* August 22, 2005. Available at: http://www.latimes.com/features/health/la-he-fibromyalgia22aug22,0,2532080.story?coll=la-home-health

25. Hensley S. **Experimental Drug May Help Multiple Sclerosis Patients Walk.** *WSJ.* May 22, 2008. Available at: http://blogs.wsj.com/health/2008/05/22/experimental-drug-may-help-multiple-sclerosis-patients-walk/

26. Keehan SP, Cuckler GA, Sisko AM, et al. **National Health Expenditure Projections: Modest Annual Growth Until Coverage Expands And Economic Growth Accelerates.** *Health Aff.* 2012; 31(7):1600-1612. Available at: http://content.healthaffairs.org/content/31/7/1600.abstract

27. Cundiff D. **Pay Health Care Aides to Jump-Start the Economy.** Health Beat; February 6, 2009. http://www.healthbeatblog.com/2009/02/pay-health-care-aides-to-jumpstart-the-economy.html.

28. Tavares M. *Financing Dental Care.* PH210x United States Health Policy. McDonough J, ed. Edx: HarvardX. Boston, MA. 2014. Accessed June 1, 2014 https://courses.edx.org/courses/HarvardX/PH210x/1T2014/courseware/ aa06792b81e149939610aa2329aa2c97/d7b46015669e440cb9d02834e162a9fc/

29. Daitz B. **Filling a Need (and a Tooth) in America's Poorest Pockets.** *NY Times.* April 12, 2005. Available at: http://www.nytimes.com/2005/04/12/ health/12teet.html?pagewanted=all&position=

30. Oral Health in America: A Report of the Surgeon General. National Institute of Dental and Craniofacial Research, National Institutes of Health U.S. Department of Health and Human Services, 2014 Rockville, MD. http://www.nidcr. nih.gov/DataStatistics/SurgeonGeneral/ Accessed June 26, 2014

Chapter 7

1. Krista Tippett. **The Private Faith of Jimmy Carter.** Speaking of Faith from American Public Radio. 2007. Available at: http://speakingoffaith.publicradio. org/programs/jimmycarter/. Accessed October 14, 2009

2. About WIC. Food and Nutrition Service of the USDA. April 2014. Available at: http://www.fns.usda.gov/sites/default/files/WIC-Fact-Sheet.pdf. Accessed June 26, 2014

3. Adolescent Fertility Rate (Births per 1000 Women Ages 15-19). United Nations Population Division, World Population Prospects. . 2014. Accessed November 13, 2014

4. Women, Infants, and Chilfren Program (WIC) encyclopedia.com. Available at: http://www.encyclopedia.com/doc/1G2-3404000918.html. Accessed October 20, 2009

5. Frieden J. **Pay and Practice: Birth Control Cases Advance.** MedPage Today; Dec 30, 2013. http://www.medpagetoday.com/Washington-Watch/ Reform/43621

6. Liptak A. **Supreme Court Rejects Contraceptives Mandate for Some Corporations Justices Rule in Favor of Hobby Lobby.** *NY Times.* June 30, 2014. Available at: http://www.nytimes.com/2014/07/01/us/hobby-lobby-case-supreme-court-contraception.html?_r=0

7. "Listening Beyond Life and Choice" an Interview with "Catholics for Choice" founder Frances Kissling and David P. Gushee, Distinguished Professor of Christian Ethics at Mercer University. "Being" on National Public

Radio. January 20, 2011. Available at: http://blog.onbeing.org/post/2758920753/frances-kissling-on-the-limits-of-common-ground-a. Accessed June 26, 2014

Chapter 8

1. Singer E. **That Placebo Punch - Scientists are Learning to Harness the Power of Sham Treatments -- Without the Trickery**. *LA Times*. December 12, 2005. Available at: http://www.latimes.com/features/health/la-he-placebo-12dec12,0,3405707.story?coll=la-home-health

2. Timmermans S, Mauck A. **The Promises and Pitfalls of Evidence-Based Medicine**. *Health Aff (Millwood)*. 2005; **24**(1):18-28. Available at: http://content.healthaffairs.org/content/24/1/18.long

3. Tannenbaum SJ. **Evidence and Expertise: The Challenge of the Outcomes Movement to Medical Professionalism**. *Academic Medicine*. 1999; **74**:757. Available at: http://journals.lww.com/academicmedicine/pages/articleviewer.aspx?year=1999&issue=07000&article=00008&type=abstract

4. Eddy DM. **Evidence-Based Medicine: a Unified Approach**. *Health affairs (Project Hope)*. 2005; **24**(1):9-17. Available at: http://content.healthaffairs.org/content/24/1/9.long

5. Muir-Gray JA. **Evidence-Based Health Care**. Edinburgh: Churchill Livingstone; 1997.

6. Harris G. **Senator Grassley Seeks Financial Details From Medical Groups**. *NY Times*. December 7, 2009. Available at: http://www.nytimes.com/2009/12/07/health/policy/07grassley.html?ref=health

7. Wolfe S, Sasich LD, Lurie P. **Worse Pills, Best Pills**. Public Citizen Health Research Group. 2014. Available at: http://www.worstpills.org/. Accessed July 17, 2014

8. Flier J. **In Speech to Grads, Dean Flier Urges Openness to Change, Readiness for Action**. The President and Fellows of Harvard College. June 5, 2008. Available at: http://hms.harvard.edu/public/news/flier_commencement/flier_060608.html. Accessed September 2, 2009

9. Groopman J, Hartzband P. **Sorting Fact From Fiction on Health Care**. *Wall Street Journal*. August 31, 2009. Available at: http://online.wsj.com/article/SB10001424052970203706604574378542143891778.html

10. Kohn LT, Corrigan JM, Donaldson MS. **To Err Is Human: Building a Safer Health System**. Institute of Medicine. National Academy Press. September 1,

1999. Available at: http://www.nap.edu/books/0309068371/html/index.html. Accessed May 3, 2004

11. Cundiff DK. **Table 1. Consequences of Tests and Treatments That Don't Work: from Money Driven Medicine--Tests and Treatments That Don't Work.** 345-6. Long Beach, CA; 2006. http://thehealtheconomy.com/MDM/ChaptersMDM.pdf

12. **National Health Expenditure Projections 2012-2022 Forecast Summary.** Center for Medicare and Medicaid Services U.S. Department of Health and Human Services, Washington, D.C. http://www.cms.gov/Research-Statistics-Data-and-Systems/Statistics-Trends-and-Reports/NationalHealthExpendData/downloads/proj2012.pdf Accessed June 19, 2014

13. Shojania KG, Sampson M, Ansari MT, Ji J, Doucette S, Moher D. **How Quickly Do Systematic Reviews Go Out of Date? A Survival Analysis.** *Ann Intern Med.* 2007; **147**(4):224-233. Available at: http://www.annals.org/cgi/content/abstract/147/4/224

14. **American Cancer Society Guidelines for the Early Detection of Cancer.** American Cancer Society. Available at: http://www.cancer.org/healthy/findcancerearly/cancerscreeningguidelines/american-cancer-society-guidelines-for-the-early-detection-of-cancer. Accessed February 20, 2014

15. **NCI Statement on Mammography Screening.** National Cancer Institute. February 21, 2002. Available at: http://www.cancer.gov/newscenter/news-fromnci/2002/mammstatement31jan02. Accessed February 20, 2014

16. **Breast Cancer: Screening.** U.S. Preventive Services Task Force U.S. Department of Health & Human Services, 2009 Washington, D.C. http://www.uspreventiveservicestaskforce.org/uspstf/uspsbrca.htm Accessed November 15, 2014

17. Bankhead C. **Do Mammograms for Younger Women Save Lives?** MedPage Today® February 18, 2014. http://www.medpagetoday.com/HematologyOncology/BreastCancer/44263

18. Kolata G. **In Reversal, Panel Urges Mammograms at 50, Not 40.** *NY Times.* November 16, 2009. Available at: http://www.nytimes.com/2009/11/17/health/17cancer.html?hp

19. Martin DF, Maguire MG, Fine SL. **Identifying and Eliminating the Roadblocks to Comparative-Effectiveness Research.** *N Engl J Med.* 2010; **363**(2):105-107. Available at: http://www.nejm.org/doi/full/10.1056/NEJMp1001201

20. **News Release: Avastin and Lucentis are Equivalent in Treating Age-Related Macular Degeneration**. National Institutes of Health. Department of Health and Human Services, 2012 Washington, DC. http://www.nih.gov/news/health/apr2012/nei-30a.htm Accessed June 19, 2014

21. **Ranibizumab and Bevacizumab for Neovascular Age-Related Macular Degeneration**. *New England Journal of Medicine*. 2011; **364**(20):1897-1908. Available at: http://www.nejm.org/doi/full/10.1056/NEJMoa1102673

22. Martin DF, Maguire MG, Fine SL, et al. **Ranibizumab and Bevacizumab for Treatment of Neovascular Age-related Macular Degeneration: Two-Year Results**. *Ophthalmology*. 2012; **119**(7):1388-1398. Available at: http://linkinghub.elsevier.com/retrieve/pii/S0161642012003211?showall=true

23. **Myth 5. Cost Control and Quality will Emerge from Comparative Effectiveness Research**. Take Back Medicine. August 10, 2009. Available at: http://www.takebackmedicine.com/health-care-reform-myths/2009/8/10/myth-5-cost-control-and-quality-will-emerge-from-comparative.html. Accessed September 23, 2009

24. **Comparative Effectiveness Research May Not Lead to Lower Health Costs or Improve Health**. RAND Corporation. September 8, 2009. Available at: http://www.rand.org/news/press/2009/09/08/. Accessed October 2, 2009

25. Kassirer JP. **Tainted Medicine - Financial Conflicts of Interest are Raising Some Upsetting Questions Aabout the Trustworthiness of Research**. *LA Times*. April 6, 2008. Available at: http://www.latimes.com/features/health/medicine/la-op-kassirer6apr06,0,2076818.story

26. Rabin RC. **Awareness: Clinical Trial Rule Is Widely Ignored**. *NY Times*. September 4, 2009. Available at: http://www.nytimes.com/2009/09/08/health/08aware.html?ref=health

27. Corbie-Smith G, Thomas SB, St George DM. **Distrust, , and Research**. *Arch Intern Med*. 2002; **162**(21):2458-2463. Available at: http://health-equity.pitt.edu/354/1/Distrust,_Race_and_Research_%28Archives_of_Internal_Medicine%29.pdf

28. Marsa L. **Clinical Trials are Suffering**. *LA Times*. December 2, 2002. Available at: http://articles.latimes.com/2002/dec/02/health/he-trials2

29. Thomas C. **Why Big Pharma Now Outsources its Clinical Trials Overseas**. Ethical Nag: Marketing Ethics for the Easily Swayed. July 10, 2011. Available at: http://ethicalnag.org/2011/07/10/clinical-trials-outsourced-oversea/. Accessed July 17, 2014

Chapter 9

1. National Research Council. **Best Care at Lower Cost: The Path to Continuously Learning Health Care in America**Washington, D.C. 2013. Available at: http://nap.edu/catalog.php?record_id=13444 Access date

2. Fisher ES, Bynum JP, Skinner JS. **Slowing the Growth of Health Care Costs -- Lessons from Regional Variation.** *N Engl J Med.* 2009; **360**(9):849-852. Available at: http://www.nejm.org/doi/full/10.1056/NEJMp0809794

3. Liptak A. **Supreme Court Rejects Contraceptives Mandate for Some Corporations Justices Rule in Favor of Hobby Lobby.** *NY Times.* June 30, 2014. Available at: http://www.nytimes.com/2014/07/01/us/hobby-lobby-case-supreme-court-contraception.html?_r=0

4. MacDorman MF, Menacker F, Declercq E. **Trends and Characteristics of Home and Other Out-of-Hospital Births in the United States, 1990–2006.** *National Vital Statistics Reports* 2010; **58**(11). Available at: http://www.cdc.gov/nchs/data/nvsr/nvsr58/nvsr58_11.PDF

5. Johnson KC, Daviss B-A. **Outcomes of Planned Home Births with Certified Professional Midwives: Large Prospective Study in North America.** *BMJ.* 2005; **330**(7505):1416. Available at: http://bmj.bmjjournals.com/cgi/content/full/330/7505/1416

6. Diao D, Wright JM, Cundiff DK, Gueyffier F. **Pharmacotherapy for Mild Hypertension.** *Cochrane Database of Systematic Reviews.* 2012; (Issue 8):CD006742. Available at: http://onlinelibrary.wiley.com/doi/10.1002/14651858.CD006742.pub2/abstract

7. Heidenreich PA, Trogdon JG, Khavjou OA, et al. **Forecasting the Future of Cardiovascular Disease in the United States.** *Circulation.* 2011. Available at: http://circ.ahajournals.org/content/early/2011/01/24/CIR.0b013e31820a55f5.full.pdf

8. **Truth and Consequences: Health R & D Spending in the U.S. (FY 11-12).** Research America. Available at: http://www.researchamerica.org/uploads/healthdollar12.pdf. Accessed September 27, 2014

9. **National Health Expenditure Projections 2012-2022 Forecast Summary.** Center for Medicare and Medicaid Services U.S. Department of Health and Human Services, Washington, D.C. http://www.cms.gov/Research-Statistics-Data-and-Systems/Statistics-Trends-and-Reports/NationalHealthExpendData/downloads/proj2012.pdf Accessed June 19, 2014

Chapter 10

1. Therolf G. **Innocents Betrayed: County Dithered, Children Died**. *Los Angeles Times*. June 14, 2009. Available at: http://www.latimes.com/news/local/la-me-child-abuse14-2009jun14,0,2562843.story?page=1

2. Therolf G. **Two Women Sentenced for Brutally Abusing South L.A. Boy**. *LA Times*. September 5, 2009. Available at: http://www.latimes.com/news/local/la-me-child-abuse5-2009sep05,0,7957503.story

3. Therolf G, Christensen K. **Innocents Betrayed: A Times Investigation**. *LA Times*. April 21, 2009. Available at: http://www.latimes.com/news/local/la-me-innocents-betrayed-sg,0,3660047.storygallery

4. Starfield B, Shi L, Macinko J. **Contribution of Primary Care to Health Systems and Health**. *The Milbank Quarterly*. 2005; **83**(4):457–502. Available at: http://www.commonwealthfund.org/usr_doc/starfield_milbank.pdf

5. Therolf G, Christensen K. **Innocents Betrayed: Files Detail Deaths of 14 Children**. *Los Angeles Times*. April 21, 2009. Available at: http://www.latimes.com/news/local/la-me-child-death,0,2767521.story

6. Wexler R. **L.A.'s Beleaguered Foster Care Kids**. *LA Times*. September 16, 2009. Available at: http://www.latimes.com/news/opinion/commentary/la-oe-wexler16-2009sep16,0,523314.story

7. Holt-Lunstad J, Smith TB, Layton JB. **Social Relationships and Mortality Risk: A Meta-analytic Review**. *PLoS Medicine*. 2010; **7**(7): http://www.plosmedicine.org/article/info%3Adoi%2F10.1371%1372Fjournal.pmed.1000316

8. Berkman L, Syme S. **Social Networks, Host Resistance, and Mortality: A Nine-Year Followup of Alameda County Residents**. *American Journal of Epidemiology*. 1979; **109**:186–204. Available at: http://aje.oxfordjournals.org/content/109/2/186.long

9. Schoenbach V, Kaplan, B., Freedman, L., and Kleinbaum, D. **Social Ties and Mortality in Evans County, Georgia**. *American Journal of Epidemiology*. 1986; **123**:577–591. Available at: http://aje.oxfordjournals.org/content/123/4/577.long

10. Berkman LF. **Social Networks and Social Support**. 2002 Gale Encyclopedia of Public Health. Accessed October 28, 2010

11. Mayer SE. **What Money Can't Buy: Family Income and Children's Life Chances**: Harvard University Press; 1998. http://www.hup.harvard.edu/catalog.php?isbn=9780674587342

12. Brooks D. **The Limits of Policy**. *NY Times*. May 3, 2010. Available at: http://www.nytimes.com/2010/05/04/opinion/04brooks.html?src=me&ref=homepage

13. Eckholm E. **Trying to Explain a Drop in Infant Mortality.** *NY Times.* November 26, 2009. Available at: http://www.nytimes.com/2009/11/27/us/27infant.html?_r=2&ref=health

14. **Rudolf Virchow on Pathology Education from the "Path Guy".** The Group for Resesarch in Pathology Education, . Available at: http://www.pathguy.com/virchow.htm. Accessed August 9, 2014

15. McDonough J. **HarvardX: PH210x United States Health Policy,** 2014. *EdX* [Massive Open Online Course (MOOC)] Available at: https://courses.edx.org/courses/HarvardX/PH210x/1T2014/courseware/0586deb43aea411e87a9593ed7f64851/4a3a847a09024a1e81228fb3d1887246/.

16. Chantrill C. **Time Series Chart of U.S. Government Spending.** USGovernmentSpending.com. 2014. Available at: http://www.usgovern-mentspending.com/charts.html. Accessed April 17, 2014

17. **President's Budget Request Fiscal Year 2015.** VA Office of the Budget Veterans Administration, Washington, D.C. http://www.va.gov/budget/products.asp Accessed August 7, 2014

18. Luhby T. **How long should we help the unemployed?** CNN. April 23, 2010. Available at: http://money.cnn.com/2010/04/23/news/economy/extending_unemployment_benefits/

19. Zarembo A. **Disability system for veterans strays far from its official purpose.** *LA Times.* November 16, 2014. Available at: http://www.latimes.com/nation/la-me-adv-disability-politics-20141116-story.html#page=1

20. **2012 State of the Line: Analysis of Workers' Compensation Results.** National Council on Compensation Insurance. 2013. Available at: https://www.ncci.com/documents/AIS-2013-SOTL-Article.pdf. Accessed April 3, 2014

21. Dilger RJ, Boyd E: **Block Grants: Perspectives and Controversies.** Congressional Research Service U.S. Congress, 2013 Washington, D.C. . https://www.fas.org/sgp/crs/misc/R40486.pdf Accessed February 26, 2014

22. Konrad W. **An Aide for the Disabled, a Companion, and Nice and Furry.** *NY Times.* August 21, 2009. Available at: http://www.nytimes.com/2009/08/22/health/22patient.html?hpw

23. Berry MF, Reynoso C, Braceras JC, et al. **Broken Promises: Evaluating the Native American Health Care System.** U.S. Commission on Civil Rights. September 2004. Available at: http://www.usccr.gov/pubs/nahealth/nabroken.pdf. Accessed December 4, 2009

24. Belluck P. **New Hopes on Health Care for American Indians**. *NY Times*. December 1, 2009. Available at: http://www.nytimes.com/2009/12/02/health/02indian.html?ref=health

Chapter 11

1. **Common Good: The Problem--Drowning in Law**. 2011. Available at: http://www.commongood.org/pages/the-problem. Accessed May 13, 2014

2. **Disturbing Trend: From Rule of Law to Rule of Lawyers**. High Beam Research. January 1, 2003. Available at: http://www.highbeam.com/doc/1P3-280971741.html. Accessed June 27, 2014

3. McClellan MB. **Is the Tide Turning on Torts?** Ideas in Action. March 16, 2004. Available at: http://www.ideasinactiontv.com/tcs_daily/2004/03/is-the-tide-turning-on-torts.html. Accessed December 19, 2010

4. **U.S. Tort Costs: 2011 Update Trends and Findings on the Cost of the U.S. Tort System**. Towers Perrin Tillinghaus. 2012. Available at: http://www.towerswatson.com/en/Insights/IC-Types/Survey-Research-Results/2012/01/2011-Update-on-US-Tort-Cost-Trends. Accessed May 13, 2014

5. Corso R, Shores E. **Public Trust of Civil Justice**: Prepared for Common Good; June 20, 2005. Available at: http://www.commongood.org/ Access date June 27, 2014

6. Kohn LT, Corrigan JM, Donaldson MS. **To Err Is Human: Building a Safer Health System**. Institute of Medicine. National Academy Press. September 1, 1999. Available at: http://www.nap.edu/books/0309068371/html/index.html. Accessed May 3, 2004

7. Levinson DR: **Adverse Events in Hospitals: National Incidence Among Medicare Beneficiaries**. OFFICE OF INSPECTOR GENERAL, Department of Health and Human Services, 2010 Washington, D.C. https://oig.hhs.gov/oei/reports/oei-06-09-00090.pdf Accessed June 27, 2014

8. Thomas EJ, Studdert DM, Newhouse JP, et al. **Costs of medical injuries in Utah and Colorado**. *Inquiry*. 1999; **36**(3):255-264. Available at: http://www.ncbi.nlm.nih.gov/pubmed/10570659

9. Thomas EJ, Studdert DM, Burstin HR, et al. **Incidence and Types of Adverse Events and Negligent Care in Utah and Colorado**. *Med Care*. 2000; **38**(3):261-271. Available at: http://www.ncbi.nlm.nih.gov/pubmed/10718351

10. **Partnership for Patients: Better Care, Lower Costs.** Center for Medicare and Medicaid Services, U.S. Department of Health & Human Services, Washington, D.C. http://partnershipforpatients.cms.gov/ Accessed June 27, 2014

11. Graham R, Mancher M, Wolman DM, Greenfield S, Steinberg E: **Standards for Developing Trustworthy Clinical Practice Guidelines (CPGs).** Institute of Medicine, U.S. Department of Health and Human Services. http://iom.edu/ Reports/2011/Clinical-Practice-Guidelines-We-Can-Trust/Standards.aspx Accessed June 27, 2014

12. Cundiff D, Agutter P, Malone P, Pezzullo J. **Diet as Prophylaxis and Treatment for Venous Thromboembolism?** *Theoretical Biology and Medical Modelling.* 2010; 7(31). Available at: http://www.tbiomed.com/content/7/1/31

13. Lundberg G. **Stop Routinely Anticoagulating Hospital Patients.** MedPage Today. December 27, 2011. Available at: http://www.medpagetoday.com/ Columns/30403

14. Garrett AD. **Guidelines Discourage Routine Use of Heparin Prophylaxis in Hospitals.** *Drug Topics.* 2012; 156(1):35. Available at: http://connection.ebscohost.com/c/articles/70640513/ guidelines-discourage-routine-use-heparin-prophylaxis-hospitals

15. McKee J. **SCIP VTE Measures Changing in 2014.** 2013 American Academy of Orthopaedic Surgeons. Available at: http://www.aaos.org/news/aaosnow/nov13/ cover2.asp. Accessed June 26, 2014

16. Lederle FA, Zylla D, MacDonald R, Wilt TJ. **Venous Thromboembolism Prophylaxis in Hospitalized Medical Patients and Those With Stroke: A Background Review for an American College of Physicians Clinical Practice Guideline.** *Annals of Internal Medicine.* 2011; 155(9):602-615. Available at: http://www.annals.org/content/155/9/602.abstract

17. Mello MM, Brennan TA. **Deterrence of Medical Errors: Theory and Evidence for Malpractice Reform.** *Tex Law Review.* 2002; 80:1595-1637. Available at: http://www.law.stanford.edu/publications/ deterrence-of-medical-errors-theory-and-evidence-for-malpractice-reform

18. Jackson I. **Medical Malpractice Costs Drop To New Low, as Medical Care Costs Soar.** About Lawsuits; August 16th, 2013. http://www.aboutlawsuits.com/ medical-malpractice-costs-drop-new-low-51717/

19. Mello M. **The Accuracy of the Medical Malpractice System: What the Evidence Tells Us: Malpractice Insurers' Medical Error Prevention and Surveillance Study (MIMEPS).** Harvard School of Public Health. Available at:

http://www.upenn.edu/ldi/mello_accuracy.malpactrice.system.pdf. Accessed November 19, 2007

20. Underwood A. **Would Tort Reform Lower Costs?** *NY Times.* August 31, 2009. Available at: http://prescriptions.blogs.nytimes.com/2009/08/31/would-tort-reform-lower-health-care-costs/

21. Hunter JR, Cassell-Stiga G, Doroshow J. **True Risk: Medical Liability, Malpractice Insurance and Health Care.** Americans for Insurance Reform. July 22, 2009. Available at: http://centerjd.org/air/TrueRiskF.pdf

22. Holzer B. **Turning a Blind Eye To Problem Doctors.** Public Citizen. July/August 2009. Available at: http://www.citizen.org/prezview/articles. cfm?ID=18761. Accessed October 27, 2009

23. **National Practitioner Databank.** Health Resources and Services Administration, U.S. Department of Health and Human Services. http://www.npdb.hrsa.gov/topNavigation/aboutUs.jsp Accessed June 26, 2014

24. Studdert DM, Mello MM, Sage WM, et al. **Defensive Medicine Among High-Risk Specialist Physicians in a Volatile Malpractice Environment.** *JAMA.* **293**(21):2609-2617. Available at: http://jama.ama-assn.org/cgi/content/abstract/293/21/2609

25. Studdert DM, Mello MM, Sage WM, DesRoches CM, Peugh J, Zapert K, Brennan TA. **Defensive Medicine Among High-Risk Specialist Physicians in a Volatile Malpractice Environment.** *JAMA.* 2005; **293**(21):2609-2617. Available at: http://jama.ama-assn.org/cgi/content/abstract/293/21/2609

26. **National Health Expenditure Projections 2012-2022 Forecast Summary.** Center for Medicare and Medicaid Services U.S. Department of Health and Human Services, Washington, D.C. http://www.cms.gov/Research-Statistics-Data-and-Systems/Statistics-Trends-and-Reports/NationalHealthExpendData/downloads/proj2012.pdf Accessed June 19, 2014

27. **First Do No Harm: A Consumer Response to the Medical Lobby's Campaign to Limit the Legal Rights of Injured Patients-Executive Summary.** 2002 The Center for Medical Consumers and The New York Public Interest Research Group. Available at: http://medicalconsumers.org/2002/12/31/consumer-response-to-the-malpractice-crises/. Accessed June 5, 2004

28. Kravitz RL, Rolph JE, Petersen L. **Omission-Related Malpractice Claims and the Limits of Defensive Medicine.** *Medical Care Research and Review.* 1997; **54**(4):456-471. Available at: http://mcr.sagepub.com/content/54/4/456.abstract

29. Mello MM, Chandra A, Gawande AA, Studdert DM. **National Costs Of The Medical Liability System**. *Health Affairs*. 2010; **29**(9):1569-1577. Available at: http://content.healthaffairs.org/content/29/9/1569.full.pdf+html

30. **Medical Liability Reform Fast Facts**. American Medical Association. Mar 03, 2003. Available at: http://www.ama-assn.org/ama/pub/article/6282-7342.html. Accessed June 4, 2004

31. **HHS Weekly Report**. US Department of Health and Human Services. 19-25 January 2003. Available at: http://hhs.gov/news/newsletter/weekly/archive/19jan03.htm#1. Accessed June 5, 2004

32. Kessler DP, McClellan M. **Do Doctors Practice Defensive Medicine?** *Quarterly Journal of Economics*. 1996; **111**:353-390. Available at: http://qje.oxfordjournals.org/content/111/2/353.abstract

33. Krauthammer C. **Health-Care Reform: A Better Plan**. *Washington Post*. August 7, 2009. Available at: http://www.washingtonpost.com/wp-dyn/content/article/2009/08/06/AR2009080602933.html?sub=AR

34. Orszag P. **Malpractice Methodology**. *NY Times*. October 20, 2010. Available at: http://www.nytimes.com/2010/10/21/opinion/21orszag.html?hp

35. McGlynn EA, Asch SM, Adams J,. **The Quality of Health Care Delivered to Adults in the United States**. *N Engl J Med*. 2003; **348**(26):2635-2645. Available at: http://www.nejm.org/doi/full/10.1056/NEJMsa022615

36. Shojania KG, Sampson M, Ansari MT, Ji J, Doucette S, Moher D. **How Quickly Do Systematic Reviews Go Out of Date? A Survival Analysis**. *Ann Intern Med*. 2007; **147**(4):224-233. Available at: http://www.annals.org/cgi/content/abstract/147/4/224

37. Cundiff DK. **An Insider's Perspective on LAC+USC Medical Center - Rebuilding LAC+USC Medical Center Is a Mistake**. *LA Times op ed.* 11/13/1997. Available at: http://articles.latimes.com/1997/nov/24/local/me-57224

38. Cundiff DK. letter to Gina Clemmons: Chief of the U.S. Health Care Financing Administration **Re: LA County + Department of Health Services Restructuring**. March 9, 1998. http://thehealtheconomy.com/WD/app197.pdf

39. Cundiff DK. **Whistleblower Doctor--The Politics and Economics of Pain and Dying** Lighening Source Books; 2010. http://www.amazon.com/Whistleblower-Doctor-The-Politics-Economics-Dying/dp/0976157136

40. **Is Physician Peer Review A Broken System?** California Legislative Hearing. March 9, 2009. Available at: http://www.allianceforpatientsafety.org/ca-senate-report.pdf

41. Seago JA, Benroth R, McDougall B, Fernandez M, Giberson A, Daniel P. **Comprehensive Study of Peer Review in California: Final Report.** 2008 Lumetra under contract with the Medical Board of California. Available at: http://www.mbc.ca.gov/publications/peer_review.pdf. Accessed December 19, 2010

42. Schoenbaum SC, Bovbjerg RR. **Malpractice Reform Must Include Steps To Prevent Medical Injury.** *Ann Intern Med.* 2004; **140**(1):51-53. Available at: http://www.annals.org/cgi/content/abstract/140/1/51

43. Reason J. **Human error: models and management.** *BMJ.* 2000; **320**:768-770. Available at: http://www.bmj.com/content/320/7237/768

44. **Liability: Patient-Centered and Safety-Focused, Nonjudicial Compensation.** In: J. M. Corrigan, A. Greiner, and S. M. Erickson,, ed. *Fostering Rapid Advances in Health Care: Learning from System Demonstrations.* Washington, D.C.: National Academy Press; 2003:81- 90. http://books.nap.edu/books/0309087074/html/81.html#pagetop.

45. Thomas EJ, Studdert DM, Newhouse JP. **Costs of Medical Injuries in Utah and Colorado.** *Inquiry.* 1999; **36**(3):255-264. Available at: http://www.ncbi.nlm.nih.gov/pubmed/10570659

46. **The Great Medical Malpractice Hoax: NPDB Data Continue to Show Medical Liability System Produces Rational Outcomes.** Public Citizen Congress Watch. January 2007. Available at: http://www.citizen.org/publica-tions/release.cfm?ID=7497#1. Accessed February 17, 2010

47. Brennan TA, Leape LL, Laird NM, et al. **Incidence of Adverse Eevents and Negligence in Hospitalized Patients: Results of the Harvard Medical Practice Study I.** *Qual Saf Health Care.* 2004; **13**(2):145-151. Available at: http://qhc.bmjjournals.com/cgi/content/abstract/13/2/145

48. Leape L, Brennan T, Laird N, et al. **The Nature of Adverse Events in Hospitalized Patients. Results of the Harvard Medical Practice Study II.** *N Engl J Med.* 1991; **324**(6):377-384. Available at: http://content.nejm.org/cgi/content/abstract/324/6/377

49. Cundiff D. **Cut Hospitalizations to Reduce Hospital Related Medical Errors.** KevinMD.com. May 25, 2011. Available at: http://www.kevinmd.com/

blog/2011/05/cut-hospitalizations-reduce-hospital-related-medical-errors. html#more-53463

50. Garson A Jr., Engelhard CL. **The Economics of Dying**. Governing the States and Localities; March 31, 2009. http://www.governing.com/topics/health-human-services/The-Economics-of-Dying.html

51. Carson EA, Golinelli D. **Prisoners in 2012: Trends in Admissions and Releases, 1991-2012**. Bureau of Justice Statistics. December 19, 2013. Available at: http://www.bjs.gov/index.cfm?ty=pbdetail&iid=4842. Accessed May 13, 2014

52. Chantrill C. **Time Series Chart of U.S. Government Spending**. USGovernmentSpending.com. 2014. Available at: http://www.usgovern-mentspending.com/charts.html. Accessed April 17, 2014

53. **Cutting Correctly: New Prison Policies for Times of Fiscal Crisis**. Center on Juvenile and Criminal Justice. 2001. Available at: http://www.cjcj.org/uploads/cjcj/documents/cut_cor.pdf

54. Torrey EF, Kenn AD, Eslinger D, Lamb R, Pavle J. **More Mentally Ill Persons Are in Jails and Prisons Than Hospitals: A Survey of the States**: Treatment Advocacy Center and National Sheriffs' Association; 2010. Available at: http://www.treatmentadvocacycenter.org/storage/documents/final_jails_v_hospi-tals_study.pdf Access date

55. Visher CA. **Transitions From Prison To Community: Understanding Individual Pathways**. *Annual Review of Sociology*. 2003; 29:89-113. Available at: http://www.annualreviews.org/doi/abs/10.1146/annurev.soc.29.010202.095931

56. **Federal Defender Fact Sheet**. 2013 Federal Public Defender's Office for the Central District of Illinois Available at: http://ilc.fd.org/General%20Documents/FPD%20Fact%20Sheet%206%2025%202013.pdf. Accessed November 16, 2014

57. Owens SD, Accetta E, Charles JJ, Shoemaker SE: **Indigent Defense Services in the United States, FY 2008-2012**. Office of Justice Programs Bureau of Justice Statistics U.S. Department of Justice, July 2014 Washington, D.C. http://www.bjs.gov/content/pub/pdf/idsus0812.pdf Accessed September 14, 2014

Chapter 12

1. **Historical Tables Budget of the U.S. Government**. Office of Management and Budget White House, 2014 U.S. Government Printing Office Washington, D.C. http://www.whitehouse.gov/sites/default/files/omb/budget/fy2015/assets/hist.pdf Accessed October 12, 2014

2. Edwards C. **Downsizing the Federal Government: Department of Labor.** Cato Institute. 2014. Available at: http://www.downsizinggovernment.org/labor. Accessed October 15, 2014

3. **Employment Projections: 2012-2022 Summary.** Bureau of Labor Statistics Deparment of Labor, 2013 Washington, D.C. http://www.bls.gov/news.release/ ecopro.nr0.htm Accessed June 16, 2015

4. Meyerson H. **Hard times for Workers on Labor Day 2010.** *Washington Post.* September 6, 2010. Available at: http://www.washingtonpost.com/wp-dyn/ content/article/2010/09/05/AR2010090502815.html

5. Luo M, Thee-Brenan M. **Poll Reveals Trauma of Joblessness in U.S.** *NY Times.* December 14, 2009. Available at: http://www.nytimes.com/2009/12/15/ us/15poll.html?em

6. de Rugy V. **Are Small Businesses The Engine Of Growth? AEI Working Paper #123.** 2005 American Enterprise Institute. Available at: http://168.144.164.73/ New%20Updates/AEISmallBusinessReport.pdf. Accessed May 31, 2014

7. **Economic News Release: Table A-1. Employment Status of the Civilian Population by Sex and Age.** Bureau of Labor Statistics Department of Labor, Washington, D.C. http://www.bls.gov/news.release/empsit.t01.htm Accessed September 18, 2014

8. Cundiff D. **Pay Health Care Aides to Jump-Start the Economy.** Health Beat; February 6, 2009. http://www.healthbeatblog.com/2009/02/pay-health-care-aides-to-jumpstart-the-economy.html.

9. Collins G. **None Dare Call It Child Care.** *NY Times.* October 18, 2007. Available at: http://www.nytimes.com/2007/10/18/opinion/18collins. html?ref=opinion

10. Lazzaro J. **Innovative Ways to Stimulate the Economy: A Parental Stipend for Working Families.** My Daily Finance; Dec 4, 2009 http://www.dailyfinance.com/2009/04/05/ innovative-ways-to-stimulate-the-economy-a-parental-stipend-for/

11. **Population.** U.S. Census Bureau U.S. Department of Commerce, 2014 Washington, D.C. http://www.census.gov/topics/population.html Accessed June 3, 2014

12. **GREEN JOBS: A Resource Guide for Individuals with Disabilitiess.** Office of Disability Employment Policy/NTAR Leadership Center Department of Labor, 2009 Washington, D.C. . http://www.dol.gov/odep/pdf/GreenResourceGuide. pdf Accessed July 4, 2014

13. **The Voice of Agriculture**. American Farm Bureau Federation. 2013. Available at: http://www.fb.org/index.php?fuseaction=newsroom.fastfacts. Accessed May 19, 2014

14. **The 2013 Report Card for America's Infrastructure** American Society of Civil Engineering. March 2013. Available at: http://www.infrastructurereport-card.org/a/browser-options/downloads/2013-Report-Card.pdf. Accessed March 6, 2014

15. **National Average Wage Index**. U.S. Social Security Administration, Washington, D.C. http://www.ssa.gov/oact/cola/AWI.html Accessed June 3, 2014

16. **Occupational Employment and Wages, May 2013**. Bureau of Labor Statistics U.S. Department of Labor, Washington, D.C. http://www.bls.gov/oes/current/oes_stru.htm Accessed July 4, 2014

17. Gever J, Kaufman R, Skole D, Vorosmarty C. **BEYOND OIL: The Threat to Food and Fuel in the Coming Decades**. Third Edition ed: Univ. Press Colorado; 1991.

18. Lundberg J. **A review of BEYOND OIL The Threat to Food and Fuel in the Coming Decades**. The Coming Global Oil Crisis. http://www.hubbertpeak.com/beyondoil/

19. **Annual Hours per Capita and per Worker in 2002**. Available at: http://dx.doi.org/10.1787/174615513635. Accessed December 7, 2009

20. **Premiums and Worker Contributions Among Workers Covered by Employer-Sponsored Coverage, 1999-2013**. 2014 Kaiser Family Foundation. Available at: http://kff.org/interactive/premiums-and-worker-contributions/. Accessed April 26, 2014

21. **National Health Expenditure Projections 2012-2022 Forecast Summary**. Center for Medicare and Medicaid Services U.S. Department of Health and Human Services, Washington, D.C. http://www.cms.gov/Research-Statistics-Data-and-Systems/Statistics-Trends-and-Reports/NationalHealthExpendData/downloads/proj2012.pdf Accessed June 19, 2014

22. **Working time**. Wikipedia. July 2, 2014. Available at: http://en.wikipedia.org/wiki/Working_time. Accessed July 4, 2014

23. Baker D, Hassett K. **Opinion: Work-sharing Could Work for Us**. *LA Times*. April 5, 2010. Available at: http://www.latimes.com/news/opinion/commentary/la-oe-baker5-2010apr05,0,3170018.story

24. Nagel D. **10.5 Million PreK-12 Students Will Attend Classes Online by 2014.** The Journal: Transforming Education Through Technology. 10/28/09. Available at: http://thejournal.com/Articles/2009/10/28/10.5-Million-PreK-12-Students-Will-Attend-Classes-Online-by-2014.aspx. Accessed December 6, 2009

25. **Federal School Nutrition Programs.** New America Foundation. Available at: http://febp.newamerica.net/background-analysis/federal-school-nutrition-programs. Accessed May 30, 2014

26. **What is an Actuary?** Purdue University Department of Mathematics. 2010. Available at: http://www.math.purdue.edu/academic/actuary/what.php?p=what. Accessed October 26, 2014

27. Arnst C. **Study Links Medical Costs and Personal Bankruptcy (Physicians for a National Health Program).** BusinessWeek. June 4, 2009. Available at: http://www.pnhp.org/news/2009/june/study_links_medical_.php. Accessed August 7, 2009

28. **How Many People Experience Homelessness?** The National Coalition for the Homeless. July 2009. Available at: http://www.nationalhomeless.org/factsheets/How_Many.html. Accessed October 14, 2009

29. Burt M. **Helping America's Homeless: Emergency Shelter or Affordable Housing?** Washington, D.C.: Urban Institute Press; 2001.

30. Link B, Susser E, Stueve A, Phelan J, Moore RE, Struening E. **Life-time and Five-year Prevalence of Homelessness in the United States.** *American Journal of Public Health.* 1994; **84**(12):1907–1912. Available at: http://www.ncbi.nlm.nih.gov/pmc/articles/PMC1615395/pdf/amjph00463-0037.pdf

31. **Homelessness and United States Compliance with the International Covenant on Civil and Political Rights.** Submitted to the Human Rights Committee by the National Law Center on Homelessness & Poverty. May 31, 2006. Accessed October 14, 2009

32. Abdulrahim R. **Permanent Housing for L.A.'s Homeless Saves Tax Dollars, Study Suggests.** *LA Times.* October 13, 2009. Available at: http://www.latimes.com/news/local/la-me-homeless14-2009oct14,0,6561655.story

Chapter 13

1. Pollan M. **Big Food vs. Big Insurance.** *NY Times.* September 9, 2009. Available at: http://www.nytimes.com/2009/09/10/opinion/10pollan.html?_r=1&em=&pagewanted=all

2. **Lowering Cholesterol With Therapeutic Lifestyle Changes (TLC)**. National Heart, Lung, and Blood Institute Department of Health and Human Services, 2005 Washington, D.C. http://www.nhlbi.nih.gov/health/public/heart/chol/wyntk.htm#lifestyle Accessed July 2, 2014

3. Tang JL, Armitage JM, Lancaster T, et al. **Systematic Review of Dietary Intervention Trials to Lower Blood Total Cholesterol in Free-Living Subjects** BMJ. **316**(7139):1213-1220. Available at: http://bmj.com/cgi/content/abstract/316/7139/1213

4. Hooper L, Summerbell CD, Higgins JPT, et al. **Dietary Fat Intake and Prevention of Cardiovascular Disease: Systematic Review**. BMJ. **322**(7289):757-763. Available at: http://bmj.bmjjournals.com/cgi/content/full/322/7289/757

5. Writing Group for the Women's Health Initiative Investigators. **Risks and Benefits of Estrogen Plus Progestin in Healthy Postmenopausal Women: Principal Results from the Women's Health Initiative Randomized Controlled Trial**. JAMA. 2002; **288**(3):321-333. Available at: http://dx.doi.org/10.1001/jama.288.3.321

6. Howard BV, Van Horn L, Hsia J, et al. **Low-Fat Dietary Pattern and Risk of Cardiovascular Disease: The Women's Health Initiative Randomized Controlled Dietary Modification Trial**. JAMA. **295**(6):655-666. Available at: http://jama.ama-assn.org/cgi/content/abstract/295/6/655

7. Mohandas B, Mehta JL. **Lessons from Hormone Replacement Therapy Trials for Primary Prevention of Cardiovascular Disease**. Current Opinion in Cardiology. **22**(5):434-442. Available at: http://www.ncbi.nlm.nih.gov/pubmed/17762545

8. Rosenberg M. **One Chilling Reason Americans are Increasingly Overweight**. May 30, 2014. http://www.salon.com/2014/05/30/one_chilling_reason_americans_are_increasingly_overweight_partner/

9. **History of Dietary Guidance Development in the United States and the Dietary Guidelines for Americans**. 2015 Dietary Guidelines Advisory Committee U.S. Department of Agriculture and U.S. Department of Health and Human Services, 2013 Washington, D.C. . http://www.health.gov/dietaryguidelines/2015-binder/2015/historyCurrentUse.aspx Accessed

10. Edwards C, James S, DeHaven T, O'Toole R. **Downsize the Federal Government: Agriculture**. Cato Institute. 2014. Available at: http://www.downsizinggovernment.org/agriculture. Accessed May 15, 2014

11. **5 A Day**. Food and Nutrition Service U.S. Department of Agriculture, 2013 Washington, D.C. http://www.fns.usda.gov/5-day Accessed November 2, 2014

12. **Out of Balance: Marketing of Soda, Candy, Snacks and Fast Foods Drowns Out Healthful Messages**. *Consumer Reports* September 2005. Available at: http://consumersunion.org/pdf/OutofBalance.pdf

13. Rafei UM. Text of Address by Dr. Uton Muchtar Rafei Regional Director, WHO South-East Asia Region. Paper presented at: Surveillance of Major Noncommunicable Diseases in the South-East Asia Region; February 2001; New Delhi.http://apps.searo.who.int/PDS_DOCS/B3549.pdf

14. Allegretto S, Doussard M, Graham-Squire D, Jacobs K, Thompson D, Thompson J. **Fast Food, Poverty Wages: The Public Cost of Low-Wage Jobs in the Fast-Food Industry.** Berkeley, CA UC Berkeley Labor Center; Center for Labor Research and Education, October 15, 2013. Available at: http://laborcenter.berkeley.edu/publiccosts/fastfoodpovertywages.shtml Access date November 2, 2014

15. Malanga S. **U.S. Dietary Guidelines Hard to Swallow**. *LA Times*. July 18, 2010. Available at: http://www.latimes.com/news/opinion/commentary/la-oe-malanga-dietary-guidelines-20100718,0,2205200.story

16. Mangels R, Stahler C, Wasserman D. **Vegetarian Resource Group's Comments on USDA Dietary Guidelines 2010**. The Vegetarian Resource Group Blog. July 15, 2010. Available at: http://www.vrg.org/blog/2010/07/15/vrgs-comments-on-usda-dietary-guidelines-2010/

17. Edwards C. **Agricultural Subsidies**Washington, D.C.: Cato Institute; June 2009. Available at: http://www.downsizinggovernment.org/agriculture/subsidies Access date November 2, 2014

18. **Stop Subsidizing Obesity**Washington, DC: U.S. PIRG: Public Interest Research Group. Available at: http://www.uspirg.org/issues/usp/stop-subsidiz-ing-obesity Access date

19. Pianin E. **How Billions In Tax Dollars Subsidize The Junk Food Industry**. The Fiscal Times; Jul. 25, 2012. http://www.businessinsider.com/billions-in-tax-dollars-subsidize-the-junk-food-industry-2012-7

20. Smith J. **U.S. Farm Bill Proposals Come Under Fire in Europe**. *Reuters/ Washington Post*. February 1, 2007. Available at: http://www.washing-tonpost.com/wp-dyn/content/article/2007/02/01/AR2007020100375. html?nav=rss_business/international

21. **Food, Conservation, and Energy Act of 2008.** Wikipedia. 2014. Available at: http://en.wikipedia.org/wiki/Food,_Conservation,_and_Energy_Act_ of_2008#cite_note-23. Accessed May 19, 2014

22. **The Voice of Agriculture.** American Farm Bureau Federation. 2013. Available at: http://www.fb.org/index.php?fuseaction=newsroom.fastfacts. Accessed May 19, 2014

23. **Resource revolution: Meeting the World's Energy, Materials, Food, and Water Needs:** McKinsey Global Institute; Nov 2011. Available at: http://www. mckinsey.com/insights/energy_resources_materials/resource_revolution Access date

24. Klein J. **Interview of Barack Obama, Campaigning for the Presidency in 2008.** Time Magazine. October 23, 2008. Available at: http://swampland.blogs. time.com/2008/10/23/the_full_obama_interview/. Accessed November 13, 2009

25. Murphy T. **Flex-Fuel Humans.** Resilience; Apr 25, 2012 http://www.resilience. org/stories/2012-04-25/flex-fuel-humans

26. **Water Sense: An EPA Partnership Program.** Environmental Protection Agency, 2014 Washington, D.C. http://www.epa.gov/watersense/our_water/ water_use_today.html Accessed January 10, 2014

27. Kenny JF, Barber NL, Hutson SS, Linsey KS, Lovelace JK, and Maupin MA: **Estimated Use of Water in the nited States in 2005, Circular 1344.** U.S. Department of the Interior U.S. Geological Survey, 2009 Reston, Virginia:52 p. http://pubs.usgs.gov/circ/1344/pdf/c1344.pdf Accessed January 10, 2014

28. **Tackling Perverse Subsidies in Agriculture, Fisheries and Energy**Geneva, Switzerland: International Centre for Trade and Sustainable Development Programme on Global Economic Policy and Institutions; June 2012. Available at: http://www.ictsd.org/downloads/2012/06/tackling-perverse-subsidies-in-agriculture-fisheries-and-energy.pdf Access date November 18, 214

29. Cundiff DK, Lanou AJ, Nigg CR. **Relation of Omega-3 Fatty Acid Intake to Other Dietary Factors Known to Reduce Coronary Heart Disease Risk.** Am J Cardiol. 2007; **99.**(9):1230-1233. Available at: http://www.ajconline.org/article/ S0002-9149%2807%2900143-9/abstract

30. Culp P, Glennon R. **Parched in the West but Shipping Water to China, Bale by Bale.** Wall Street Journal. Oct. 5, 2012. Available at: http://online.wsj.com/ news/articles/SB20000872396390444517304577653432417208116

31. Olson-Sawyer K. **Beef: The "King" of the Big Water Footprints.** Ecocentric: A blog about food, water, and energy 08.01.2011 GRACE

Communications Foundation. http://www.gracelinks.org/blog/1143/
beef-the-king-of-the-big-water-footprints

32. **Product Water footprint**. Water Footprint Network. 2014. Available at: http://
www.waterfootprint.org/?page=files/Animal-products. Accessed November 3,
2014

33. Mekonnen MM, Hoekstra AY. **A Global Assessment of the Water Footprint
of Farm Animal Products.** Enschede, The Netherlands: Department of
Water Engineering and Management, University of Twente; 2012. Available
at: http://www.waterfootprint.org/Reports/Mekonnen-Hoekstra-2012-
WaterFootprintFarmAnimalProducts.pdf Access date January 14, 2014

34. Hoekstra AY. **The Water Footprint of Food**: Twente Water Centre, University
of Twente, the Netherlands; 2008. Available at: http://www.waterfootprint.org/
Reports/Hoekstra-2008-WaterfootprintFood.pdf Access date January 13, 2014

35. Wood S, Sebastian K, Scherr S. **Pilot Analysis of Global Ecosystems:
Agroecosystems.** Washington, DC: International Food Policy Research Institute
and World Resources Institute; 2000. http://www.ifpri.org/sites/default/files/
publications/agroeco.pdf

36. Cassman K, Wood S. **Cultivated Systems.** *In Millennium Ecosystem
Assessment: Global Ecosystem Assessment Report on Conditions and Trends.* Vol
1. Washington, DC: Island Press; 2005:741–789. http://www.millenniumassess-
ment.org/documents/document.295.aspx.pdf

37. **Endocrine Disruption: The Fossil Fuel Connection.** TEDX. Available at:
http://endocrinedisruption.org/endocrine-disruption/the-fossil-fuel-connec-
tion. Accessed December 17, 2010

38. Jackson W. **The 50-Year Farm Bill.** *Solutions,* 1(Issue #3:). July 7, 2010.
Available at: http://thesolutionsjournal.com/node/649

39. **Livestock Impacts on the Environment.** Food and Agriculture Organization
of the United Nations. November 2006. Available at: http://www.fao.org/ag/
magazine/0612sp1.htm. Accessed August 7, 2014

40. Eckholm E. **U.S. Meat Farmers Brace for Limits on Antibiotics.** *New York
Times.* September 14, 2010. Available at: http://www.nytimes.com/2010/09/15/
us/15farm.html?_r=1&hp

41. Parker-Pope T. **From Farm to Fridge to Garbage Can.** *NY Times.*
November 1, 2010. Available at: http://well.blogs.nytimes.com/2010/11/01/
from-farm-to-fridge-to-garbage-can/?hpw

42. **Your Scraps Add Up: Reducing Food Waste Can Save Money and ResourcesSan** San Francisco, CA: Natural Resources Defense Council; 2013. Available at: http://www.nrdc.org/living/eatingwell/files/foodwaste_2pgr.pdf Access date January 13, 2014

43. **FY 2015 Budget Summary and Annual Performance Plan.** USDA Office of Budget and Program Analysis U.S. Department of Agriculture. http://www.obpa.usda.gov/budsum/FY15budsum.pdf Accessed

44. Solomon S, Qin D, Manning M, et al., eds. **IPCC Fourth Assessment Report (AR4): Climate Change 2007: The Physical Science Basis. Contribution of Working Group I to the Fourth Assessment Report of the Intergovernmental Panel on Climate Change**: Cambridge University Press http://www.ipcc.ch/publications_and_data/publications_ipcc_fourth_assessment_report_wg1_report_the_physical_science_basis.htm

45. Hillman T, Ramaswami A. **Greenhouse Gas Emission Footprints and Energy Use Benchmarks for Eight U.S. Cities.** *Environmental Science & Technology.* 2010; 44(6):1902-1910. Available at: http://dx.doi.org/10.1021/es9024194

46. Weber C, Matthews H. **Food-Miles and the Relative Climate Impacts of Food Choices in the United States Environ.** *Sci. Technol.* 2008; 42(10):3508–3513. Available at: http://pubs.acs.org/doi/pdf/10.1021/es702969f?cookieSet=1

47. Saragih H. **Why We Left Our Farms to Come to Copenhagen.** CommonDreams.org for La Via Campesina. December 8, 2009. Available at: http://www.commondreams.org/view/2009/12/08-2. Accessed July 2, 2014

48. **Climate Crisis - Copenhagen - Putting Agriculture Front and Centre in the Discussions Over Climate Change.** Grain. Available at: http://www.grain.org/fr/article/entries/4160-climate-crisis-copenhagen-putting-agriculture-front-and-centre-in-the-discussions-over-climate-change. Accessed May 18, 2014

49. **Climate Change and Agriculture.** Wikipedia. May 11, 2014. Available at: http://en.wikipedia.org/wiki/Impact_of_global_climate_changes_on_agriculture#cite_note-32. Accessed May 18, 2014

50. **Food Expenditures Overview.** Economic Research Service, USDA, U.S. Census Bureau, and the Bureau of Labor Statistics 2013 Washington, D.C. http://www.ers.usda.gov/data-products/food-expenditures.aspx#.UtKqq7Q3CvE Accessed January 12, 2014

51. **Facts about Farmworkers.** National Center for Farmworker Health. August 2012 Available at: http://www.ncfh.org/docs/fs-Facts%20about%20Farmworkers.pdf. Accessed May 19, 2014

52. **U.S. Agricultural Trade.** USDA Economic Research Service U.S. Department of Agriculture, 2013 Washington, D.C. http://www.ers.usda.gov/topics/international-markets-trade/us-agricultural-trade.aspx Accessed

53. **Administration Announces U.S. Emission Target for Copenhagen.** House TW, 2009 Washington, D.C. http://www.whitehouse.gov/the-press-office/president-attend-copenhagen-climate-talks Accessed November 18, 2014

54. **Wake Up Before It's Too Late: Make Agriculture Truly Sustainable Now For Food Security in a Changing Climate. Trade and Environment Review 2013.** United Nations Conference on Trade and Development. 18 September 2013. Available at: http://unctad.org/en/PublicationsLibrary/ditcted2012d3_en.pdf. Accessed November 13, 2014

Chapter 14

1. **Bloomberg: New York City Will Collapse Without Illegal Immigrants.** Associated Press; July 05, 2006. http://www.foxnews.com/story/2006/07/05/bloomberg-new-york-city-will-collapse-without-illegal-immigrants/

2. **Rupert Murdoch, Mayor Bloomberg Lobby For Immigration Reform, Path To 'Legal Status' For Illegal Immigrants.** Huffington Post. 06-24-10. Available at: http://www.huffingtonpost.com/2010/06/24/rupert-murdoch-mayor-bloo_n_623805.html

3. Camarota SA. **Illegal Immigrants and HR 3200: Estimate of Potential Costs to Taxpayers.** The Center for Immigration Studies. September 2009. Available at: http://www.cis.org/IllegalsAndHealthCareHR3200. Accessed September 8, 2009

4. Stimpson JP, Wilson FA, Su D. **Unauthorized Immigrants Spend Less Than Other Immigrants and US Natives on Health Care.** *Health Aff (Millwood).* 2013; **32**(7):1313-1318. Available at: http://content.healthaffairs.org/content/32/7/1313.long

5. **National Health Expenditures Aggregate, Per Capita Amounts, Percent Distribution, and Average Annual Percent Growth, by Source of Funds: Selected Calendar Years 1960-2008.** 2009 Center for Medicare and Medicaid Services. Department of Health and Human Services. Available at: http://www.cms.hhs.gov/NationalHealthExpendData/downloads/tables.pdf. Accessed February 6, 2010

6. **National Health Expenditure Projections 2012-2022 Forecast Summary.** Center for Medicare and Medicaid Services U.S. Department of Health and

Human Services, Washington, D.C. http://www.cms.gov/Research-Statistics-Data-and-Systems/Statistics-Trends-and-Reports/NationalHealthExpendData/downloads/proj2012.pdf Accessed June 19, 2014

7. Wilson D. **An Airing of Border Issues, But No Coverage for 'Illegal Immigrants'.** *NY Times.* August 29, 2009. Available at: http://prescriptions.blogs.nytimes.com/2009/08/29/an-airing-of-border-issues-but-no-coverage-for-illegal-immigrants/

8. **83% Say Proof of Citizenship Should Be Required to Get Government Health Aid.** Rasmussen Reports. September 07, 2009. Available at: http://www.rasmussenreports.com/public_content/politics/current_events/healthcare/september_2009/83_say_proof_of_citizenship_should_be_required_to_get_government_health_aid. Accessed September 08, 2009

9. **Immigrants in the United States: A Profile of America's Foreign-Born Population** Center for Immigration Studies. 2011. Available at: http://cis.org/node/3876. Accessed May 27, 2014

10. DeaneAbernethy V. **The Demographic Transition Revisited: Lessons for Foreign Aid and U.S. Immigration Policy** St. Martin's Press; 1999. http://www.virginiaabernethy.com/publishdetail.php?publishid=22

11. Ehrlich P, Ehrlich A. **The Population Explosion.** New York, N.Y.: Simon and Schuster; 1990.

12. Pimentel D, Pimentel M. **Land, Energy and Water: The Constraints Governing Ideal U.S. Population Size.** Teaneck, NJ: Negative Population Growth; 1990.

13. **Population Connection: America's Voice for Population Stabilization.** 2014. Available at: http://www.populationconnection.org/site/PageServer. Accessed November 12, 2014

14. **Total Fertility Rate.** Wikipedia. 2014. Available at: http://en.wikipedia.org/wiki/Total_fertility_rate#Replacement_rates. Accessed November 7, 2014

15. Livingston G, Cohn DV. **U.S. Birth Rate Falls to a Record Low; Decline Is Greatest Among Immigrants.** Pew Research of Social and Demographic Trends. November 29, 2012. Available at: http://www.pewsocialtrends.org/2012/11/29/u-s-birth-rate-falls-to-a-record-low-decline-is-greatest-among-immigrants/. Accessed November 7, 2014

16. Kirby D. **Effective Approaches to Reducing Adolescent Unprotected Sex, Pregnancy, and Childbearing.** *J Sex Res* 2002; **39**(1):51-57. Available at: http://www.ncbi.nlm.nih.gov/pubmed/12476257

17. Hardin G. **Foreword to Abernethy, V., Population Politics: Choices That Shape our Future**. New York, N.Y. : Plenum Press; 1993.

18. **Sweet Child of Mine: Tax Credits for Parents**. 2014 Intuit: TurboTax. Available at: https://turbotax.intuit.com/tax-tools/tax-tips/Family/Sweet-Child-of-Mine--Tax-Credits-for-Parents/INF18388.html. Accessed November 6, 2014

19. Tanner M, DeHaven T. **TANF and Federal Welfare**. Cato Institute. September 2010. Available at: http://www.downsizinggovernment.org/hhs/welfare-spending. Accessed November 6, 2014

20. Passel JS, Cohn DV. **A Portrait of Unauthorized Immigrants in the United States**. Pew Hispanic Center. 4-14-2009. Available at: http://pewhispanic.org/reports/report.php?ReportID=107. Accessed August 20, 2009

21. Bazar E. **Report: Most Illegal Immigrants' Kids are U.S. Citizens**. *USA TODAY*. 4/15/2009. Available at: http://usatoday30.usatoday.com/news/nation/2009-04-14-immigrant-report_N.htm

Chapter 15

1. **The 2013 Report Card for America's Infrastructure** American Society of Civil Engineering. March 2013. Available at: http://www.infrastructurereportcard.org/a/browser-options/downloads/2013-Report-Card.pdf. Accessed March 6, 2014

2. **The Impacts of Altering Tax --Exempt Municipal Bond Financing on Public Drinking Water & Wastewater System**. National Association of Clean Water Agencies & Association of Metropolitan Water Agencies. 2013. Available at: http://www.awwa.org/portals/0/files/legreg/documents/amwanac-wamunibondanalysisjuly2013.pdf. Accessed March 8, 2014

3. **The Outdoor Economy**. The Outdoor Industry Association. 2012. Available at: http://www.asla.org/uploadedFiles/CMS/Government_Affairs/Federal_Government_Affairs/OIA_OutdoorRecEconomyReport2012.pdf. Accessed March 8, 2014

4. Lundberg J. **Food Security, sail transport, and petroleum awareness: Radio interview with Jan Lundberg**. The Sail Transport Network August 10, 2014. Available at: http://www.sailtransportnetwork.org/. Accessed November 21, 2014

5. **National Average Wage Index**. U.S. Social Security Administration, Washington, D.C. http://www.ssa.gov/oact/cola/AWI.html Accessed June 3, 2014

Chapter 16

1. Hacker A, Dreifus C. **Colleges: Where the Money Goes**. *LA Times.* September 12, 2010. Available at: http://www.latimes.com/news/opinion/commentary/la-oe-dreifushacker-college-cost-20100912,0,6821452.story

2. Gabriel T. **A Celebratory Road Trip for Education Secretary**. *NY Times.* September 1, 2010. Available at: http://www.nytimes.com/2010/09/02/education/02duncan.html?hpw

3. Holden S. **Waiting for Superman**. *NY Times.* September 23, 2010. Available at: http://movies.nytimes.com/2010/09/24/movies/24waiting.html?hpw=&pagewanted=all

4. **The Status and Trends in the Education of Racial and Ethnic Minorities**. Institute of Education Sciences, National Center for Education Statistics, U.S. Department of Education, 2010 Washington, D.C. http://nces.ed.gov/pubs2010/2010015/#7 Accessed June 5, 2014

5. Leonhardt D. **The Case for $320,000 Kindergarten Teachers**. *NY Times.* July 27, 2010. Available at: http://www.nytimes.com/2010/07/28/business/economy/28leonhardt.html?hpw

6. Dillon S. **Method to Grade Teachers Provokes Battles**. *New York Times.* August 31, 2010. Available at: http://www.nytimes.com/2010/09/01/education/01teacher.html?hp

7. Leonhardt D. **When Does Holding Teachers Accountable Go Too Far?** *NY Times.* September 1, 2010. Available at: http://www.nytimes.com/2010/09/05/magazine/05FOB-wwln-t.html

8. Izumi LT. **Help the Parents**. *NY Times.* September 6, 2010. Available at: http://www.nytimes.com/roomfordebate/2010/09/06/assessing-a-teachers-value?hp

9. Rivera C. **This Summer's Lesson: Learning is Fun**. *Los Angeles Times.* August 23, 2010. Available at: http://www.latimes.com/news/local/la-me-freedom-schools-20100823,0,1925893.story

10. Hu W. **Brick Avon Academy, A Public School in Newark with 650 Students, Began Operating on Thursday Under its Teachers' Leadership**. *NY Times.* September 6, 2010. Available at: http://www.nytimes.com/2010/09/07/education/07teachers.html?ref=homepage&src=me&pagewanted=all

11. Winerip M. **A Chosen Few Are Teaching for America**. *New York Times.* July 11, 2010. Available at: http://www.nytimes.com/2010/07/12/education/12winerip.html

12. Taylor MC. **Academic Bankruptcy**. *NY Times*. August 14, 2010. Available at: http://www.nytimes.com/2010/08/15/opinion/15taylor. html?src=me&ref=homepage

13. Quinn M. **Student Loan Debt Increases $31 Billion to $1.1 Trillion**. Red Alert Politics; May 13, 2014. http://redalertpolitics.com/2014/05/13/student-loan-debt-increases-31-billion-1-1-trillion/

14. Edwards C. **Downsizing the Federal Government: Education**. Cato Institute. May 2014. Available at: http://www.downsizinggovernment.org/education. Accessed October 15, 2014

15. **edX: Take Great Online Courses from the World's Best Universities**. MIT and Harvard. 2014. Available at: https://www.edx.org/. Accessed August 16, 2014

16. **Khan Academy: A Free World-Class Education for Anyone Anywhere**. 2014. Available at: https://www.khanacademy.org/. Accessed August 16, 2014

Chapter 17

1. **About the Department of Defense (DOD)**. United States Department of Defense Defense.gov. http://www.defense.gov/about/ Accessed December 26, 2013

2. **War**. Wikiquote. http://en.wikiquote.org/wiki/War

3. Ryan P: **Budget Functions**. House Committee on the Budget Representatives Ho, Washington, D.C. http://budget.house.gov/budgetprocess/budgetfunctions.htm Accessed

4. **The State Department and USAID Budget**. Bureau of Public Affairs U.S. State Department, 2014 Washington, D.C. http://www.state.gov/r/pa/pl/222843.htm Accessed September 23, 2014

5. **Strengthening America's Leadership in the World Through a Strategic Investment in Development and Diplomacy**. 2014 The U.S. Global Leadership Coalition. Available at: http://www.usglc.org/about/our-mission/. Accessed September 23, 2014

6. Yaqoubi A, King L. **Afghan President Hamid Karzai Again Takes a Swipe at His Western Backers**. *Los Angeles Times*. February 9, 2011. Available at: http://www.latimes.com/news/nationworld/world/la-fg-afghan-bases-20110209,0,4504815.story

7. **Time to Stop Aid for Africa?** Africa News; Feb 5, 2009. http://blogs.reuters.com/africanews/2009/02/05/time-to-stop-aid-for-africa/

8. Russell R. **R★ Foundation**. July 2014. Available at: http://rstarfoundation.org/. Accessed August 7, 2014

9. Kristof ND. **Here's a Woman Fighting Terrorism. With Microloans**. *NY Times*. November 13, 2010. Available at: http://www.nytimes.com/2010/11/14/opinion/14kristof.html?_r=1&hp

10. **FY 2015 Budget Summary and Annual Performance Plan**. USDA Office of Budget and Program Analysis U.S. Department of Agriculture. http://www.obpa.usda.gov/budsum/FY15budsum.pdf Accessed

11. **Livestock Impacts on the Environment**. Food and Agriculture Organization of the United Nations. November 2006. Available at: http://www.fao.org/ag/magazine/0612sp1.htm. Accessed August 7, 2014

12. Silverman J. **Do Cows Pollute as Much as Cars?** How Stuff Works. Available at: http://animals.howstuffworks.com/mammals/methane-cow.htm. Accessed October 31, 2014

13. Steinfeld H, Gerber P, Wassenaar T, Castel V, Rosales M, de Haan C. **Livestock's Long Shadow**. 2006 Food and Agriculture Organization of the United Nations. Available at: ftp://ftp.fao.org/docrep/fao/010/a0701e/a0701e00.pdf. Accessed August 17, 2014

14. Schwartz JD. **Greener Pastures** *Conservation Magazine*. Summer 2011. Available at: http://conservationmagazine.org/2011/06/greener-pastures/

15. Khan A. **How to Stop Two Thirds of the Earth From Turning Into a Desert**. Regenerating Grassland. Available at: http://www.regeneratinggrassland.com/. Accessed October 31, 2014

16. Piccone T, Feinberg R, Saladrigas C. **Emerging Entrepreneurs and Middle Classes in Cuba: A Soft Landing?** Brookings Institute. 2013. Available at: http://www.brookings.edu/events/2013/11/08-entrepreneurs-middle-classes-cuba. Accessed October 31, 2014

17. **Updated Budget Projections: 2014 to 2024**. Congressional Budget Office U.S. Congress, 2014 Washington, D.C. http://www.cbo.gov/sites/default/files/cbofiles/attachments/45229-UpdatedBudgetProjections_2.pdf Accessed August 7, 2014

18. Lefort R. **Thousands March in Wwave' Against Climate Change Ahead of Copenhagen Conference**. *Telegraph of London*. Dec 5, 2009. Available at: http://www.telegraph.co.uk/earth/copenhagen-climate-change-confe/6737104/Thousands-march-in-wave-against-climate-change-ahead-of-Copenhagen-conference.html

19. Murray M. **Poll: 68% Lack Confidence U.S. Will Achieve Goals Against ISIS.** NBC NEWs/Wall Street Journal; 09/14/14. http://www.msnbc.com/msnbc/poll-68-lack-confidence-us-will-achieve-goals-against-isis

20. Manning CE. **How to Make Isis Fall on Its Own Sword: Degrade and Destroy?** . *The Guardian.* 16 September 2014. Available at: http://www.the-guardian.com/commentisfree/2014/sep/16/chelsea-manning-isis-strategy

21. **Report of the Independent International Commission of Inquiry on the Syrian Arab Republic: Rule of Terror: Living under ISIS in Syria** United Nations; November 14, 2014. Available at: http://www.ohchr.org/Documents/HRBodies/HRCouncil/CoISyria/HRC_CRP_ISIS_14Nov2014.pdf Access date November 20, 2014

22. Friedman TL. **Who Are We?** *NY Times.* NOV. 15, 2014. Available at: http://www.nytimes.com/2014/11/16/opinion/sunday/thomas-l-friedman-who-are-we.html?src=me

23. **Syria Regional Refugee Response.** United Nations High Commissioner on Refugees. October 9, 2014. Available at: http://data.unhcr.org/syrianrefugees/regional.php. Accessed October 10, 2014

24. **For Palestine Refugees in the Near East.** United Nations Relief and Works Agency. October 9, 2014. Available at: http://www.unrwa.org/. Accessed October 10, 2014

25. **United Nations seminar of Assistance to Palestinian People.** United Nations. 2 July 2014. Available at: http://unispal.un.org/unispal.nsf/47d4e277b4 8d9d3685256ddc00612265/d6a17e0116af905485257d540051ddfc?OpenDocument. Accessed October 31, 2014

Chapter 18

1. **Insurance CEOs.** Sick For Profit. 2009. Available at: http://sickforprofit.com/ceos/. Accessed October 18, 2009

2. **The Bankruptcy of General Motors.** *The Economist.* June 4, 2009. Available at: http://www.economist.com/node/13782942

3. Emanuel EJ, Wyden R. **Why Tie Health Insurance to a Job?** *Wall Street Journal.* December 10, 2008. Available at: http://online.wsj.com/article/SB122887085038593345.html

4. Reich RB. **Bust the Health Care Trusts.** *NY Times.* February 23, 2010. Available at: http://www.nytimes.com/2010/02/24/opinion/24reich.html?em

5. Nylen L. **Employer-Based System for Health Insurance Should Change, But It's Complicated, Panelists Say. Commonwealth Fund.** Commonwealth Fund. March 21, 2008. Available at: http://www.commonwealthfund.org/publications/ newsletters/washington-health-policy-in-review/2008/mar/washington-health-policy-week-in-review---march-24--2008/employer-based-system-for-health-insurance-should-change--but-its-complicated--panelists-say. Accessed May 18, 2009.

6. Roffenbender J. **Employer-Based Health Insurance: Why Congress Should Cap Tax Benefits Consistently: Backgrounder #2214.** Heritage Foundation. December 5, 2008. Available at: http://www.heritage.org/research/ reports/2008/12/employer-based-health-insurance-why-congress-should-cap-tax-benefits-consistently. Accessed May 18, 2009

7. **National Health Expenditure Projections 2012-2022 Forecast Summary.** Center for Medicare and Medicaid Services U.S. Department of Health and Human Services, Washington, D.C. http://www.cms.gov/Research-Statistics-Data-and-Systems/Statistics-Trends-and-Reports/NationalHealthExpendData/ downloads/proj2012.pdf Accessed June 19, 2014

8. Martin AB, Hartman M, Whittle L, Catlin A, the National Health Expenditure Accounts Team. **National Health Spending In 2012: Rate Of Health Spending Growth Remained Low For The Fourth Consecutive Year.** *Health Affairs.* 2014; **33**(1):67-77. Available at: http://content.healthaffairs.org/content/33/1/67. abstract

9. Woolhandler S, Campbell T, Himmelstein DU. **Health Care Aadministration in the United States and Canada: Micromanagement, Macro Costs.** *Int J Health Serv.* 2004; **34**(1):65-78. Available at: http://www.ncbi.nlm.nih.gov/ pubmed/15088673

10. **The Single-Payer Path to Genuine Health Care Reform: The United States National Health Insurance Act, H.R. 676.** Physicians for a National Health Program. Available at: http://www.pnhp.org/campaign/materials/HR%20 676%20fast%20facts.pdf. Accessed November 5, 2009

11. Fisher ES, Wennberg DE, Stukel TA, Gottlieb DJ, Lucas FL, Pinder EL. **The Implications of Regional Variations in Medicare Spending. Part 1: The Content, Quality, and Accessibility of Care.** *Ann Intern Med.* 2003; **138**(4):273-287. Available at: http://www.annals.org/cgi/content/abstract/138/4/273

12. **U.S. Census Bureau, Statistical Abstract of the United States: 2012--Table 3. Resident Population Projections: 2010 to 205.** U.S. Census Bureau Commerce

USDo, Washington, D.C. http://www.census.gov/compendia/statab/2012/ tables/12s0003.pdf Accessed November 20, 2014

13. Merlis M. **Simplifying Administration of Health Insurance**. 2009 National Academy of Social Insurance, National Academy of Public Administration, Robert Wood Johnson Foundation. Available at: http://www.nasi.org/usr_doc/ Simplifying_Administration_of_Health_Insurance.pdf. Accessed July 18, 2014

14. Keehan SP, Cuckler GA, Sisko AM, et al. **National Health Expenditure Projections: Modest Annual Growth Until Coverage Expands And Economic Growth Accelerates**. *Health Aff.* 2012; **31**(7):1600-1612. Available at: http:// content.healthaffairs.org/content/31/7/1600.abstract

15. **The John Hopkins Adjusted Clinical Groups (ACG) Case-Mix System. Johns Hopkins Bloomberg School of Public Health**. Available at: http://www. acg.jhsph.edu/

16. **FY 2014 Budget Overview Table of Contents**. Social Security Administration,, 2013 Washington, D.C. http://www.ssa.gov/budget/ FY14Files/2014BO.pdf Accessed July 14, 2015

17. Liberty Mutual Research Institute for Safety. **2012 Liberty Mutual Workplace Safety Index** www.libertymutualgroup.com/omapps/ContentServer?c=cms...ʃ

18. **Department of Veterans Affairs**. Whitehouse Budget. Available at: http:// www.whitehouse.gov/sites/default/files/omb/budget/fy2014/assets/veterans.pdf. Accessed December 3, 2013

19. **2012 State of the Line: Analysis of Workers' Compensation Results**. National Council on Compensation Insurance. 2013. Available at: https://www. ncci.com/documents/AIS-2013-SOTL-Article.pdf. Accessed April 3, 2014

20. Chantrill C. **Total Budgeted Government Revenue**. US Government Revenue. 2014. Available at: http://www.usgovernmentrevenue.com/. Accessed February 23, 2014

21. **Medicare.gov - the Official U.S. Government Site for Medicare**. Centers for Medicare & Medicaid Services, 2014 Washington, D.C. http://www.medicare. gov/your-medicare-costs/costs-at-a-glance/costs-at-glance.html Accessed April 27, 2014

22. Coots D. **The Average Medicare Part D Premium**. eHow. 2014. Available at: http://www.ehow.com/facts_6825343_average-medicare-part-premium.html. Accessed April 27, 2014

23. **Ultimate Guide to Retirement**. 2014 CNN Money. Available at: http://money. cnn.com/retirement/guide/insurance_health.moneymag/index4.htm. Accessed April 27, 2014

24. **Premiums and Worker Contributions Among Workers Covered by Employer-Sponsored Coverage, 1999-2013**. 2014 Kaiser Family Foundation. Available at: http://kff.org/interactive/premiums-and-worker-contributions/. Accessed April 26, 2014

25. **Donations Barely Rose Last Year as Individuals Held Back**. Giving USA Foundation. June 17, 2013. Available at: http://philanthropy.com/article/ Fundraisings-Recovery-Could/139801/?cid=pt&utm_source=pt&utm_ medium=en. Accessed April 27, 2014

Chapter 19

1. Goodman DC, Stukel TA, Chang C-h, Wennberg JE. **End-Of-Life Care At Academic Medical Centers: Implications For Future Workforce Requirements. 10.1377/hlthaff.25.2.521**. *Health Aff.* 25(2):521-531. Available at: http://content.healthaffairs.org/cgi/content/abstract/25/2/521

2. Fisher ES, Wennberg DE, Stukel TA, Gottlieb DJ, Lucas FL, Pinder EL. **The Implications of Regional Variations in Medicare Spending. Part 1: The Content, Quality, and Accessibility of Care**. *Ann Intern Med.* 2003; 138(4):273-287. Available at: http://www.annals.org/cgi/content/abstract/138/4/273

3. Cundiff DK. **Audit of Hospitalized Patients at LA County + USC Medical Center: from Money Driven Medicine--Tests and Treatments That Don't Work**. 427–446. Long Beach, CA; 2006. http://thehealtheconomy.com/MDM/ ChaptersMDM.pdf

4. Cundiff DK. Gina Clemons - Chief of U.S. Health Care Financing Administration **Letter regarding fraudulent Medicaid billing at LA County + USC Medical Center.** http://thehealtheconomy.com/WD/app197.pdf

5. Lopez G. **Report: The VA Ignored Whistleblowers' Warnings for Years**. Vox; June 23, 2014. http://www.vox.com/2014/6/23/5834844/ report-the-va-ignored-whistleblowers-warnings-for-years

6. Jauhar S. **A Doctor by Choice, a Businessman by Necessity**. *NY Times.* July 6, 2009. Available at: http://www.nytimes.com/2009/07/07/health/07essa.html

7. Hartzband P, Groopman J. **Money and the Changing Culture of Medicine**. *N Engl J Med.* 2009; 360(2):101-103. Available at: http://nejm-journals.blogspot. com/2009/01/money-and-changing-culture-of-medicine.html

8. Martin AB, Hartman M, Whittle L, Catlin A, the National Health Expenditure Accounts Team. **National Health Spending In 2012: Rate Of Health Spending Growth Remained Low For The Fourth Consecutive Year.** *Health Affairs.* 2014; 33(1):67-77. Available at: http://content.healthaffairs.org/content/33/1/67. abstract

9. Chantrill C. **Time Series Chart of U.S. Government Revenue.** U.S. Government Revenue. 2014. Available at: http://www.usgovernmentrevenue. com/custom_chart. Accessed April 17, 2014

10. **2012 State of the Line: Analysis of Workers' Compensation Results.** National Council on Compensation Insurance. 2013. Available at: https://www. ncci.com/documents/AIS-2013-SOTL-Article.pdf. Accessed April 3, 2014

11. **Historical Tables Budget of the U.S. Government.** Office of Management and Budget White House, 2014 U.S. Government Printing Office Washington, D.C. http://www.whitehouse.gov/sites/default/files/omb/budget/fy2015/assets/hist. pdf Accessed October 12, 2014

12. Edwards C. **Downsizing the Federal Government: Department of Labor.** Cato Institute. 2014. Available at: http://www.downsizinggovernment.org/labor. Accessed October 15, 2014

13. Edwards C, James S, DeHaven T, O'Toole R. **Downsize the Federal Government: Agriculture.** Cato Institute. 2014. Available at: http://www. downsizinggovernment.org/agriculture. Accessed May 15, 2014

14. **President's Budget Request Fiscal Year 2015.** VA Office of the Budget. Veterans Administration, Washington, D.C. http://www.va.gov/budget/products.asp Accessed August 7, 2014

15. **Retirement and Education Savings (Chapter 7): A Review of Trends and Activities in the U.S. Investment Company Industry.** *2014 Investment Company Fact Book*: Investment Company Institute; 2014. http://www.icifactbook.org/fb_ch7.html

16. Isaacs KP. **Federal Employees' Retirement System: Budget and Trust Fund Issues. Analyst in Income Security.** Congressional Research Service March 24, 2014. Available at: http://fas.org/sgp/crs/misc/RL30023.pdf. Accessed November 9, 2014

17. **Personal Savings in the United States from 2002 to 2013** Statistica: The Statistics Portal. 2014. Available at: http://www.statista.com/statistics/246261/ total-personal-savings-in-the-united-states/. Accessed November 9, 2014

18. Woolhandler S, Campbell T, Himmelstein DU. **Costs of Health Care Administration in the United States and Canada**. *N Engl J Med.* 2003; **349**(8):768-775. Available at: http://www.nejm.org/doi/full/10.1056/NEJMsa022033

19. Woolhandler S, Campbell T, Himmelstein DU. **Health Care Administration in the United States and Canada: Micromanagement, Macro Costs.** *Int J Health Serv.* 2004; **34**(1):65-78. Available at: http://www.ncbi.nlm.nih.gov/pubmed/15088673

20. **The Healthcare Imperative: Lowering Costs and Improving Outcomes: Workshop Series Summary.** *Excess Administrative Costs* National Academy of Sciences. 2010 http://www.ncbi.nlm.nih.gov/books/NBK53942/

21. Pecquet J. **Community Health Centers Seen as Key to Reducing Emergency Room Cost**. Healthwatch. 05/11/11. Available at: http://thehill.com/blogs/healthwatch/other/160555-community-health-centers-seen-as-key-to-reducing-emergency-room-cost

22. Chantrill C. **Time Series Chart of U.S. Government Spending**. USGovernmentSpending.com. 2014. Available at: http://www.usgovern-mentspending.com/charts.html. Accessed April 17, 2014

23. Wilson R. **Health Care Spending Still Rising for States and Cities**. January 31, 2014. http://www.washingtonpost.com/blogs/govbeat/wp/2014/01/31/health-care-spending-still-rising-for-states-and-cities/

24. Petterson SM, Liaw WR, Phillips RL, Rabin DL, Meyers DS, Bazemore AW. **Projecting US Primary Care Physician Workforce Needs: 2010-2025.** *The Annals of Family Medicine.* 2012; **10**(6):503-509. Available at: http://www.an-nfammed.org/content/10/6/503.abstract

25. **MGMA Survey: Physician Compensation Includes Quality and Patient Satisfaction Components.** Medical Group Management Association. June 12, 2013. Available at: http://www.mgma.com/about/mgma-press-room/press-releases/physician-compensation-includes-quality-and-patient-satisfaction-component. Accessed April 14, 2014

26. Hartman B. **Can NPs and PAs Fill the Primary Care Gap?** MedPage Today; Sep 17, 2013 http://www.medpagetoday.com/PublicHealthPolicy/WorkForce/41678

27. **U.S. Census Bureau, Statistical Abstract of the United States: 2012--Table 3. Resident Population Projections: 2010 to 2050.** U.S. Census Bureau

Commerce USDo, Washington, D.C. http://www.census.gov/compendia/ statab/2012/tables/12s0003.pdf Accessed November 20, 2014

28. Schock A: **H.R. 1201: Training Tomorrow's Doctors Today Act**. US House of Representatives, 2013 Washington, DC. https://www.govtrack.us/congress/ bills/113/hr1201 Accessed August 10, 2014

29. Nelson B: **S. 577: Resident Physician Shortage Reduction Act of 2013**. US Senate 2013 Washington, DC. https://www.govtrack.us/congress/bills/113/s577 Accessed July 19, 2015

30. Herz EJ, Tilson S. **Medicaid and Graduate Medical Education**. Congressional Research Service: Health Care Financing, Domestic Social Policy Division. June 20, 2008. Available at: http://assets.opencrs.com/rpts/RS22852_20080401.pdf. Accessed October 15, 2009

31. Wynn B, Guarino C, Morse L, Cho M. **Alternative Ways of Financing Graduate Medical Education. Report to the Office of the Assistant Secretary for Planning and Evaluation, Department of Health and Human Services**Santa Monica, CA: RAND Health; May 2006. Available at: http://aspe. hhs.gov/health/reports/06/AltGradMedicalEdu/report.pdf Access date

32. Keehan SP, Cuckler GA, Sisko AM, et al. **National Health Expenditure Projections: Modest Annual Growth Until Coverage Expands And Economic Growth Accelerates**. *Health Aff*. 2012; **31**(7):1600-1612. Available at: http:// content.healthaffairs.org/content/31/7/1600.abstract

33. **AAMC Remains Concerned About Shortage of Residency Positions Despite Successful Match Day**. Association of American Medical Colleges. March 21, 2014. Available at: https://www.aamc.org/newsroom/newsre-leases/374000/03212014.html. Accessed April 15, 2014

34. Starfield B, Fryer GE, Jr. **The Primary Care Physician Workforce: Ethical and Policy Implications**. *Ann Fam Med*. **5**(6):486-491. Available at: http://www. annfammed.org/cgi/content/abstract/5/6/486

35. Youngclaus JJ, Fresne JA. **Physician Education Debt and the Cost to Attend Medical School 2012 Update**. 2013 Association of American Medical Colleges. Available at: https://www.aamc.org/download/328322/data/statedebtreport.pdf. Accessed April 15, 2014

36. **Medical Student Education: Debt, Costs, and Loan Repayment Fact Card**. 2013 Association of American Medical Colleges. Available at: https://www.aamc. org/download/152968/data/debtfactcard.pdf. Accessed April 17, 2014

Chapter 20

1. Kolata G. **Tackling the Mystery of How Much It Costs.** *NY Times.* August 18, 2009. Available at: http://www.nytimes.com/2009/08/19/health/policy/19fees.html?ref=health

2. Keehan SP, Cuckler GA, Sisko AM, et al. **National Health Expenditure Projections: Modest Annual Growth Until Coverage Expands And Economic Growth Accelerates.** *Health Aff.* 2012; **31**(7):1600-1612. Available at: http://content.healthaffairs.org/content/31/7/1600.abstract

3. Hartman M, Martin A, Nuccio O, Catlin A, the National Health Expenditure Accounts Team. **Health Spending Growth At A Historic Low In 2008.** *Health Aff.* **29**(1):147-155. Available at: http://content.healthaffairs.org/cgi/content/abstract/29/1/147

4. Cundiff DK. **Invasive Cardiology Procedures – A $160 Billion Placebo: from Money Driven Medicine--Tests and Treatments That Don't Work.** 137-148. Long Beach, CA; 2006. http://thehealtheconomy.com/MDM/ChaptersMDM.pdf

5. Pittman D. **Focus on Medicare Cost Drivers, Congress Told.** MedPage Today; May 21, 2013. http://www.medpagetoday.com/PublicHealthPolicy/Medicare/39315

6. Fisher ES, Bynum JP, Skinner JS. **Slowing the Growth of Health Care Costs -- Lessons from Regional Variation.** *N Engl J Med.* 2009; **360**(9):849-852. Available at: http://www.nejm.org/doi/full/10.1056/NEJMp0809794

7. Leonhardt D. **Making Health Care Better.** *NY Times.* November 3, 2009. Available at: http://www.nytimes.com/2009/11/08/magazine/08Healthcare-t.html?_r=1&pagewanted=all

8. Adler J, Interlandi J. **The Hospital That Could Cure Health Care: Cleveland Clinic is Both Highly Effective and Fiercely Efficient. So Why are Its Methods so Rare?** *Newsweek.* Nov 27, 2009. Available at: http://www.newsweek.com/id/224585/page/1

9. Leonhardt D. **Health Care Rationing Rhetoric Overlooks Reality. NY Times.** *NY Times.* June 17, 2009. Available at: http://www.nytimes.com/2009/06/17/business/economy/17leonhardt.html?em

10. Wilper AP, Woolhandler S, Lasser KE, McCormick D, Bor DH, Himmelstein DU. **Health Insurance and Mortality in US Adults.** *American Journal of Public Health.* 2009; **99**(12):2289-2295. Available at: http://www.pnhp.org/excess-deaths/health-insurance-and-mortality-in-US-adults.pdf

11. Weissman JS, Schneider EC, Weingart SN. **Comparing Patient-Reported Hospital Adverse Events with Medical Record Review: Do Patients Know Something That Hospitals Do Not?** *Ann Intern Med.* 2008; **149**(2):100-108. Available at: http://annals.org/article.aspx?articleid=741736

12. **Hospital-Acquired Infection.** Wikipedia. April 22, 2014. Available at: http://en.wikipedia.org/wiki/Hospital-acquired_infection. Accessed April 29, 2014

13. Jauhar S. **To Curb Repeat Hospital Stays, Pay Doctors.** *NY Times.* November 30, 2009. Available at: http://www.nytimes.com/2009/12/01/health/01essay.html?_r=1&emc=eta1

14. **Four Million Hospital Admissions Potentially Unnecessary.** Agency for Healthcare Research and Quality Archive U.S. Department of Health and Human Services, Rockville , MD. http://archive.ahrq.gov/news/newsletters/research-activities/dec10/1210RA22.html Accessed June 27, 2014

15. Cundiff DK. **Table 1. Consequences of Tests and Treatments That Don't Work: from Money Driven Medicine--Tests and Treatments That Don't Work.** 345-6. Long Beach, CA; 2006. http://thehealtheconomy.com/MDM/ChaptersMDM.pdf

16. Leff B, Burton L, Mader SL. **Hospital at Home: Feasibility and Outcomes of a Program To Provide Hospital-Level Care at Home for Acutely Ill Older Patients.** *Ann Intern Med.*; **143**(11):798-808. Available at: http://www.annals.org/content/143/11/I-56.long

17. Gross J. **Why House Calls Save Money.** *NY Times.* January 12, 2009. Available at: http://newoldage.blogs.nytimes.com/2009/01/12/why-house-calls-save-money/?hp

18. Jencks SF, Williams MV, Coleman EA. **Rehospitalizations among Patients in the Medicare Fee-for-Service Program.** *N Engl J Med.* 2009; **360**(14):1418-1428. Available at: http://content.nejm.org/cgi/content/abstract/360/14/1418

19. Jauhar S. **Referral System Turns Patients Into Commodities.** *NY Times.* May 25, 2009. Available at: http://www.nytimes.com/2009/05/26/health/26essa.html?_r=1&emc=eta1

20. Forrest CB. **Primary Care Gatekeeping and Referrals: Eeffective Filter or Failed Experiment?** *BMJ.* Mar 29, 2003; **326**(7391):692–695. Available at: http://www.ncbi.nlm.nih.gov/pmc/articles/PMC152368/

21. Pollack A. **Questioning a $30,000-a-Month Cancer Drug.** *NY Times.* December 4, 2009. Available at: http://www.nytimes.com/2009/12/05/health/05drug.html?_r=1&hp=&pagewanted=all

22. Geiger K, Hamburger T. **A Broader Definition of Healthcare.** *LA Times.* December 6, 2009. Available at: http://www.latimes.com/news/nation-and-world/la-na-alternative-meds6-2009dec06,0,6914799.story

23. Yi D. **U.S. Employers Look Offshore for Healthcare.** *LA Times.* July 30, 2006. Available at: http://articles.latimes.com/2006/jul/30/business/fi-outsource30

24. Leung R. Vacation, Adventure And Surgery? 60 Minutes-CBS News. September 4, 2005. http://www.cbsnews.com/news/vacation-adventure-and-surgery/

25. Keckley PH. **Medical Tourism: Update and Implications. Deloitte Center for Health Solutions.** 2009 Deloitte Center for Health Solutions. Available at: http://www.deloitte.com/assets/Dcom-UnitedStates/Local%20assets/docu-ments/us_chs_medicaltourism_111209_web.pdf. Accessed April 29, 2014

26. Singer N. **Health Bills Aim a Light on Doctors' Conflicts.** *NY Times. http://www.nytimes.com/2009/11/04/health/policy/04sunshine.html.* November 3, 2009

27. Martin AB, Hartman M, Whittle L, Catlin A, the National Health Expenditure Accounts Team. **National Health Spending In 2012: Rate Of Health Spending Growth Remained Low For The Fourth Consecutive Year.** *Health Affairs.* 2014; **33**(1):67-77. Available at: http://content.healthaffairs.org/content/33/1/67.abstract

28. **National Health Expenditure Projections 2013-2023 Forecast Summary Major Findings for National Health Expenditures.** U.S. Department of Health and Human Services, 2014 Washington, D.C. http://www.cms.gov/Research-Statistics-Data-and-Systems/Statistics-Trends-and-Reports/NationalHealthExpendData/Downloads/Proj2013.pdf Accessed

29. **Updated Budget Projections: Fiscal Years 2013 to 2023.** http://www.cbo.gov/sites/default/files/cbofiles/attachments/44172-Baseline2.pdf

30. Cuckler GA, Sisko AM, Keehan SP, et al. **National Health Expenditure Projections, 2012–22: Slow Growth Until Coverage Expands And Economy Improves.** *Health Affairs.* 2013; **32**(10):1820-1831. Available at: http://content.healthaffairs.org/content/early/2013/09/13/hlthaff.2013.0721.abstract

Chapter 21

1. Ryan P. **A Roadmap for America's Future: Description of the Legislation.** Available at: http://www.roadmap.republicans.budget.house.gov/. Accessed July 18, 2010

2. U.S. Companies Now Stashing $2 Trillion Overseas. NBC News. November 19, 2014. http://www.nbcnews.com/business/economy/u-s-companies-now-stashing-2-trillion-overseas-n247256

3. Pomerleau K. **Summary of Latest Federal Income Tax Data**. December 18, 2013. Available at: http://taxfoundation.org/article/summary-latest-federal-income-tax-data. Accessed February 26, 2014

4. Blades M. **Median Wage for U.S. Workers is Nearly $1000 Less Than in 2007 When the Great Recession Began**. Daily Kos LaborRSS; Nov 06, 2013. http://www.dailykos.com/story/2013/11/06/1253593/-Median-U-S-wage-now-as-high-as-in-1998-and-nearly-1-000-less-than-in-2007-when-recession-began#

5. Baxandall P, Smith D. **Picking Up the Tab in 2013: Average Citizens and Small Businesses Pay the Price for Offshore Tax Havens**. U.S. PIRG: the federation of state Public Interest Research Groups. April 2013. Available at: http://www.uspirg.org/sites/pirg/files/reports/Picking_Up_the_Tab_2013_USPIRG.pdf. Accessed June 4, 2014

6. Pomerleau K, Lundeen A. **The U.S. Has the Highest Corporate Income Tax Rate in the OECD**. Tax Foundation. January 27, 2014. Available at: http://tax-foundation.org/blog/us-has-highest-corporate-income-tax-rate-oecd. Accessed June 4, 2014

7. **American Corporations Tell IRS the Majority of Their Offshore Profits Are in 12 Tax Havens** Citizens for Tax Justice. May 27, 2014. Available at: http://ctj.org/ctjreports/2014/05/american_corporations_tell_irs_the_majority_of_their_offshore_profits_are_in_12_tax_havens.php#.U4-l8CjLNR4. Accessed June 4, 2014

8. Chantrill C. **Time Series Chart of U.S. Government Revenue**. U.S. Government Revenue. 2014. Available at: http://www.usgovernmentrevenue.com/custom_chart. Accessed April 17, 2014

9. **Price Elasticity of Demand**. Wikipedia. October 30, 2014. Available at: http://en.wikipedia.org/wiki/Price_elasticity_of_demand. Accessed November 22, 2014

10. **Smoking-Attributable Mortality, Years of Potential Life Lost, and Productivity Losses—United States, 2000–2004**. *MMWR Highlights*. 2008; 57(45):1226-1228. Available at: http://www.cdc.gov/tobacco/data_statistics/mmwrs/byyear/2008/mm5745a3/highlights.htm

11. **Smoking and Tobacco Use**. Center for Disease Control and Prevention Health and Human Services, 2013 Washington, D.C.. http://www.cdc.gov/tobacco/ data_statistics/fact_sheets/fast_facts/ Accessed January 11, 2014

12. **Consumption of Cigarettes and Combustible Tobacco—United States, 2000–2011**. Center for Disease Control and Prevention Health and Human Services, 2013 Washington, D.C.. http://www.cdc.gov/tobacco/data_statistics/ mmwrs/byyear/2012/mm6130a1/highlights.htm Accessed January 11, 2014

13. **Trends in State and Federal Cigarette Tax and Retail Price—United States, 1970–2011**. Center for Disease Control and Prevention Health and Human Services, 2013 Washington, D.C. http://www.cdc.gov/tobacco/data_statistics/ tables/economics/trends/index.htm Accessed January 11, 2014

14. Jha P, Peto R. **Global Effects of Smoking, of Quitting, and of Taxing Tobacco**. *New England Journal of Medicine*. 2014; **370**(1):60-68. Available at: http://www.nejm.org/doi/full/10.1056/NEJMra1308383

15. **2014 Surgeon General's Report: The Health Consequences of Smoking—50 Years of Progress**. Center for Disease Control and Prevention U.S. Department of Health & Human Services, Washington, D.C. http://www.cdc.gov/tobacco/ data_statistics/sgr/50th-anniversary/index.htm Accessed November 22, 2014

16. Midanik L, Chaloupka F, Saitz R, et al. **Alcohol-Attributable Deaths and Years of Potential Life Lost--United States, 2001**. *MMWR*. 2004; **53**(37):866-870. Available at: http://www.cdc.gov/mmwr/preview/mmwrhtml/mm5337a2. htm

17. **Alcohol and Public Health: Alcohol-Related Disease Impact**. Center for Disease Control and Prevention: National Center for Chronic Disease Prevention and Health Promotion, Division of Population Health U.S. Department of Health and Human Services, 2013 Washington, D.C. http://apps. nccd.cdc.gov/DACH_ARDI/Default/Default.aspx Accessed July 22, 2014

18. Gabay M, Goplerud E, Joubran K, Laura-Jacobus-Kantor. **Treatment of Alcohol Medical Consequences/Related Insurance Administration Costs**. George Washington University Medical Center. December, 2007. Available at: http://www.alcoholcostcalculator.org/business/about/?page=note. Accessed June 28, 2014

19. **National Health Expenditure Projections 2012-2022 Forecast Summary**. Center for Medicare and Medicaid Services U.S. Department of Health and Human Services, Washington, D.C. http://www.cms.gov/Research-Statistics-

Data-and-Systems/Statistics-Trends-and-Reports/NationalHealthExpendData/downloads/proj2012.pdf Accessed June 19, 2014

20. **Preventing Excessive Alcohol Consumption: Increasing Alcohol Taxes**. The Guide to Community Preventive Services. http://www.thecommunityguide.org/alcohol/increasingtaxes.html

21. Pogue TF, Sgontz LG. **Taxing to Control Social Costs: The Case of Alcohol**. *American Economic Review.* 1989; **79**:235–243

22. **Food Expenditures Overview**. Economic Research Service, USDA, U.S. Census Bureau, and the Bureau of Labor Statistics 2013 Washington, D.C. http://www.ers.usda.gov/data-products/food-expenditures.aspx#.UtKqq7Q3CvE Accessed January 12, 2014

23. **CDC Reports Excessive Alcohol Consumption Cost the U.S. $224 Billion in 2006**. Center for Disease Control and Prevention U.S. Department of Health and Human Services, 2011 Washington, D.C. . http://www.cdc.gov/media/releases/2011/p1017_alcohol_consumption.html Accessed June 29, 2014

24. Bouchery EE, Harwood HJ, Sacks JJ, Simon CJ, Brewer RD. **Economic Costs of Excessive Alcohol Consumption in the U.S., 2006**. *American Journal of Preventive Medicine.* 2011; **41**(5):516-524. Available at: http://linkinghub.elsevier.com/retrieve/pii/S0749379711005381?showall=true

25. Elder RW, Lawrence B, Ferguson A, et al. **The Effectiveness of Tax Policy Interventions for Reducing Excessive Alcohol Consumption and Related Harms**. . *American Journal of Preventive Medicine.* 2010; **38**(2):217–229. Available at: http://www.thecommunityguide.org/alcohol/EffectivenessTaxPolicyInterventionsReducingExcessiveAlcoholConsumptionRelatedHarms.pdf

26. Beider P, Tawil N, Moore D, Hitchner R: **Future Investment in Drinking Water and Wastewater Infrastructure** Congressional Budget Office 2002 Washington, D.C. http://www.cbo.gov/sites/default/files/cbofiles/ftpdocs/39xx/doc3983/11-18-watersystems.pdf Accessed June 29, 2014

27. Stallworth H: **Water and Wastewater Pricing**. Economist, Office of Wastewater Management, Agency USEP, 2009 Washington, D.C. http://water.epa.gov/infrastructure/sustain/upload/2009_05_26_waterinfrastructure_pricings_waterpricing_final2.pdf Accessed June 29, 2014

28. Kenny JF, Barber NL, Hutson SS, Linsey KS, Lovelace JK, and Maupin MA: **Estimated Use of Water in the nited States in 2005, Circular 1344**. U.S.

Department of the Interior U.S. Geological Survey, 2009 Reston, Virginia:52 p. http://pubs.usgs.gov/circ/1344/pdf/c1344.pdf Accessed January 10, 2014

29. **Plastics: Wastes - Resource Conservation - Common Wastes & Materials.** Environmental Protection Agency, 2014 Washington, D.C. http://www.epa.gov/epawaste/conserve/materials/plastics.htm Accessed January 16, 2014

30. **About Plastics.** SPI: The Plastics Industry Trade Association. Available at: http://www.plasticsindustry.org/aboutplastics/?navItemNumber=1008. Accessed January 16, 2014

31. Moore C. **Plastic Ocean.** New York: Avery an imprint of Penguin Books; 2011. http://www.plasticoceanthebook.com/plasticoceanthebook.html

32. Blake M. **The Scary New Evidence on BPA-Free Plastics: And the Big Tobacco-Style Campaign to Bury It.** *Mother Jones.* April 2014. Available at: http://www.motherjones.com/environment/2014/03/tritan-certichem-eastman-bpa-free-plastic-safe

33. Kroft S. **How Speed Traders Are Changing Wall Street.** CBS News 60 Minutes. Oct. 10, 2010. Available at: http://www.cbsnews.com/news/is-the-us-stock-market-rigged/

34. Salmon F. **Wall Street's Dead End.** *NY Times.* February 13, 2011. Available at: http://www.nytimes.com/2011/02/14/opinion/14Salmon.html?_r=0

35. **Banking, Finance, & Insurance: Stocks and Bonds, Equity Ownership.** The 2011 Statistical Abstract: The National Data Book, U.S. Census Bureau. Available at: http://www.census.gov/compendia/statab/cats/banking_finance_insurance/stocks_and_bonds_equity_ownership.html

36. DeFazio P, Welch P, Sutton B, et al. **H.R.1068 - Let Wall Street Pay for Wall Street's Bailout Act of 2009.** The House of Representatives. February 13, 2009. Available at: http://www.opencongress.org/bill/111-h1068/text

37. Rowland R. **Congress Proposing Transaction Tax On Stock Trades.** The Blog of HORAN Capital Advisors. March 01, 2009. Available at: http://disciplinedinvesting.blogspot.com/2009/03/congress-proposing-transaction-tax-on.html

38. Hill EW, Levin MG. **How Many Guns are in the United States?: Americans Own between 262 Million and 310 Million Firearms.** College of Urban Affairs Cleveland State University. March 28, 2013. Available at: http://www.urban.csuohio.edu/publications/hill/GunsInTheUS_Hill_032813.pdf. Accessed August 13, 2014

39. **Who is Most Likely to be Targeted by Gun Violence?** Office of Justice Programs Department of Justice, 2010 Washington, D.C. http://www.nij.gov/ topics/crime/gun-violence/Pages/affected.aspx Accessed January 18, 2014

40. Stoneman D. **If We Don't Address Poverty, We Won't Reduce Gun Violence.** *Huffington Post.* 07/01/2013 Available at: http://www.huffingtonpost.com/ dorothy-stoneman/poverty-gun-violence_b_3528888.html

41. **Firearms and Ammunition Industry: Economic Impact Report 2012** 2014 National Shooting Sports Foundation. Available at: http://nssf.org/impact/. Accessed January 18, 2014

42. Baus CD. **Gun Background Checks Set New Record in 2013.** Buckeye Firearms Association. January 15, 2014. Available at: http://www.buckeyefire-arms.org/node/9277. Accessed January 18, 2014

43. Cook PJ, Ludwig J. **Gun Violence: The Real Costs.** New York, NY: Oxford University Press; 2000.

44. **Gun Violence.** National Institute of Justice, U.S. Department of Justice, Washington, D.C. . http://www.nij.gov/topics/crime/gun-violence/Pages/ welcome.aspx Accessed January 17, 2014

45. **Why Should Taxpayers Give Big Banks $83 Billion a Year?** *Bloomberg News.* Feb 20, 2013. Available at: http://www.bloomberg.com/news/2013-02-20/why-should-taxpayers-give-big-banks-83-billion-a-year-.html

46. **Report to the House Committee on Ways and Means on Present Law and Suggestions for Reform Submitted to the Tax Reform Working Groups.** Joint Committee on Taxation U.S. House of Representatives, Washington, D.C. https://www.jct.gov/publications.html?func=startdown&id=4517 Accessed January 20, 2014

47. Rubin R. **Biggest Banks Said to Face Asset Tax in Republican Plan.** Bloomberg Personal Finance; Feb 25, 2014. http://www.bloomberg.com/ news/2014-02-25/biggest-banks-said-to-face-asset-tax-in-republican-plan.html

48. **Telecommunications Industry Market Research** Plunket Research Ltd. Available at: http://www.plunkettresearch.com/telecommunications-market-research/industry-and-business-data. Accessed January 18, 2014

49. **Broadband Industry Stats: The Story Behind the Statistics.** 2013 US Telecom. Available at: http://www.ustelecom.org/broadband-industry/ broadband-industry-stats. Accessed January 18, 2014

50. **Media and Children**. American Academy of Pediatrics. Available at: http://www.aap.org/en-us/advocacy-and-policy/aap-health-initiatives/pages/media-and-children.aspx. Accessed January 21, 2014

51. Council on Communications Media. **Children, Adolescents, and the Media**. *Pediatrics*. 2013; **132**:958-961. Available at: http://pediatrics.aappublications.org/content/early/2013/10/24/peds.2013-2656.full.pdf+html

52. **Children and Electronic Media**. *The Future of Children*. 2008; **18**(1):1-259. Available at: http://futureofchildren.org/futureofchildren/publications/docs/18_01_FullJournal.pdf

53. Puzzanghera J, Mitchell R. **Obama Strongly Endorses Tough Net Neutrality Rules**. *LA Times*. November 11, 2014. Available at: http://www.latimes.com/business/la-fi-obama-net-neutrality-20141111-story.html#page=1

54. **Monopoly and Competition in Twenty-First Century Capitalism**. *Monthly Review*, **62**(11). Available at: http://monthlyreview.org/2011/04/01/monopoly-and-competition-in-twenty-first-century-capitalism/

55. McSherry C, Tien L, Stoltz M, Gillula J, Glaser A: **In the Matter of Protecting and Promoting the Open Internet: Electronic Frontier Foundation's Comments Regarding Proposed Rulemaking**. Federal Communications Commission, July 15, 2014 Washington, D.C. https://www.eff.org/files/2014/07/15/efffcccomments7152014.pdf Accessed

56. **U.S. International Trade Data: Latest U.S. International Trade in Goods and Services Report** U.S. Census Bureau U.S. Department of Commerce, 2014 Washington, D.C. http://www.census.gov/foreign-trade/data/ Accessed June 3, 2014

57. **Total Energy Supply and Disposition Summary**. Energy Information Administration U.S. Department of Energy, 2014 Washington, D.C. http://www.eia.gov/forecasts/aeo/er/pdf/0383er%282014%29.pdf Accessed June 29, 2014

Chapter 22

1. Quinn J. **Energy Independence - The Big Lie**. Financial Sense Newsletter; 11/14/2011. http://www.financialsense.com/node/6886

2. **World Energy Outlook 2013**. International Energy Agency 2014. Available at: https://www.iea.org/publications/freepublications/publication/name,44381,en.html. Accessed May 15, 2014

3. Klare M. **It's Official--The Era of Cheap Oil Is Over**. *The Nation*. June 11, 2009. Available at: http://www.thenation.com/doc/20090629/klare

4. **Annual Energy Outlook 2014**. U.S. Energy Information Administration Department of Energy, 2014 Washington, D.C. http://www.eia.gov/oiaf/aeo/tablebrowser/#release=AEO2014&subject=0-AEO2014&table=1-AEO2014&region=0-0&cases=full2013full-d102312a,ref2014-d102413a Accessed July 22, 2014

5. **CPI Inflation Calculator**. Bureau of Labor Statistics. 2014. Available at: http://www.bls.gov/data/inflation_calculator.htm. Accessed October 12, 2014

6. **Short-Term Energy Outlook**. US Energy Information Administration Department of Energy, 2014 Washington, D.C. http://www.eia.gov/forecasts/steo/report/natgas.cfm Accessed July 22, 2014

7. **Energy Kid's Page- Energy Calculator: Common Units and Conversions. Energy Information Administration**. Department of Energy. Available at: http://www.eia.doe.gov/kids/energy.cfm?page=about_energy_conversion_calculator-basics#unitsexplained. Accessed December 7, 2010

8. **Total Energy Supply and Disposition Summary**. Energy Information Administration U.S. Department of Energy, 2014 Washington, D.C. http://www.eia.gov/forecasts/aeo/er/pdf/0383er%282014%29.pdf Accessed June 29, 2014

9. **Fossil Fuel Subsidy Reform: Building momentum at Rio and beyond: Side Event Summary**: International Institute for Sustainable Development; 2012. Available at: http://www.iisd.org/gsi/sites/default/files/ffs_sideevent_rio_beyond_meetingreport.pdf Access date

10. Clements B, Coady D, Fabrizio S, et al. **Energy Subsidy Reform: Lessons and Implications**: International Monetary Fund; January 29, 2013. Available at: https://www.imf.org/external/np/pp/eng/2013/012813.pdf Access date

11. Tankersley J. **Copenhagen Climate Talks will Hinge on Economics**. *LA Times*. December 7, 2009. Available at: http://articles.latimes.com/2009/dec/07/world/la-fg-climate-economy7-2009dec07

12. Shear MD, Eilperin J. **McCain Seeks to End Offshore Drilling Ban**. *Washington Post*. June 17, 2008. Available at: http://www.washingtonpost.com/wp-dyn/content/article/2008/06/16/AR2008061602731.html?sid=ST2008061700079

13. **Tell Your Senators A Climate Bill That is "Worse Than Nothing" is Not Good Enough** CLIMATE SOS. Available at: http://www.climatesos.org/. Accessed December 13, 2009

14. **Each Country's Share of CO2 Emissions**. Union of Concerned Scientists. Available at: http://www.ucsusa.org/global_warming/science_and_impacts/ science/each-countrys-share-of-co2.html. Accessed December 12, 2009

15. **Most Voters Still See Finding New Energy Sources As More Important Than Conservation**. Rasmussen Reports. October 10, 2010. Available at: http://www. rasmussenreports.com/public_content/politics/current_events/environment_ energy/most_voters_still_see_finding_new_energy_sources_as_more_impor- tant_than_conservation

16. Smith G. **U.S. Seen as Biggest Oil Producer After Overtaking Saudi Arabia**. Bloomberg News; Jul 4, 2014. http://www.bloomberg.com/news/2014-07-04/u- s-seen-as-biggest-oil-producer-after-overtaking-saudi.html

17. Kaufman L. **In Kansas, Climate Skeptics Embrace Cleaner Energy**. *New York Times*. October 18, 2010. Available at: http://www.nytimes.com/2010/10/19/ science/earth/19fossil.html?_r=1&hp

18. Conti J, Holtberg P, Beamon JA, et al.: **The International Energy Outlook 2013**. U.S. Energy Information Administration (EIA) U.S. Department of Energy, 2013 Washington, D.C. http://www.eia.gov/forecasts/ieo/ pdf/0484%282013%29.pdf Accessed November 22, 2014

19. Grunwald M. **How the Stimulus Is Changing America**. Time in partnership with CNN. Aug. 26, 2010. Available at: http://www.time.com/time/nation/ article/0,8599,2013683,00.html

20. **Hidden Costs of Energy:Unpriced Consequences of Energy Production and Use**: The National Academies Press; 2010. http://www.nap.edu/openbook. php?record_id=12794

21. **Current Dollar and Real Gross Domestic Product**. Bureau of Economic Analysis, U.S. Department of Commerce, 2013 Washington, D.C. www.bea.gov/ national/xls/gdplev.xls Accessed January 15, 2015

22. Weber C, Matthews H. **Food-Miles and the Relative Climate Impacts of Food Choices in the United States Environ**. *Sci. Technol.* 2008; 42(10):3508– 3513. Available at: http://pubs.acs.org/doi/pdf/10.1021/es702969f?cookieSet=1

23. Saragih H. **Why We Left Our Farms to Come to Copenhagen**. CommonDreams.org for La Via Campesina. December 8, 2009. Available at: http://www.commondreams.org/view/2009/12/08-2. Accessed July 2, 2014

24. **The Price-Anderson Act**. Center for Nuclear Science and Technology Information. 2005. Available at: http://www.nuclearconnect.org/wp-content/

uploads/2014/07/54_PriceAnderson_Background.pdf. Accessed October 27, 2014

25. **Price-Anderson Act: The Billion Dollar Bailout for Nuclear Power Mishaps** Public Citizen. 2004. Available at: http://www.citizen.org/documents/Price%20 Anderson%20Factsheet.pdf. Accessed October 27, 2014

26. Starr S. **Costs and Consequences of the Fukushima Daiichi Disaster** Available at: http://www.psr.org/environment-and-health/environmental-health-policy-institute/responses/costs-and-consequences-of-fukushima.html

27. **Carbon Footprint Calculator.** Nature Conservancy. Available at: http://www.nature.org/greenliving/carboncalculator/index.htm. Accessed December 10 2009

28. **Another Pump Price Hike**. Fuels News, Prices & Analysis; May 5, 2014. http://www.cspnet.com/fuels-news-prices-analysis/fuels-analysis/articles/another-pump-price-hike

Chapter 23

1. **The 2013 Annual Report of the Board of Trustees of the Federal Old-Age and Survivors Insurance and Federal Disability Insurance Trust Funds**. Social Security Administration, 2013 Government Printing Office Washington, D.C. http://www.ssa.gov/oact/TR/2013/tr2013.pdf Accessed July 9, 2014

2. Smith AW. **Government Owes $2.7 Trillion to Social Security**. May 23, 2013. Available at: http://www.fedsmith.com/2013/05/23/government-owes-2-7-trillion-to-social-security/. Accessed June 11, 2014

3. Chantrill C. **Time Series Chart of U.S. Government Spending**. USGovernmentSpending.com. 2014. Available at: http://www.usgovern-mentspending.com/charts.html. Accessed April 17, 2014

4. Chantrill C. **Time Series Chart of U.S. Government Revenue.** U.S. Government Revenue. 2014. Available at: http://www.usgovernmentrevenue.com/custom_chart. Accessed April 17, 2014

5. Villarreal P. **Social Security and Medicare Projections: 2009.** National Center for Policy Analysis. June 11, 2009. Available at: http://www.ncpa.org/pub/ba662. Accessed December 3, 2009

6. Smith CH. **How To Fix Social Security: A 4-Point Plan That Faces the Brutal Realities**. of two minds.com. January 19, 2011. Available at: http://www.oftwo-minds.com/blogjan11/Social-Security-fixes01-11.html

7. Calmes J. **Obama Deficit Panel Gets Some Competition**. *NY Times*. November 16, 2010. Available at: http://www.nytimes.com/2010/11/17/us/politics/17fiscal. html?hpw

8. Calmes J. **Obama Warns Against Idea of Privatizing Social Security**. *NY Times*. August 14, 2010. Available at: http://www.theledger.com/ article/20100814/news/8145015

9. Blades M. **Median Wage for U.S. Workers is Nearly $1000 Less Than in 2007 When the Great Recession Began**. Daily Kos LaborRSS; Nov 06, 2013. http:// www.dailykos.com/story/2013/11/06/1253593/-Median-U-S-wage-now-as-high-as-in-1998-and-nearly-1-000-less-than-in-2007-when-recession-began#

10. **Calculators: Online Calculator**. Social Security Administration, 2014 Washington, D.C http://www.socialsecurity.gov/retire2/AnypiaApplet.html Accessed July 24, 2014

11. Edwards C, DeHaven T. **Social Security Administration**. Cato Institute. 2013. Available at: http://www.downsizinggovernment.org/social-security-administration. Accessed June 11, 2014

12. Biggs AG, Sarney M, Tamborini CR: **A Progressivity Index for Social Security: Issue Paper No. 2009-01**. Office of Retirement and Disability Policy Administration USSS, January 2009 Washington, D.C. http://www.ssa.gov/ policy/docs/issuepapers/ip2009-01.html Accessed November 12, 2014

13. **National Debt**. Just Facts. June 4, 2014. Available at: http://www.justfacts. com/nationaldebt.asp. Accessed June 11, 2014

14. **Historical Tables Budget of the U.S. Government**. Office of Management and Budget White House, 2014 U.S. Government Printing Office Washington, D.C. http://www.whitehouse.gov/sites/default/files/omb/budget/fy2015/assets/hist. pdf Accessed October 12, 2014

15. Baker D. **State and Local Pension Funds Face a Shortfall Equal to 0.3 Percent of GDP**. Truthout; 20 September 2014. http://truth-out.org/opinion/ item/26331

16. Fritz M. **Pension Reform or Else**. *LA Times*. January 18, 2011. Available at: http://www.latimes.com/news/opinion/la-oe-fritz-pension-reform-20110118,0,6116807.story?track=rss

17. Riordan R, Rubalcava A. **How Pensions Can Get Out of the Red**. *NY Times. http://www.nytimes.com/2010/09/16/opinion/16riordan.html?ref=opinion.* September 15, 2010

18. **"Annuity" Definition** Merriam Webster's Dictionary. Available at: http://www. merriam-webster.com/dictionary/annuity. Accessed October 23, 2014

19. Morrissey M. **Move Public Employees Into 401(k)s? Private Sector Workers were Herded into 401(k)-Style Plans Long Ago. Why Should New Government Employees Keep Their Traditional Pensions?** *NY Times.* February 27, 2011. Available at: http://www.nytimes.com/roomfordebate/2011/02/27/ why-not-401ks-for-public-employees/a-cash-cow-for-wall-street

20. Ghilarducci T. **Move Public Employees Into 401(k)s?...A Bad Deal for Taxpayers.** *NY Times.* February 27, 2011. Available at: http://www.nytimes.com/roomfordebate/2011/02/27/ why-not-401ks-for-public-employees/401ks-a-bad-deal-for-taxpayers

21. **The Pension Benefits Guarantee Corporation.** Unfunded Liabilities and the Coming Class War. September 21, 2009. Available at: http://unfundedliabilities-andclasswar.blogspot.com/2009/09/pension-benefits-guarantee-corporation. html. Accessed October 14, 2010

22. Geus AD. **The Living Company: Habits for Survival in a Turbulent Business Environment. Prologue: The Lifespan of a Company.** Boston, MA: Harvard Business Press Books; 2002. http://www.businessweek.com/chapter/degeus.htm

23. **Retirement and Education Savings (Chapter 7): A Review of Trends and Activities in the U.S. Investment Company Industry.** *2014 Investment Company Fact Book*: Investment Company Institute; 2014. http://www.icifact-book.org/fb_ch7.html

24. Rauh JD. **Move Public Employees Into 401(k)s?... Start Paying or Stop Promising.** *NY Times.* February 27, 2011. Available at: http://www.nytimes. com/roomfordebate/2011/02/27/why-not-401ks-for-public-employees/ start-paying-or-stop-promising

25. John DC. **Move Public Employees Into 401(k)s?...Automatic Enrollment Is the Key.** *NY Times.* February 27, 2011. Available at: http://www.nytimes. com/roomfordebate/2011/02/27/why-not-401ks-for-public-employees/ automatic-enrollment-is-the-key

Chapter 24

1. **The Financial Services Industry in the United States.** Select USA. Available at: http://selectusa.commerce.gov/industry-snapshots/financial-services-industry-united-states. Accessed July 6, 2014

2. **Community Affairs: Financial Literacy Resource Directory**. Controller of the Currency: Administrator of National Banks U.S. Department of Treasury, 2010 Washington, D.C. http://www.occ.treas.gov/cdd/finlitresdir.htm#FLEC Accessed June 7, 2014

3. **President's Advisory Council on Financial Literacy**. Financial Literacy and Education Commission U.S. Dept. of the Treasury, 2008. http://www.treasury. gov/resource-center/financial-education/Documents/Starting%20Early%20 Research%20Priorities%20May%202013.pdf Accessed June 7, 2014

4. Ketchum RG, Barr MS. **Financial Capability in the United States National Survey—Executive Summary**. FINRA Investor Education Foundation. December 2009. Available at: http://www.finrafoundation.org/web/groups/ foundation/@foundation/documents/foundation/p120535.pdf. Accessed August 7, 2010

5. Bottari M. **Bailed-Out Banks Finance Predatory Payday Lenders**. Center for Media and Democracy: PR Watch. September 16, 2010. Available at: http:// www.prwatch.org/node/9456. Accessed June 7, 2014

6. Eichenbaum P. **Debit-card Fee Cap May Ding Credit Card Lenders**. *Bloomberg News*. Jan. 09, 2011. Available at: http://www.kansas.com/2011/01/09/1665859/ debit-card-fee-cap-may-ding-credit.html

7. **Study: Credit Card Penalty Fees Fell in 2010**. CreditCards.com. Available at: http://www.creditcards.com/credit-card-news.php. Accessed February 3, 2011

8. Touryalai H. **$1 Trillion Student Loan Problem Keeps Getting Worse**. *Forbes*. 2/21/2014. Available at: http://www.forbes.com/sites/ halahtouryalai/2014/02/21/1-trillion-student-loan-problem-keeps-getting- worse/

9. Quinn M. **Student Loan Debt Increases $31 Billion to $1.1 Trillion**. Red Alert Politics; May 13, 2014. http://redalertpolitics.com/2014/05/13/ student-loan-debt-increases-31-billion-1-1-trillion/

10. **GDP Turns up in Second Quarter** Bureau of Economic Analysis U.S. Department of Commerce, 2014 Washington, D.C. http://www.esa.doc.gov/ Blog/2014/09/26/gdp-turns-second-quarter Accessed October 2, 2014

11. **Legacies, Clouds, Uncertainties--Chapter 2: Country and Regional Perspectives**. World Economic Outlook (WEO): International Monetary Fund; October 2014. Available at: http://www.imf.org/external/pubs/ft/weo/2014/02/ Access date October 15, 2014

12. Williams JC. **The Federal Reserve's Mandate and Best Practice Monetary Policy: Presentation to the Marian Miner Cook Athenaeum, Claremont McKenna College Claremont, California.** Federal Reserve Bank of San Francisco. Feb. 13, 2012. Available at: http://www.frbsf.org/our-district/press/presidents-speeches/williams-speeches/2012/february/williams-federal-reserve-mandate-best-practice-monetary-policy/#_ftn1. Accessed October 29, 2014

13. **Historical Inflation Rates: 1914-2014.** U.S. Inflation Calculator. October 22, 2014. Available at: http://www.usinflationcalculator.com/inflation/historical-inflation-rates/. Accessed October 29, 2014

14. Reinhart CM, Rogof KS. **Shifting Mandates: The Federal Reserve's First Centennial.** *American Economic Review: Papers & Proceedings.* 2013; **103**(3):48-54. Available at: http://scholar.harvard.edu/files/rogoff/files/shifting_mandates_aer.pdf

15. **Federal Reserve Act.** Board of Governors of the Federal Reserve System. August 16, 2013 Available at: http://www.federalreserve.gov/aboutthefed/fract.htm. Accessed October 29, 2014

16. Amadeo K. **The History of Recessions in the United States.** About News and Issues. 2014. Available at: http://useconomy.about.com/od/grossdomesticproduct/a/recession_histo.htm. Accessed October 29, 2014

17. Rosnick D. **The Adult Recession: Age-Adjusted Unemployment at Post-War Highs.** Center for Economic and Policy Research. July 2010. Available at: http://www.cepr.net/documents/publications/ur-2010-07.pdf. Accessed October 29, 2014

18. Kostohryz JA. **Recession Risk: The Threat Of Rising Interest Rates.** Seeking Alpha. Dec. 8, 2012. Available at: http://seekingalpha.com/article/1052821-recession-risk-the-threat-of-rising-interest-rates. Accessed October 29, 2014

19. **How Did the Fed Change its Approach to Monetary Policy in the Late 1970s and Early 1980s?** Federal Reserve Bank of San Francisco. January 2003. Available at: http://www.frbsf.org/education/publications/doctor-econ/2003/january/monetary-policy-1970s-1980s. Accessed October 29, 2014

20. Michel NJ, Moore S. **Quantitative Easing, The Fed's Balance Sheet, and Central Bank Insolvency: Backgrounder #2938 on Economy**Washington, D.C.: Heritage Foundation; August 14, 2014. Available at: http://www.heritage.org/research/reports/2014/08/quantitative-easing-the-feds-balance-sheet-and-central-bank-insolvency Access date November 23, 2014

21. **What is Larry Summers' Criticism of the Fed?** Center for Economic and Policy Research. 11 November 2013 Available at: http://www.cepr.net/index. php/blogs/beat-the-press/what-is-larry-summers-criticism-of-the-fed. Accessed October 25, 2014

22. Haldane AG, Madouros V. **What is the Contribution of the Financial Sector?** Vox; November 22, 2011. http://www.voxeu.org/article/what-contribution-financial-sector

23. **Financial Accounts of the United States.** Federal Reserve Statistical Release, 2014 Washington, D.C. http://www.federalreserve.gov/releases/z1/Current/z1r-2.pdf Accessed July 11, 2014

24. Chantrill C. **Time Series Chart of U.S. Government Spending.** USGovernmentSpending.com. 2014. Available at: http://www.usgovern-mentspending.com/charts.html. Accessed April 17, 2014

25. **Savings vs. Credit Union, What are the Trade Offs?** Better Trades. 2012. Available at: http://www.bettertrades.org/better-trade-offs/savings-vs-creditunion.asp. Accessed October 14, 2014

26. **Differences between Banks, Credit Unions and Savings Institutions.** State of Wisconsin Department of Financial Institutions. Available at: http://www.wdfi.org/wca/consumer_credit/credit_guides/differencesbankscreditunions-savingsinstitutions.htm. Accessed October 14, 2014

27. Black WK. **The Best Way to Rob a Bank Is to Own One: How Corporate Executives and Politicians Looted the S&L Industry:** University of Texas Press 2005. http://www.amazon.com/The-Best-Way-Rob-Bank/dp/0292721390

28. Holland J. **Hundreds of Wall Street Execs Went to Prison During the Last Fraud-Fueled Bank Crisis.** Moyers and Company; September 17, 2013. http://billmoyers.com/2013/09/17/hundreds-of-wall-street-execs-went-to-prison-during-the-last-fraud-fueled-bank-crisis/

29. Nocera J. **The States Take on Foreclosures.** *NY Times.* October 29, 2010. Available at: http://www.nytimes.com/2010/10/30/business/30nocera.html?_r=1&hp

30. **More Than Nine Million U.S. Properties Remain Seriously Underwater In Q2.** The National Mortgage Professional; 30 Jul 2014. http://www.ormortgages.org/page-1666066/3057169

31. Gudell S. **Negative Equity Causing Housing Gridlock, Even as it Slowly Recedes.** Zillow Real Estate Research Blog; August 25, 2014 http://www.zillow.com/research/2014-q2-negative-equity-report-7465/

32. Ausick P. **Underwater Mortgage Levels Continue to Drop.** 24/7 Wall Street; June 5, 2014 http://247wallst.com/housing/2014/06/05/underwater-mortgage-levels-continue-to-drop/

33. Ritholtz B. **Another Look at Underwater Mortgages: Ritholtz Chart.** Bloomberg View; 7 Jul 24, 2014. http://www.bloombergview.com/articles/2014-07-24/another-look-at-underwater-mortgages-ritholtz-chart

34. **CPI Inflation Calculator.** Bureau of Labor Statistics. 2014. Available at: http://www.bls.gov/data/inflation_calculator.htm. Accessed October 12, 2014

35. **Home Value and Homeownership Rates: Recession and Post-Recession Comparisons From 2007–2009 to 2010–2012.** U.S. Census Bureau U.S. Department of Commerce, Nov 2013 Washington, D.C. . http://www.census.gov/prod/2013pubs/acsbr12-20.pdf Accessed November 23, 2014

36. **American's Rental Housing: Evolving Markets and Needs.** 2013 Joint Center for Housing Studies of Harvard University, Harvard Graduate School of Design and Harvard Kennedy School. Available at: http://www.jchs.harvard.edu/sites/jchs.harvard.edu/files/jchs_americas_rental_housing_2013_1_0.pdf. Accessed October 11, 2014

37. Husock H. **Public Housing and Rental Subsidies.** Cato Institute. June 2009. Available at: http://www.downsizinggovernment.org/hud/public-housing-rental-subsidies. Accessed October 27, 2014

38. **United States Housing Bubble.** Wikipedia. 22 September 2014. Available at: http://en.wikipedia.org/wiki/United_States_housing_bubble. Accessed October 11, 2014

39. **Reforming America's Housing Finance System: Written Testimony of Dr. Dwight M. Jaffee.** June 10, 2013. Available at: http://www.haas.berkeley.edu/groups/online_marketing/facultyCV/papers/jaffee_testimony.pdf

40. Herman K. **Federal Housing Policy at the Crossroads – What's at Stake?** Washington State Housing Finance Commission; January 2014. http://www.wshfc.org/newsletter/2014.01.index.htm

41. Edwards C, DeHaven T. **Department of Housing and Urban Development.** Downsizing the Federal Government from the Cato Institute. May 2010. Available at: http://www.downsizinggovernment.org/housing-and-urban-development. Accessed October 11, 2014

42. Grumet J, Anderson J, Hoagland GW. **Housing--America's Future: New Directions for National Policy.** Bipartisan Policy Center. February 2013.

Available at: http://bipartisanpolicy.org/sites/default/files/BPC_Housing%20 Report_web_0.pdf. Accessed October 11, 2014

43. Calabria MA. **The Role of Mortgage Finance in Financial (In)Stability (Working Paper No. 23)**. September 12, 2014. Available at: http://www.cato. org/publications/working-paper/role-mortgage-finance-financial-instability. Accessed October 11, 2014

44. **Downsizing the Federal Government: Department of Housing and Urban Development (HUD)**. Cato Institute. 2014. Available at: http://www.down-sizinggovernment.org/hud. Accessed October 15, 2014

45. Gandel S. **By Every Measure, the Big Banks are Bigger**. Forbes Magazine; September 13, 2013. http://fortune.com/2013/09/13/by-every-measure-the-big-banks-are-bigger/

46. Calabria MA. **Monetary Policy and the State of the Economy: Testimony to House Committee on Financial Services.** February 11, 2014 Washington, D.C., Congressional Record. http://www.cato.org/publications/testimony/monetary-policy-state-economy

47. **Savings and Loan Crisis**. Wikipedia. Available at: http://en.wikipedia.org/wiki/Savings_and_loan_crisis. Accessed October 28, 2014

48. **What are B Corps**. 2014. Available at: https://www.bcorporation.net/what-are-b-corps/the-non-profit-behind-b-corps. Accessed August 18, 2014

49. **Personal Saving as a Percentage of Disposable Personal Income.** Economic Research Department: Federal Reserve Bank of Saint Louis. September 26, 2014. Available at: http://research.stlouisfed.org/fred2/series/A072RC1Q156SBEA. Accessed October 28, 2014

50. **Updated Budget Projections: 2014 to 2024.** Congressional Budget Office U.S. Congress, 2014 Washington, D.C. http://www.cbo.gov/sites/default/files/cbofiles/attachments/45229-UpdatedBudgetProjections_2.pdf Accessed August 7, 2014

51. Blades M. **Median Wage for U.S. Workers is Nearly $1000 Less Than in 2007 When the Great Recession Began.** Daily Kos LaborRSS; Nov 06, 2013. http://www.dailykos.com/story/2013/11/06/1253593/-Median-U-S-wage-now-as-high-as-in-1998-and-nearly-1-000-less-than-in-2007-when-recession-began#

52. Pomerleau K. **Summary of Latest Federal Income Tax Data**. December 18, 2013. Available at: http://taxfoundation.org/article/summary-latest-federal-income-tax-data. Accessed February 26, 2014

53. Lundberg J. **Time to Leave GDP Behind: Eco-Economists Support Activists' Dreams**. Culture Change; January 17,2014. http://www.culturechange.org/cms/content/view/903/65/

Chapter 25

1. McKibben D. **Fired Official Gets $1.7 Million**. *LA Times*. April 9, 2005. Available at: http://articles.latimes.com/2005/apr/09/local/me-norby9

2. Lawder D. **U.S. Veterans Deal to Provide $17 Billion to Ease Medical Wait Times**. Reuters; Jul 28, 2014 http://www.reuters.com/article/2014/07/28/us-usa-veterans-funding-idUSKBN0FX1PO20140728

3. Rubin A. **The Accurate Numbers as to Social Security and Medicare Solvency**. The Rubins. 8/2/14. Available at: http://www.therubins.com/socsec/solvency.htm. Accessed October 7, 2014

4. **President's Budget Request Fiscal Year 2015**. VA Office of the Budget. Veterans Administration, Washington, D.C. http://www.va.gov/budget/products.asp Accessed August 7, 2014

5. **New Research from EBRI: Average Couple Today Needs $295,000 for Retiree Health Expenses**. EBRI News. July 20, 2006. Available at: http://www.ebri.org/pdf/PR_742_20July06.pdf. Accessed August 21, 2009

6. Cuckler GA, Sisko AM, Keehan SP, et al. **National Health Expenditure Projections, 2012–22: Slow Growth Until Coverage Expands And Economy Improves**. *Health Affairs*. 2013; **32**(10):1820-1831. Available at: http://content.healthaffairs.org/content/early/2013/09/13/hlthaff.2013.0721.abstract

7. Chantrill C. **Time Series Chart of U.S. Government Spending**. USGovernmentSpending.com. 2014. Available at: http://www.usgovernmentspending.com/charts.html. Accessed April 17, 2014

8. **U.S. Charitable Giving Estimated to be $307.65 Billion in 2008**. GivingUSA Foundation. 2009. Available at: http://www.givingusa.org/press_releases/gusa/GivingReaches300billion.pdf. Accessed August 29, 2009

9. **Ultimate Guide to Retirement**. 2014 CNN Money. Available at: http://money.cnn.com/retirement/guide/insurance_health.moneymag/index4.htm. Accessed April 27, 2014

Chapter 26

1. **National Health Expenditure Projections 2012-2022 Forecast Summary**. Center for Medicare and Medicaid Services U.S. Department of Health and

Human Services, Washington, D.C. http://www.cms.gov/Research-Statistics-Data-and-Systems/Statistics-Trends-and-Reports/NationalHealthExpendData/downloads/proj2012.pdf Accessed June 19, 2014

2. Chantrill C. **Time Series Chart of U.S. Government Spending.** USGovernmentSpending.com. 2014. Available at: http://www.usgovernmentspending.com/charts.html. Accessed April 17, 2014

3. **Updated Budget Projections: 2014 to 2024.** Congressional Budget Office Congress of the United States, 2014 Washington, D.C. http://www.cbo.gov/sites/default/files/cbofiles/attachments/45229-UpdatedBudgetProjections_2.pdf Accessed September 27, 2014

4. **Housing's Contribution to Gross Domestic Product (GDP).** National Association of Home Builders. 2014. Available at: http://www.nahb.org/generic.aspx?genericContentID=66226. Accessed October 12, 2014

5. **CPI Inflation Calculator.** Bureau of Labor Statistics. 2014. Available at: http://www.bls.gov/data/inflation_calculator.htm. Accessed October 12, 2014

6. **The Financial Services Industry in the United States.** Select USA. Available at: http://selectusa.commerce.gov/industry-snapshots/financial-services-industry-united-states. Accessed July 6, 2014

7. **U.S. Tort Costs: 2011 Update Trends and Findings on the Cost of the U.S. Tort System.** Towers Perrin Tillinghaus. 2012. Available at: http://www.towerswatson.com/en/Insights/IC-Types/Survey-Research-Results/2012/01/2011-Update-on-US-Tort-Cost-Trends. Accessed May 13, 2014

8. **Table 3-3: U.S. Gross Domestic Product (GDP) Attributed to Transportation-Related Final Demand (Current billions of dollars)** Bureau of Transportation Statistics U.S. Department of Transportation, 2014 Washington, D.C. http://www.rita.dot.gov/bts/sites/rita.dot.gov.bts/files/publications/national_transportation_statistics/html/table_03_03.html Accessed October 31, 2014

9. **Broadband Industry Stats: The Story Behind the Statistics.** 2013 US Telecom. Available at: http://www.ustelecom.org/broadband-industry/broadband-industry-stats. Accessed January 18, 2014

10. **Postsecondary Revenues by Source.** National Center for Educational Statistics U.S. Department of Education, 2014 Washington, D.C. http://nces.ed.gov/programs/coe/indicator_cud.asp Accessed November 12, 2014

11. **10 Facts About K-12 Education Funding**. U.S. Department of Education, Washington, D.C. http://www2.ed.gov/about/overview/fed/10facts/index.html Accessed

12. **Public School Expenditures**. April 2014. Available at: http://nces.ed.gov/ fastfacts/display.asp?id=66. Accessed September 27, 2014

13. **Financing Postsecondary Education in the United States** National Center for Educational Statistics U.S. Department of Education, Washington, D.C. http:// nces.ed.gov/programs/coe/indicator_tua.asp Accessed September 27, 2014

14. **Food Expenditures Overview**. Economic Research Service, USDA, U.S. Census Bureau, and the Bureau of Labor Statistics 2013 Washington, D.C. http://www.ers.usda.gov/data-products/food-expenditures.aspx#.UtKqq7Q3CvE Accessed January 12, 2014

15. **Historical Tables Budget of the U.S. Government**. Office of Management and Budget White House, 2014 U.S. Government Printing Office Washington, D.C. http://www.whitehouse.gov/sites/default/files/omb/budget/fy2015/assets/hist. pdf Accessed October 12, 2014

16. Noss A: **Household Income: 2012**. U.S. Census Bureau U.S. Department of Commerce, September 2013 Washington, D.C. http://www.census.gov/ prod/2013pubs/acsbr12-02.pdf Accessed November 1, 2014

17. Vespa J, Lewis JM, Kreider RM: **Population Characteristics: America's Families and Living Arrangements**. Census Bureau U.S. Department of Commerce, 2013. http://www.census.gov/prod/2013pubs/p20-570.pdf Accessed July 11, 2014

Index

A

Abortion vii, ix, xiii, 57, 128-132, 159, 253, 256, 259

Accountable care organizations (ACOs) 6, 7, 14, 21, 49-51, 54, 60, 199

Acupuncture 50, 121, 351

Afghanistan 292, 301

Agriculture vii, xi, 10, 38, 80, 207-209, 218, 220-247, 258, 260, 266, 267, 291, 294, 295, 298, 300, 301, 306, 329, 370, 396, 399, 405, 434, 458, 460, 464, 465

Alcohol xii, xiv, 35, 37, 44, 58, 60, 109-111, 118, 167, 177, 188, 217, 364, 367-369, 378, 385, 447

Alternative and complimentary services 13, 16, 21, 50, 75, 107, 109, 120-121, 127, 138, 142, 143, 156, 215, 320, 329, 351, 352

Alzheimer's disease 101, 141, 314, 347, 452

Autism 121, 331

B

Benefit companies ("B" companies) 301, 439

Benefit packages for health care 7, 8, 16, 18, 19, 49, 53-56, 59, 107, 153-155, 214, 265, 309

Block grants 18, 26, 31, 41, 171-175, 204, 214, 284, 317, 218, 322, 337, 440

C

Capitated funding 14, 126

Carbon footprint 232, 383, 387, 395, 401, 402

Cardiovascular diseases 3, 48, 75, 78, 159, 233, 352

Center for Medicare and Medicaid Services (CMS) 15, 31, 52, 82, 99, 355

Children x, 4, 19, 20, 48, 80, 81, 125, 126, 128, 131, 132, 163-167, 173, 176, 202, 205-7, 211, 212, 216, 218, 224, 250, 252-260, 266, 268, 278-281, 286, 294, 317, 321, 322, 332, 353, 359, 378-382, 386, 391, 407, 410, 417, 421, 423, 439, 454

Chronic disease 3, 8, 69, 75, 81, 147, 220, 222-225, 227, 228, 242, 246, 247, 278

Climate change 235, 238, 246, 247, 252, 297, 300, 370, 389, 391-396, 404, 424

Communitarianism x, 3, 7, 9, 45, 46, 60, 458, 459

Conservatives xi, xiii, xiv, 5, 33, 39, 80, 93, 152, 186, 190, 198, 203, 226, 240, 250, 251, 262, 263, 300, 357, 358, 361, 380, 395, 406, 408, 412, 428

Consumption taxes (or "sin taxes") x, xv, 35, 36, 41, 44, 46, 117, 124, 207, 211, 218, 232, 237, 240, 241, 247, 256, 266, 274, 284, 300, 301, 316, 317, 318, 329, 333, 357-386, 395, 396, 410, 423, 424, 439, 440, 444, 446, 447, 456, 457, 462

Co-operative (definition by International Co-operative Alliance) 6, 7

Corporate income taxes xiv, 28, 30, 35, 36, 46, 203, 205, 208, 275, 357-361, 365, 386, 444

Cost control x, 6, 11, 13, 14, 65, 152, 154, 158, 173, 190, 340-356

Credit unions and savings and loan banks 9, 32- 34, 241, 275, 311, 328, 330, 352, 411, 415-418, 420, 425, 429, 431, 435-443, 446-450

Crime prevention 198, 200

Criminal justice 10, 27, 114

Culture xvi, 2-4, 30, 46, 73, 74, 167, 190, 193, 199, 278, 326, 394, 433, 453, 459, 463

D

Death panels 93, 107

Defensive medicine 184-186, 190, 193, 199, 200, 349

Democrats xiii, 47, 172, 173, 377, 380, 412, 435, 436

Dental care 17, 124-127, 319, 456

Development assistance 209, 257, 261, 291, 292, 461

Direct practice primary care providers (or boutique providers) vii, 10-14, 35, 55, 60, 62-79, 96, 175, 213, 333, 334, 336, 338, 339, 345, 348, 349, 355, 455, 457, 461

Disability insurance 193, 194, 199, 316

E

Electronic communications 378-379

Employee benefits xiv, 46, 203, 205, 208, 212, 219

Employer mandate 19, 49, 203, 218, 308

End-of-life palliative care vii, 13, 70, 85-108, 325, 326, 344

Energy, (non-renewable and renewable) 207, 208, 209, 231, 237, 239, 241, 242, 245, 247, 273, 304, 305, 383, 384, 386-405, 423, 440, 464

Enterprise medical malpractice liability vii, 22, 23, 25, 179-185, 199, 216, 349, 446, 463

Entitlements xiii, 10, 20, 32, 33, 35, 45, 60, 172, 407, 408

Entrepreneurs xiii, 10, 20, 32, 33, 35, 45, 60, 172, 407, 408

Environment ix, x, xiv, 2, 3, 31, 35, 36, 48, 110, 117, 166, 167, 205, 211, 230, 231, 234, 236, 237, 246, 247, 276, 357, 369, 371, 386, 387, 400-401, 445

Equities trading 371-373

Evidence-based medicine vii, 15, 70, 75, 133-150, 153, 187, 215

Experimental treatments 109, 121, 127, 134, 148, 149

Exports 230, 233, 235, 242-245, 256, 271, 291, 295, 383, 393, 397, 400, 404

F

Federal debt xv, 411, 444

Federal deficit spending xiv, 36

Federal Reserve Bank (FED) 426, 427, 441, 442, 447

Fee-for-service 21, 55, 56, 72, 119, 126, 331, 333, 350

Financial literacy and education 31, 219, 420, 421, 423, 449

Financial security viii, 25, 31, 32, 48, 154, 409, 417, 418, 419-450

Financial services 10, 19, 20, 21, 31, 32, 34, 35, 50, 60, 193, 198, 212-214, 216, 219, 245, 310-322, 328, 329, 331, 350, 411, 413, 418-450, 458, 460, 463, 465

Fisher, Edward (Dr.) 341, 342, 350

Food and Agriculture Organization (FAO) 235, 236, 295-297

Food and Drug Administration (FDA) 15, 52, 107, 122, 136, 143, 146, 149, 215, 236, 351

Food security 229, 237, 246, 258, 294-295, 387, 391

Food services 10, 80, 239, 241, 245, 266, 352, 460, 464

Food Stamps (Supplemental Nutrition Assistance Program) 20, 29, 172, 224, 225, 228, 260, 263, 317, 322

Fossil fuel xii, xiv, 3, 35, 208, 220, 230-247, 257, 267, 296, 297, 304, 370, 384, 388-390, 392-405, 424, 463, 464

Free-market x, 3, 8, 45, 214, 285, 459, 464

Friedman, Milton 32, 304, 343

G

Global budgets 7, 48, 315

Grand Bargain #1 Accountable Care Cooperatives (ACCs) Centerpiece of the Grand Bargains 6

Grand Bargain #2 "Direct Practice" Primary Care Providers for All 10, 11

Grand Bargain #3 Direct Practice PCPs to Provide Primary Care in "Patient-Centered Medical Homes" 11, 12

Grand Bargain #4 Direct Practice PCPs will Assume Responsibility for ACC Cost Control 13

Grand Bargain #5 Replace Government Health Care Guidelines and Regulations with ACC Self-Regulation 15

Grand Bargain #6 ACCs to Provide Long-Term Care 16

Grand Bargain #7 ACCs to Provide Oral Health Care 17

Grand Bargain #8 Merge ACC Health Care with Social Services 17

Grand Bargain #9 Comprehensive Payment System Reform with ACC Providers Deciding Medical Coverage 19

Grand Bargain #10 Reduce Administrative Complexity in Health Care and Retrain Redundant Workers 21

Grand Bargain #11 ACCs to Adopt an "Enterprise" Liability Medical Malpractice System 22

Grand Bargain #12 ACCs to Provide Disability, Unemployment, and Workers' Compensation Benefits 25

Grand Bargain #13 ACCs to Foster Legal System 27

Grand Bargain #14 ACCs to Provide Jobs for Members 28

Grand Bargain #15 Raise Minimum Wage to $15/Hour 29

Grand Bargain #16 ACCs to Provide Members Financial Education and Counseling 30

Grand Bargain #17 ACCs to Administer Social Security for Members 32

Grand Bargain #18 ACCs to Administer Pension Plans for Members 33

Grand Bargain #19 Taxing Consumption More Than Income 35

Grand Bargain #20 Comprehensive Immigration 37

Grand Bargain #21 ACCs to Lead Experimentation with the Education System 38

Grand Bargain #22 ACC Members to Enhance National Security as Development Workers 39

Grand Bargain #23 ACCs to Self-Insure Against Bankruptcy 429

Grand Bargain #24 ACC-Affiliated Credit Unions/S&Ls to Enter the Housing Market and to Manage Pensions 436

Grand Bargain #25 Veterans Health and Social Services to be Shifted from the Veterans Administration to ACCs 174

Grand Bargain #26 ACCs to Replace the Indian Health Service in Providing Health and Social Services 174

Grand Bargain #27 Right to Life Proponents and Right to Choose Advocates May Choose ACCs in Accordance with Their Beliefs 131

Grand Bargain #28 New Public Infrastructure Investments—$3.6 Trillion from 2016-2025 274

Grand Bargain #29 Preventing Violence by Fixing Mental Health Care and Taxing Guns 115, 373

Great Recession 33, 34, 201, 202, 211, 217, 252, 283, 308, 310, 332, 420, 421, 422, 427, 428, 432, 434, 436, 448, 451

Guns ix, xiii, xiv, 10, 35, 37, 44, 112-117, 364, 373-377, 385

H

Health care premiums 7, 9, 20, 36, 124, 219, 256, 265, 319-321, 355

Health policy xi, 1, 55, 65, 71, 106, 143, 145, 151, 308, 341, 343, 350

HIV/AIDS 97, 250, 254, 291, 331

Home mortgage crisis 9, 416, 427, 430, 431, 436

Hospice or palliative care iii, xi, xii, 69, 75, 85-108, 126, 187, 195, 215, 324, 325, 346

Housing 20, 31, 60, 132, 170, 172, 173, 197, 206, 216, 217, 260, 317, 322, 416, 416, 427-431, 434-443, 447, 448, 454, 456, 460, 462, 463

I

Immigration viii, 9, 10, 37, 38, 219, 248-269, 386, 446, 465

Imports 35, 242-245, 290, 383-384, 388, 389, 394, 400, 404

Inequality or income and/or wealth ix, 9, 32, 35, 45, 46, 48, 217, 220, 263, 298, 358, 400, 458, 463

Income taxes viii, xiv, xv, 28, 30, 35-37, 41, 46, 203, 205, 207, 208, 259, 275, 317, 357-386, 393, 420, 424, 430, 444, 446, 447, 455-457

Indian Health Service 174, 176, 177, 317

Infant mortality 17, 66, 168, 177, 257, 258, 336

Infrastructure vii, ix, xv, 41, 46, 207, 208, 209, 218, 260, 267, 270-276, 298, 300, 305, 306, 332, 359, 365, 366, 397, 450, 460, 462

Internal Revenue Service (IRS) 36, 358, 420

Investors xi, 6, 50, 204, 308, 361, 362, 371, 372, 425, 431, 432, 433, 436, 440, 444, 448, 449

Islamic State of Iraq and Syria (ISIS) 302, 304, 397

J

Jauhar, Sandeep (Dr.) 326, 327, 346, 348, 349

L

LA County + USC Medical Center xi, xii, 88, 92, 93, 95, 96, 103, 248, 324-326, 419

Legal system reform (tort reform) 7, 27, 179-200, 216, 446

Liberals xi, xiv, 5, 33, 39, 152, 203, 262, 300, 357, 358, 380, 407, 411, 412, 428

Livestock 232, 235, 236, 238, 241, 295-297

Longevity 17, 66, 165, 166, 177

Long-term care 13, 16-17, 58, 60, 109, 122-124, 127, 166, 174, 178, 205, 313, 319,
    451, 453, 454, 456

M

Medicaid xii, xiii, 14, 15, 19, 20, 29, 51, 52, 55, 66, 82, 92, 93, 99, 107, 125, 155, 177,
    188, 250, 263, 317, 322, 324, 325, 326, 332, 334, 351, 355, 453

Medical insurance companies x, 10, 13, 19, 20, 83, 94, 145, 214, 307-323

Medical malpractice See "Enterprise medical malpractice liability"

Medical research 8, 14, 54, 135, 146-148, 157, 160, 161, 312, 331, 344, 354, 406

Medical students 62-67, 73-77, 92, 96, 108, 136, 336, 337

Medical tourism 353-354

Medicare xiii, 14, 15, 19, 51-55, 66, 68, 72, 82, 93, 94, 99, 101, 104-106, 121, 126, 143,
    151, 152, 195, 310, 317, 318, 319, 322, 334, 347, 348, 351, 355, 360, 361, 453-457

Mental health 73, 109, 113-119, 126, 165, 198, 202, 280, 373-375

Minimum wage xiv, 29, 30, 36, 123, 203, 204, 206, 208, 210- 211, 219, 226, 240, 241,
    260, 263, 264, 359, 361, 409, 410, 447, 462, 464

Monetary policies 428, 435, 441, 443, 448, 450

N

National Center for Quality Assurance 12, 77

National debt ix, 41, 276, 444

National defense ix, 40, 41, 46, 60, 209, 218, 290, 298, 299

National security xiii, 4, 39, 40, 41, 207, 208, 219, 231, 245, 246, 256, 288-306, 359,
    365, 387, 393, 394, 396, 398, 446, 461

Net-neutrality 380

Nurse practitioners 10, 11, 53, 66, 77, 86, 165, 213, 215, 255, 333, 342

Nutrition 17, 58, 63, 68, 80, 89, 90, 91, 117, 120, 128, 132, 163, 165, 221, 223, 224,
    226, 227, 246, 247, 260, 344

O

Obama, Barack (President) 231, 390

Obamacare (see "Patient Protection and Accountable Care Act (ACA)" xiii, xiv, 6, 7, 11, 14, 20, 21, 47, 49, 54, 64, 82, 83, 93, 129, 152, 177, 199, 250, 308, 310, 317, 343, 354

Obesity 3, 48, 63, 78, 80-82, 140, 170, 176, 177, 224-227, 231, 235, 278, 370, 378, 465

Ornish, Dean (Dr.) 78, 79, 81, 82, 120

P

Patient Protection and Accountable Care Act (ACA) xiii, 47, 93, 94, 113, 152, 343, 351 (also see Obamacare)

Payment system reform 14, 19

Pensions 33, 34, 213, 311, 330, 332, 400, 406-418, 425, 437, 444

Personal debt 3, 423

Philanthropic spending 322

Physician assistants 10, 77, 215, 255, 333, 338, 339

Physician assisted suicide/euthanasia debate xi, 102-103

Plastic products xiv, 35, 37, 44, 89, 364, 370-371, 383, 384, 385, 404, 423, 440

Policy experts 1, 14, 55, 106, 185, 281, 308, 341, 441, 442, 450

Population growth vii, 66, 248-269, 306

Postgraduate medical training 334-335

Poverty 2, 31, 40, 48, 58, 164, 165, 167, 171, 173, 177, 211, 215, 216, 217, 218, 232, 252, 257, 258, 260, 291, 293, 295, 299, 301, 304, 322, 343, 348, 373, 373, 454, 465

Pregnancy 121, 131, 132, 253, 254, 256, 342, 352

Preventive medicine ix, 7, 13, 21, 56, 60, 69, 78-84, 109, 126, 139, 147, 157, 166, 171, 301, 311, 329

Price transparency 340-341, 345, 353

Prison 27, 110, 111, 163, 174, 196-200, 209, 278, 302, 374

Q

Quality of life 17, 29, 38, 48, 75, 108, 166, 210, 271, 277, 402, 463

Quantitative easing 427, 428, 435, 442, 447, 449, 462

R

Randomized controlled trials 15, 120, 122, 134, 147, 148, 149, 158-161, 312

Rationing health care 144, 258, 343-345, 354-355

Regulation of health care vii, x, 15-17, 21, 24, 28, 31, 51, 91, 94, 99, 100, 113, 135, 145, 146, 148, 150, 151-162, 184, 185, 338, 358

Religion xi, 4, 56, 131, 289

Republicans xii, xiii, 47, 80, 171, 173, 357, 377, 380, 394, 408, 412, 435, 436

Ryan, Paul (Congressman) 357, 358, 365

S

Sebelius, Nancy (former Secretary of Health and Human Services) 83, 181

Single-payer medical care 309, 310

Social indicators of health 17, 38, 154, 168, 277, 348

Social justice x, 244, 439, 450

Social Security Disability 25, 26, 111, 315, 316, 409, 410, 418

Social Security Trust funds 32, 33, 330, 407, 410, 411, 443, 444, 446, 449

Soft power 3, 4

Spiritual practices 115, 352

Substance abuse 23, 110-118, 165, 171, 173, 197, 198, 216, 217, 278, 331, 352

Sustainable development 2, 269, 297, 300-302, 306, 389

T

Tax sheltered funds 36, 46, 208, 209, 359, 360

Terrorism 9, 40, 288, 289, 291, 293, 294, 295, 298, 301

Third World people 40, 208, 244, 257, 258, 261, 261, 290-292, 295, 297-301, 303, 306, 399, 444, 460

Tobacco xii, xiv, 2, 35, 37, 44, 364, 366-367, 378, 385

Too-big-to-fail banks xiv, 35, 377, 378, 416, 422, 425, 432, 435, 436, 439

Trade deficit 308, 388, 392, 394, 397, 398, 400

Transportation 10, 31, 43, 44, 177, 211, 231, 238, 240, 274, 275, 301, 348, 363, 364, 387, 396, 398, 401, 405, 454, 456, 460, 463, 464

U

U.S. Department of Health and Human Services (HHS) 15, 84, 94, 114, 181, 186, 188, 229, 314, 329, 331

U.S. Preventive Services Task Force 83, 142, 368

Unemployment insurance 25, 26, 28, 170, 174, 219, 329, 360, 361, 365

United Nations Food and Agriculture Organization 235-236, 295-297

Universal health care xii, 16, 258, 349

Acknowledgments

I owe huge debts of gratitude to many people that helped me over the seven years of researching and writing this book.

Physicians that critiqued my work and encouraged me included William Lamers, MD (pioneering hospice physician), George Lundberg, MD (former chief editor of *JAMA* and the *Medscape Journal of Medicine*), Barbara Starfield, MD (Distinguished Professor of Public Health at the Johns Hopkins Medical School). Paul Agutter, MD, Colm Malone, MD, and John Pezzullo, PhD, coauthored a key evidence-based medicine article with me on anticoagulants in venous thromboembolism.

Jan Lundberg (CultureChange.org) edited the book. Jan suggested the content for the cover. He encouraged me for years. I added at least 100 pages to the manuscript during the first round of editing because of his challenges to my thinking and insightful comments. Other editors included David Kennedy, Leyla Ali, PharmD. Eddie Young crafted a beautiful book cover.

Friends that sent useful articles relating to the book included Peter Darroch, Jane Bock, Dale Bock, my cousin Richard Duval, Jack Berro, and Pamela Mokler.

Family members that had to cope with and adapt to my lack of a day job while writing this book included my daughters Amanda Cundiff, Molly Thompson, and Chelsea Cundiff and their men Greg Freemon, Andy Thompson, and Dan Morris.

The patients, nurses, interns and residents, faculty, and administrators of LA County + USC Medical Center gave me the experiences in palliative care, general internal medicine, and medical bureaucracy that helped form my perspectives on the material in this book. My thanks and blessings to them all.

Of all the people for me to acknowledge, my granddaughters are most special, because they will be most affected by the subjects in this book. May Olivia Freemon and Ruby Thompson inherit a sustainable planet inhabited by healthy, peaceful people.